HANDBOOK OF SYMPTOMS OF KEY DISEASES

Dr. Kashieca Yap

ALLIED HEALTH PRESS

Handbook of Symptoms of Key Diseases

Author: **Dr. Kashieca Yap**

Allied Health Press
4164 Lakeshore Road
Burlington ON L7L 1A4
Canada
www.alliedhealthpress.com
Email: orders@arclereducation.com

ISBN: 978-1-77956-263-0

ABOUT THE AUTHOR

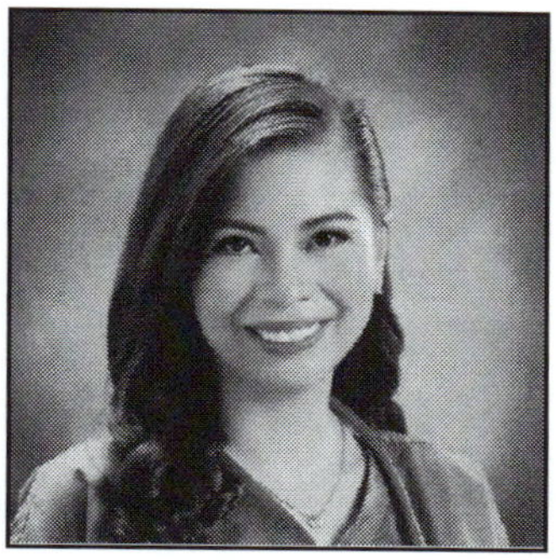

Kashieca Yap, M.D., is a devoted medical doctor and medical writer. She currently works as a general practice physician in a rural town, where she handles adult and pediatric cases, infectious diseases, and chronic medical conditions. Kashieca also lectures on mental health, clinical pharmacology, physiology, and psychiatry and is an enthusiastic researcher and medical writer. She obtained her medical degree from Cebu Doctor's University College of Medicine and further developed her clinical skills at a large public hospital. Alongside her professional endeavors, Kashieca dedicates her time to volunteering at NGOs and medical missions, reaching out to people in geographically isolated areas. Her unwavering passion for medicine and her strong desire to serve people is a testament to her compassion and skill as a healthcare professional.

Word Roots, Prefixes, and Suffixes by Chapter

Chapter 1 Symptoms of Heart Disease

Endo-: Inside, within
Exo-: Outside, outer
Hemi-: Half
Hyper-: Excessive, above normal
Hypo-: Below, under, deficient
Trans-: Across, beyond, through
-ectomy: Surgical removal
-ostomy: Surgical opening
-pathy: Disease, disorder
-graph:Instrument for recording
-plasty: Surgical repair or reconstruction

Chapter 2 Symptoms of Breast Disease

-itis: inflammation, infection
-mastia: breast or mammary gland
-plasia: growth or proliferations
-algia: pain
Intra-: within

Chapter 3 Symptoms of Lung Disease

Pulmo-: Pertaining to the lungs
Pneumo-: Related to air or lungs
-pnea: Breathing or respiration
-ectomy: Surgical removal or excision
Broncho-: Pertaining to the bronchial tubes
-logy: Study or science of
Dys-: Abnormal or difficult
-osis: Abnormal condition or disease
Thoraco-: Related to the chest or thorax

Chapter 4 Symptoms of Mental Illness or Emotional Problems

aut/o: self
iatr/o: treatment
ment/o: mind
psych/o: mind
schist/o: split
schiz/o: split
somat/o: body
(prefix) cata: down

Chapter 5 Symptoms of Female Reproductive Health Problems

-algia: Pain
cervic/o: Cervix
colp/o: Vagina
-cyesis: Pregnancy
endometri/o: Endometrium
episi/o: Vulva
gyn/o, gynec/o: Woman

Chapter 6 Symptoms of Stomach and Digestive Diseases

abdomin/o: Abdomen, abdominal
an/o: Anus
antr/o: Antrum
gastr/o: Stomach
dys-: Painful, abnormal, difficult, labored
endo-: Within, in
-cele: Hernia, protrusion

Chapter 7 Symptoms of Cancer

neuro-: nerve
osteo-: bone
carcin-: cancer
-oma: tumor, swelling
-opsy: viewing, process of viewing
-sarcoma: malignant tumor
-thorax: chest cavity, chest
-emia: a condition of the blood

Chapter 8 Symptoms of Diabetes and Hypertension

Ab: away from

Anti-: opposite, against

Bi: two

Calc-: relating to calcium

cyt-: cell

Cyto-: prefix denoting cell or cytoplasm

Dia-: through, throughout

Dis-: reversed or separated

Chapter 9 Symptoms of Joint Disease

endo-: inside

epi-: upon

hypo-: below

inter-: between, among

intra-: within

-lysis, -lyso: destruction

neuro-: nerve

-oid: resembles

-osis: pathologic condition

Chapter 10 Symptoms of Eating Disorders and Weight Problems

Fibr/o-: Fiber

Gluco-, Glyco-: Glucose; Sugar

Adip/o-: Fat

Cutane-: Skin

epat/o-, Hepatico-: Liver

abdomin-: abdomen

Table of Contents

LIST OF FIGURES

LIST OF TABLES

PREFACE

The diagnosis of diseases is a leading area of research that involves multiple disciplines. Physiological diseases, such as cancer and diabetes, have frequently been regarded as the most serious and widespread diseases that affect humans all over the world. These diseases are not contagious to other people. Typically, this is brought on by a lack of physical activity, unhealthy eating habits, and the consumption of alcohol, drugs, and smoking. Certain diseases, such as diabetes, dental caries, and asthma, are more prevalent in younger populations that are living in the "western" way of life. The increased incidence of these diseases is not related to age, which is why the terms cannot be used interchangeably for all diseases.

Around forty million people are killed annually by noncommunicable diseases (NCDs), which accounts for approximately seventy percent of all deaths worldwide. A noncommunicable disease (NCD) is a chronic condition that cannot be passed on from one individual to another. Both genetics and physiology, as well as environmental and behavioral factors, all play a role in the development of these conditions. In addition to cancer, the most common types of noncommunicable diseases are cardiovascular diseases and chronic respiratory diseases. As a result of the strong connection between lifestyle choices and noncommunicable diseases (NCDs) like cardiovascular diseases (CVD), stroke, diabetes, and certain types of cancer, these diseases are frequently referred to as lifestyle diseases. Cardiovascular diseases, which include heart attacks and strokes, are responsible for 17.7 million deaths annually, making it the most fatal disease in the world according to the World Health Organization. According to estimates, approximately 8.8 million people lose their lives to cancer every year. This is followed by respiratory diseases, which claim approximately 3.9 million lives annually, and diabetes, which has a morbidity rate of 1.6 million people annually. Among all noncommunicable diseases (NCDs), these four categories of illnesses are the most prevalent causes of death. Tobacco use, unhealthy diet, insufficient physical activity, and toxic alcohol consumption are the four behavioral risk factors that are responsible for a significant portion of the development of noncommunicable diseases (NCDs). WHO reports that countries with low and middle incomes, as well as the poorest people in all countries, are the most severely affected by deaths caused by noncommunicable diseases (NCDs). It is a vicious cycle of risk in which those who are poor are increasingly exposed to behavioral risk factors for noncommunicable diseases (NCDs), and in turn, such diseases may play a significant role in driving people and their families towards poverty. Individuals are the first to be affected, and eventually entire nations are impacted as well.

This book provides a concise summary of the fundamental principles underlying the symptoms and transmission of key diseases, while also highlighting a significant number of the agent, host, and environmental determinants of these diseases that are of particular significance to workers in the field of public health. Additionally, fundamental principles of disease diagnosis, control, and prevention are examined in this book. The audience for this handbook primarily consists of medical professionals, including general practitioners, specialists, and medical students, who require a comprehensive and reliable reference to aid in diagnosing various conditions. It is also a valuable resource for nursing staff and other healthcare providers involved in patient care, as it offers a detailed overview of symptoms associated with numerous diseases. Additionally, the handbook can be useful for medical researchers and educators looking for a concise yet thorough compilation of symptomatology to support their studies and teaching efforts. Its clear, structured format makes it accessible not only to experienced clinicians but also to those at the beginning of their medical careers.

Chapter

SYMPTOMS OF HEART DISEASE

1

Contents

Introduction

Heart disease encompasses a range of conditions that can impact your heart. Coronary artery disease (CAD) is the most prevalent and well-known heart disease. The disease process creates a waxy accumulation in the coronary arteries. This is the most common cause of a myocardial infarction, also known in layman as a heart attack.

Other issues that can occur in the heart include issues with the electrical system (e.g., arrhythmias), heart valves (e.g., valvular heart disease), and heart muscle (e.g., cardiomyopathy).

The heart pumps blood which provides oxygen and nutrients necessary for your body's systems to function. Any issue about blood delivery has an impact on all bodily systems. Most heart conditions can be prevented or treated with good lifestyle choices, medications, and medical interventions.

Orientation and Directional Terms

Term	Definition	Illustration
Angina	A type of chest pain caused by reduced blood flow to the heart.	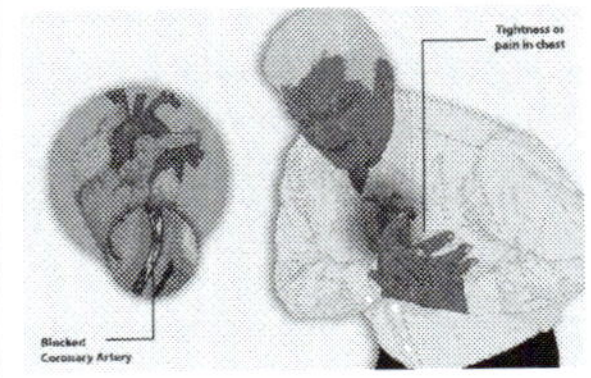
Echocardiograms	An echocardiogram uses sound waves to show how blood flows through the heart and heart valves. Sensors attached to the chest and sometimes the legs check the heart rhythm during the test. The test can help a healthcare provider diagnose heart conditions.	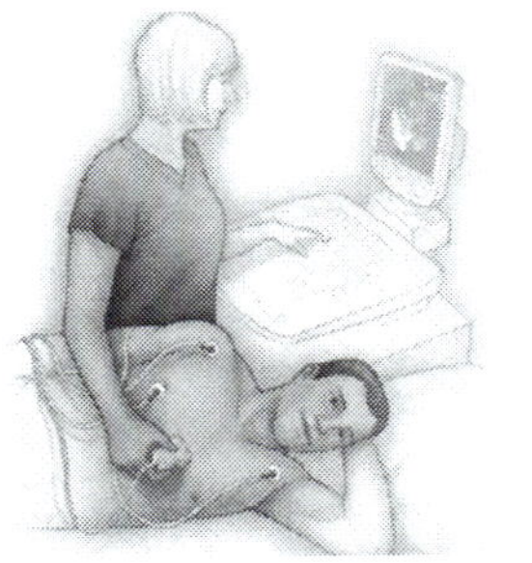
Heart muscle	The heart muscle is unique from other muscle types due to its branches and striations. It is involuntary and pushes blood through the lungs and the rest of the body.	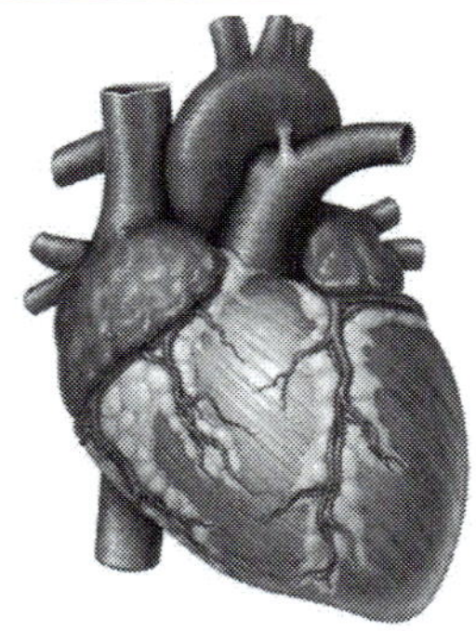
Dizziness	Altered sense of balance and place, possibly described as lightheaded, feeling faint or as if head is spinning.	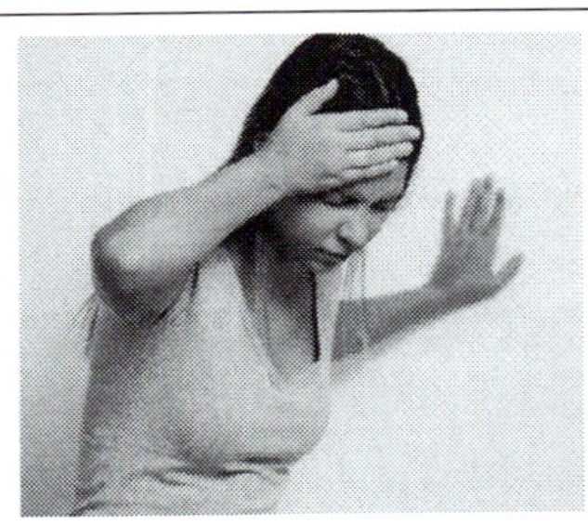
Atrial fibrillation	An irregular heart rhythm that begins in your heart's upper chambers (atria). Symptoms include fatigue, heart palpitations, trouble breathing and dizziness.	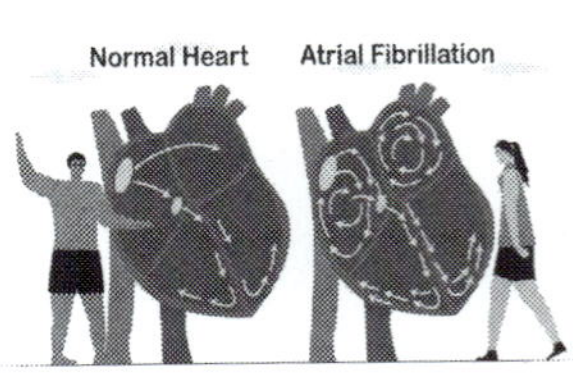

1.1. Heart Disease

Heart disease is a general term that includes conditions like coronary artery disease, arrhythmias, congenital heart defects and heart failure. High blood pressure, high cholesterol, smoking, obesity, diabetes, sedentary lifestyle, and family history are risk factors for heart disease.

Coronary artery disease, in which plaque accumulation narrows the arteries supplying blood to the heart muscle, is one of the most common types. This constriction may result in a heart attack if a plaque bursts or in angina (chest pain).

Heart failure is the result of the heart's inability to pump blood efficiently, which causes fluid to accumulate in the lungs and other tissues. Arrhythmias throw off the heart's normal rhythm and can result in palpitations, lightheadedness, or even cardiac arrest.

Abnormal heart valves can be acquired or congenital, and they impede the heart's ability to pump blood properly.

A healthy lifestyle that includes regular exercise, a balanced diet low in saturated fats and salt, maintaining a healthy weight, managing stress, abstaining from tobacco, and taking prescribed medications as directed are some prevention and management techniques. A variety of tests, including blood work, electrocardiograms, echocardiograms, stress tests, cardiac catheterization, and evaluation of the patient's medical history, are frequently used in the diagnosis process. The course of treatment for a given condition varies based on its type and severity but may involve lifestyle modifications, medications, medical procedures like bypass surgery or angioplasty, implanted devices like pacemakers or defibrillators, and cardiac rehabilitation programs. The fact that heart disease is still the world's leading cause of morbidity and death despite tremendous advances in diagnosis and treatment highlights the continued significance of public health programs, research, and education focused on early detection and prevention (Mozaffarian et al., 2016; Benjamin et al., 2019).

1.1.1. Symptoms

The symptoms of heart disease vary depending on the kind. The main blood vessels that supply the heart muscle are impacted by the common heart condition known as coronary artery disease. Typically, coronary artery disease is brought on by cholesterol buildup (plaques) in the heart arteries. The term atherosclerosis (ath-ur-o-skluh-RO-sis) refers to the accumulation of these plaques. Blood supply to the heart and other organs is decreased by atherosclerosis. Angina or a stroke could result from it. Gender differences may exist in the symptoms of coronary artery disease. Men are prone to experiencing chest pain, for example. Other symptoms like nausea, extreme fatigue, and shortness of breath are more common in women in addition to chest discomfort.

Symptoms of coronary artery disease can include:

- Chest pain, chest tightness, chest pressure and chest discomfort (angina)
- Shortness of breath
- Pain in the neck, jaw, throat, upper belly area or back
- Pain, numbness, weakness or coldness in the legs or arms if the blood vessels in those body areas are narrowed

1.1.2. Causes

Heart disease is complex and common throughout the world due to a wide range of factors, both modifiable and non-modifiable. One of the main causes is atherosclerosis, a disorder marked by the accumulation of plaque in the arteries, which can restrict or obstruct the heart's ability to pump blood. Plaque is made up of calcium, fat, cholesterol, and other materials that build up over time as a result of many conditions including high blood pressure, high cholesterol, smoking, diabetes, and inflammation. These risk factors have the potential to harm the arterial wall, which will encourage plaque buildup and raise the risk of coronary artery disease. High blood pressure, or hypertension, is another important contributing factor. This puts stress on the heart because it requires it to beat harder to pump blood throughout the body. Extended high blood pressure can cause the heart muscle to thicken and stiffen, which can hinder heart function and raise the risk of heart attack, stroke, and heart failure. Sedentary lifestyles and obesity also play a significant role in the development of heart disease risk factors, including high blood pressure, high cholesterol, and type 2 diabetes. Overweight can worsen insulin resistance and inflammation, which raises the risk of cardiovascular disease, especially around the abdomen.

Dietary factors are also important; diets high in cholesterol, sodium, saturated and trans fats, and refined sugars raise the risk of heart disease. On the other hand, diets high in whole grains, fruits, vegetables, lean meats, and healthy fats can help reduce the risk. Furthermore, because smoking damages blood vessels, lowers oxygen delivery to tissues, increases blood pressure, and hastens the development of arterial plaque, it continues to be a significant modifiable risk factor for heart disease. A person's susceptibility to heart disease can be increased by specific genetic conditions and familial traits. Genetic predisposition and family history also play a part. Cardiovascular risk can also be increased by other variables like stress, binge drinking, sleep apnea, and some underlying medical conditions like autoimmune disorders or chronic kidney disease. To lessen the burden of heart disease and enhance general cardiovascular health, it is crucial to identify and treat these complex causes through lifestyle changes, medication management, and preventive interventions. To address the underlying causes of heart disease and lower its prevalence worldwide, public health initiatives that promote awareness, education, and access to preventive care are essential.

1.1.3. Heart Disease Symptoms Caused by Irregular Heartbeats (Heart Arrhythmias)

Arrhythmias can present with a wide range of symptoms.

- **Palpitations**. Palpitations are a common symptom. It is the awareness of one's heartbeat. It can be described as experiencing rapid, fluttering, or pounding heartbeats in the chest, throat, or neck. There may be a sense of unease or anxiety along with palpitations.
- **Angina**. Angina is another symptom. This is described as a tightness, pressure, or squeezing sensation in the chest that is often described as discomfort or pain. This can mimic the symptoms of a heart attack.
- **Shortness of breath.** Irregular heart rhythms can hinder the heart's ability to pump blood efficiently to meet the body's demand for oxygen. Shortness of breath, especially during physical activity or exertion, is another common symptom. This is also called dyspnea.

- **Dizziness or lightheadedness**. Too little blood flow to the brain can cause dizziness or lightheadedness, especially when one is standing up quickly or exerting themselves.
- **Syncope or presyncope**. The heart's rhythm can become noticeably erratic, resulting in syncope, also known as a fainting spell or presyncope, which is a feeling that one is about to pass out.
- **Fatigue**. A decrease in the amount of oxygen delivered to tissues and organs due to inefficient heart pumping can also cause fatigue or weakness.
- **Tachycardia**. Racing heartbeats.
- **Bradycardia**. A slowed heart rate.

Arrhythmias, especially when chronic and untreated, result in complications such as heart failure or stroke. People who have atrial fibrillation, a common arrhythmia marked by fast and erratic heartbeats, are more likely to experience blood clots.

These blood clots can travel to the brain and cause a stroke or travel to the lungs to cause a pulmonary embolism. Sudden weakness or numbness on one side of the body, trouble speaking or understanding speech, changes in vision, and excruciating headaches are signs of a stroke.

Certain arrhythmias such as premature ventricular contractions might not manifest any symptoms at all and might only be discovered through standard diagnostic procedures or medical examinations, such as electrocardiograms (ECGs or EKGs), Holter monitoring, or event monitoring.

1.1.4. Heart Disease Symptoms Caused by Congenital Heart Defects

Congenital heart defects are structural abnormalities present at birth, affecting the heart's chambers, valves, walls, or blood vessels. Some individuals may remain asymptomatic, while others may experience significant complications. Among the common symptoms are:

- **Cyanosis**. A bluish tint to the skin, lips, or nail beds, caused by reduced oxygen levels in the blood. This occurs when there is a defect that allows oxygen-poor blood to mix with oxygen-rich blood, bypassing the lungs.
- **Dyspnea**. Shortness of breath, particularly during feeding or exertion, can occur due to reduced oxygen supply to the body's tissues.
- **Tachypnea**. Rapid breathing, especially in infants, may also be observed.
- **Failure to thrive.** Poor feeding and inadequate weight gain in infants may result from fatigue and increased energy expenditure due to the heart's inefficiency in pumping blood. Difficulty with feeding may manifest as excessive sweating, especially around the forehead, during feeding sessions.
- **Heart murmurs**. Abnormal sounds heard during a physical examination, may be present and can indicate turbulent blood flow through the heart due to structural abnormalities.
- **Cardiac symptoms**. In some cases, *palpitations, chest pain,* or *fainting*

episodes may occur, particularly as the individual grows older and the demands on the heart increase.

- **Edema**. Swelling of the legs, abdomen, or other areas of the body due to fluid buildup.
- **Hepatomegaly.** Liver enlargement and abdominal distension. Other symptoms may include:

Some congenital heart defects can lead to complications such as heart failure, arrhythmias, infective endocarditis (infection of the heart lining), and stroke. It is important to note that the severity and timing of symptoms can vary widely, with some defects being detected soon after birth during routine newborn screenings or prenatal ultrasounds, while others may go undetected until later in life. Prompt medical evaluation is essential if any symptoms suggestive of congenital heart defects are present, as early diagnosis and intervention can help prevent complications and improve long-term outcomes. Treatment options may include medications, minimally invasive procedures, or surgery to repair or alleviate the defect's effects on heart function. Long-term management and monitoring are often necessary to ensure optimal heart health and quality of life.

Serious congenital heart defects usually are noticed soon after birth. Congenital heart defect symptoms in children could include:

- Pale gray or blue skin or lips (cyanosis)
- Swelling in the legs, belly area or areas around the eyes
- In an infant, shortness of breath during feedings, leading to poor weight gain

Less-serious congenital heart defects are often not diagnosed until later in childhood or during adulthood. Symptoms of congenital heart defects that usually aren't immediately life-threatening include:

- Easily getting short of breath during exercise or activity
- Easily tiring during exercise or activity
- Swelling of the hands, ankles or feet

1.1.5. Heart Disease Symptoms Caused by Diseased Heart Muscle (Cardiomyopathy)

Cardiomyopathy refers to a disease of the heart muscle, where the heart becomes enlarged, thickened, or stiffened, impairing its ability to pump blood effectively. The symptoms of cardiomyopathy can vary depending on the type of cardiomyopathy, the underlying cause, and the severity of the condition.

Early stages of cardiomyopathy may not cause noticeable symptoms. As the condition worsens, symptoms may include:

- **Shortness of breath**, especially during physical activity or when lying flat, due to fluid buildup in the lungs (pulmonary congestion) caused by the heart's inability to pump blood efficiently.
- **Fatigue or weakness** may also be present, as the heart's diminished pumping capacity can lead to reduced oxygen delivery to the body's tissues and organs.
- **Edema.** Swelling of the legs, ankles, feet, or abdomen may occur due to fluid retention caused by impaired circulation and increased pressure within the blood vessels.
- **Palpitations.** Some individuals may experience palpitations, which are sensations of rapid, fluttering,

or pounding heartbeats, as the heart's electrical system becomes disrupted by the underlying muscle abnormalities.

- **Angina.** Chest pain or discomfort, often described as a tightness, pressure, or squeezing sensation, may occur, particularly during physical exertion or emotional stress, due to inadequate blood supply to the heart muscle (ischemia).
- **Dizziness or lightheadedness** may occur, especially when standing up quickly or exerting oneself, due to reduced blood flow to the brain.
- **Syncope or presyncope.** Fainting or near-fainting episodes can occur in severe cases, particularly when the heart's pumping function is severely impaired.

In some cases, symptoms of cardiomyopathy may resemble those of heart failure, such as coughing or wheezing, especially when lying down, and difficulty with breathing at night (paroxysmal nocturnal dyspnea).

Additionally, symptoms of underlying conditions that contribute to cardiomyopathy, such as high blood pressure, diabetes, or thyroid disorders, may also be present. It should be noted that some individuals with cardiomyopathy may not experience any symptoms, especially in the early stages of the disease.

However, as the condition progresses, symptoms may become more pronounced and debilitating. Prompt medical evaluation is essential if any symptoms suggestive of cardiomyopathy are present, as early diagnosis and treatment can help slow the progression of the disease, alleviate symptoms, and improve outcomes.

1.1.6. Heart Disease Symptoms Caused By Heart Valve Problems (Valvular Heart Disease)

Valvular heart disease refers to conditions that affect the heart's valves, impairing their function and disrupting blood flow within the heart. The aortic, mitral, pulmonary, and tricuspid valves are the four valves in the heart. To pump blood through the heart, they open and close. There are numerous ways to harm the heart valves. A heart valve can be narrowed or obstructed (i.e., valve stenosis), prolapsed (i.e., valve prolapse), leaking (i.e., valve regurgitation), or weakened (i.e., valve insufficiency).

The symptoms of valvular heart disease vary depending on the type of valve affected, the severity of the valve dysfunction, and whether the condition is causing obstruction (stenosis) or leakage (regurgitation) of blood flow. Depending on which valve isn't working properly, heart valve disease symptoms generally include:

- Chest pain
- Fainting (syncope)
- Fatigue
- Irregular heartbeat
- Shortness of breath
- Swollen feet or ankles

1.1.7. Management and Treatment

Heart disease is managed and treated using a multimodal approach that aims to improve overall cardiovascular health, reduce symptoms, prevent complications, and address underlying risk factors. A key component of management is changing one's lifestyle, which includes eating a heart-healthy diet high in fruits, vegetables, whole grains, lean proteins, and healthy fats and low in saturated, trans, and cholesterol fats and sodium. It is also recommended that individuals engage in muscle-strengthening activities on two or more days per week, in addition to 150 minutes of moderate-intensity aerobic exercise or 75 minutes of vigorous-intensity exercise per week. It is critical to stop smoking because tobacco use raises the risk of heart disease and aggravates pre-existing cardiovascular conditions. Other crucial elements of lifestyle management include keeping a healthy weight, reducing stress through mindfulness or relaxation exercises, and getting enough good sleep.

Treatment for heart disease often involves pharmacological interventions, where drugs are used to address different aspects of cardiovascular health. Statins to lower cholesterol, beta-blockers to lower blood pressure and heart rate, ACE inhibitors or angiotensin receptor blockers (ARBs) to lower blood pressure and improve heart function, diuretics to reduce fluid retention, and anticoagulants to prevent blood clots in people with atrial fibrillation or other high-risk conditions are among the commonly prescribed medications. Each person's unique risk factors, comorbidities, and treatment objectives are taken into account when managing their medications, and both efficacy and possible side effects are closely monitored.

For some people with advanced or complex heart disease, surgical interventions may be required. These operations try to fix structural irregularities, replace or repair damaged heart valves, repair or replace damaged heart muscle, or implant devices that control the heart's rhythm. Common interventions include valve repair or replacement surgery to treat valvular heart disease, pacemaker or defibrillator implantation to regulate heart rhythm, percutaneous coronary intervention (PCI) with balloon angioplasty and stent placement to open blocked arteries, coronary artery bypass grafting (CABG) surgery to reroute blood flow around blocked arteries, and heart transplant for end-stage heart failure when other treatments have failed.

In the period following treatment, cardiac rehabilitation programs are essential because they offer patients recovering from heart disease or cardiac procedures education, counseling, and support in addition to structured exercise training. To maximize recovery and lower the risk of subsequent cardiovascular events, these programs seek to increase overall well-being, lower risk factors, encourage medication adherence, and improve physical fitness. Cardiologists, nurses, dietitians, exercise physiologists, and other medical specialists work together in multidisciplinary care teams to provide comprehensive, individualized care that is suited to the needs of each patient. The management and treatment of heart disease aim to improve quality of life, lessen the burden of cardiovascular disease on individuals and society as a whole, and improve outcomes through a combination of pharmacological interventions, invasive procedures, and rehabilitation programs (Mozaffarian et al., 2016; Benjamin et al., 2019).

1.2. Coronary Artery Disease

According to the Centers for Disease Control and Prevention, coronary artery disease is the most prevalent form of heart disease among adults in the country. Cholesterol, a waxy material from animal sources in the diet, accumulates inside the coronary artery lining and forms plaque. In coronary artery disease, the main blood vessels supplying the heart are blocked by plaque build up. This disrupts the blood and nutrient supply to the heart muscle. When the heart does not receive enough oxygen-rich blood, the signs and symptoms of CAD appear. It frequently takes decades to manifest. Breathlessness and angina (chest pain) are symptoms of reduced blood flow to the heart in people with coronary artery disease. Some people may have mild symptoms and are diagnosed with ischemic heart disease. However, these symptoms may go unnoticed until a total blockage of blood supply causes an acute myocardial infarction. When the tiny blood vessels in the heart sustain damage to their inner walls, coronary microvascular disease develops. Women are more likely to have coronary microvascular disease. CAD can be avoided by leading a heart-healthy lifestyle.

1.2.1. Forms of Coronary Artery Disease

CAD encompasses a spectrum of conditions that affect the arteries supplying blood to the heart muscle, leading to reduced blood flow and oxygen delivery to the heart. The primary forms of CAD include:

1. **Atherosclerosis**: Atherosclerosis is the most common form of CAD and occurs when fatty deposits, cholesterol, calcium, and other substances accumulate within the walls of the coronary arteries, forming plaques. These plaques can narrow the arteries, restricting blood flow to the heart muscle and increasing the risk of heart attack or angina.
2. **Coronary Artery Stenosis**: Stenosis refers to the narrowing of the coronary arteries due to the buildup of plaque, leading to partial or complete obstruction of blood flow. This reduction in blood flow can impair the heart's ability to pump effectively and increase the risk of myocardial infarction (heart attack) or ischemia (insufficient blood supply to the heart muscle).
3. **Coronary Artery Spasm**: Coronary artery spasm, also known as vasospastic angina or Prinzmetal's angina, occurs when the coronary arteries constrict or spasm, temporarily reducing blood flow to the heart muscle. These spasms can occur spontaneously or be triggered by various factors such as stress, exposure to cold temperatures, or certain medications. A coronary artery spasm can cause chest pain, shortness of breath, and potentially life-threatening arrhythmias.
4. **Coronary Microvascular Disease**: Coronary microvascular disease affects the smaller arteries and arterioles that branch off from the main coronary arteries. In this condition, the walls of these tiny blood vessels become damaged or dysfunctional, impairing blood flow regulation and delivery of oxygen to the heart muscle. Coronary microvascular disease may present with symptoms such as chest pain, fatigue, and shortness of breath, particularly in women and individuals with risk factors such as diabetes or hypertension.
5. **Non-Obstructive Coronary Artery Disease**: Non-obstructive CAD refers to the presence of coronary artery disease without significant narrowing or blockage of the coronary arteries. In some cases, individuals may experience symptoms of CAD despite having minimal or no blockages on angiography. Non-obstructive CAD can be challenging to diagnose and manage, as the underlying mechanisms may involve endothelial dysfunction, inflammation, or abnormalities in coronary microcirculation.

These forms of CAD can present with a range of symptoms, including chest pain or discomfort (angina), shortness of breath, fatigue, palpitations, and in severe cases, heart attack or sudden cardiac arrest. Early detection, risk factor modification, lifestyle changes, and appropriate medical management are essential for preventing and managing CAD and reducing the risk of complications.

1.2.2. Causes

Plaque, a mixture of fat, cholesterol, and other materials, begins to adhere to the walls of your blood vessels as early as childhood. It gradually accumulates within the arteries causing narrowing and hardening of the arteries, known in medically as "atherosclerosis." Plaque may occasionally shatter or rupture. Consequently, a blood clot will form as platelets attempt to mend the artery. Similar to debris in an obstructed drainpipe, this accumulation obstructs the unimpeded passage of blood via the arteries. The heart receives nutrition and oxygen from the blood. Insufficient blood flow to the heart muscle causes myocardial ischemia, which can cause angina and dyspnea. A heart without enough oxygen may weaken. An arrhythmia, or irregular heartbeat, may result from this. Moreover, it may result in heart failure, which is characterized by the heart's inability to adequately pump blood throughout the body to meet demands. Peripheral artery disease is the term for the condition that results in restricted blood flow to the arms and legs. You may experience a heart attack if a plaque gets so big that it restricts blood flow to the heart muscle. However, the majority of the time, smaller plaques burst to cause heart attacks.

When plaque accumulates and narrows or obstructs the coronary arteries, CAD results. Although statins and other treatment options can help, plaque can cause a heart attack. Coronary heart disease, or CAD, is often brought on by plaques formed by cholesterol accumulation on the arterial walls. These plaques can cause inflammation and hardening of the blood vessel walls, or they can narrow the arteries, decreasing heart-related blood flow. Sometimes a clot will impede blood flow, leading to life-threatening complications. The network of blood vessels that cover the surface of the heart and supply it with oxygen is made up of coronary arteries. The heart might not get enough oxygen-rich blood if these arteries narrow, especially when exercising. Smoking, having high cholesterol, and other factors raise the chance of getting the illness.

1.2.3. Symptoms of Coronary Artery Disease

Initial symptoms might not be recognized, or they might only show up during periods of high heart rate, such as exercise. As the coronary arteries narrow further, the heart receives less and less blood, which can lead to worsening or more frequent symptoms.

Coronary artery disease signs and symptoms can include:

- **Chest pain (angina).** Your chest might feel constrictive or under pressure. Some claim that it feels as though someone is pressing against their chest. Usually, the left or center side of the chest feels the pain. Angina can be brought on by activity or intense feelings. The triggering event usually ends minutes later, at which point the pain usually subsides. Some people, particularly women, may experience sudden, intense pain in the back, arm, or neck.
- **Shortness of breath.** You may feel like you can't catch your breath.
- **Fatigue.** If the heart can't pump enough blood to meet your body's needs, you may feel unusually tired.

Myocardial infarction or a heart attack is the end-result of a totally blocked coronary artery. The lack of oxygen supplying the heart muscle causes this part of the heart to become damaged. Sweating, shortness of breath, shoulder or arm pain, and crushing chest pain or pressure are the classic signs and symptoms of a heart attack. Less common symptoms that women may experience include fatigue, nausea, and jaw or neck pain. Certain heart attacks have no outward symptoms or indicators.

1.2.4. Risk Factors

The hallmark of coronary artery disease is atherosclerosis-related cardiac issues. Atherosclerosis, a kind of arteriosclerosis, is a persistent inflammatory condition of the arteries that results in the buildup of cholesterol plaques, also known as atheromatous plaques, on the arterial walls. Atherosclerosis is a result of several established risk factors associated with CAD. The following are risk factors for coronary artery disease (CAD): smoking, diabetes, hypertension, abnormally high blood pressure, abnormally high blood levels of cholesterol and other fats (dyslipidemia), type 2 diabetes, and being overweight or obese (carrying excess body fat as a result of inactivity and poor diet). High blood pressure, smoking, diabetes, obesity, high blood cholesterol, poor diet, depression, family history, psychological stress, and excessive alcohol consumption are a few more risk factors. In approximately half of cases, genetics play a role. About 36% of cases are linked to smoking, and 20% of cases are linked to obesity. A single daily cigarette smoker nearly doubles their risk of developing CAD. 7 to 12% of cases have been linked to inactivity. Risk may increase if exposed to the herbicide Agent Orange. Independent risk factors also include rheumatologic conditions like psoriasis, psoriatic arthritis, systemic lupus erythematosus, and rheumatoid arthritis.

Workplace stress seems to be a small factor, accounting for around 3% of cases. According to one study, women who experienced no stress at work had larger blood vessels, which slowed the advancement of atherosclerosis. On the other hand, females who were under a lot of stress at work saw a reduction in blood vessel diameter and a marked acceleration of the disease's progression. The personality traits of time urgency, competitiveness, hostility, and impatience, collectively known as the type A behavior pattern, are associated with a higher risk of coronary heart disease.

1.2.4.1. Blood Fats

The amount of cholesterol in the blood is influenced by the types of fats that are consumed in the diet, such as trans unsaturated, trans, and saturated fats. Plants are the source of unsaturated fats (such as oils). Unsaturated fats come in two varieties: trans and cis isomers. Trans unsaturated fats have a linear molecular structure, whereas trans unsaturated fats are bent. Saturated fats have a linear molecular structure and come from animal sources, such as animal fats. When consumed in excess and other positive measures towards physical health are not met, unsaturated trans and saturated fats easily accumulate and stack at the arterial walls due to their linear configurations. Since fats and cholesterol are insoluble in blood, they combine with proteins to create lipoproteins, which are then transported. Blood cholesterol levels are raised by low-density lipoproteins (LDL), which carry cholesterol from the liver to the rest of the body. The body produces more LDL when saturated fats are consumed, which raises blood cholesterol levels. Since high-density lipoproteins (HDL) seek out and return excess cholesterol to the liver for elimination, they are regarded as "good" lipoproteins. Trans fats also cause the body to produce more LDL and less HDL, which dramatically raises blood cholesterol levels. Atherosclerosis is caused by elevated blood cholesterol levels. Increased blood levels of low-density lipoprotein (LDL) cause deposits of LDL particles to build up inside the walls of the arteries, causing plaques to form and obstruct blood flow. As a result of atherosclerosis in the coronary arteries, the heart's blood supply is reduced, which can lead to heart attacks (myocardial infarctions), angina pectoris, and dyspnea. These symptoms are typically relieved with rest.

1.2.4.2. Genetics

The heritability of coronary artery disease has been estimated between 40% and 60%. Genome-wide association studies have identified over 160 genetic susceptibility loci for coronary artery disease.

1.2.4.3. Transcriptome

Transcripts associated with CAD (TRACs) – FoxP1, ICOSLG, IKZF4/Eos, SMYD3, TRIM28, and TCF3/E2A that are likely markers of regulatory T cells (Treg), consistent with known reductions in Tregs in CAD.

The majority of the RNA alterations are connected to ciliary and endocytic transcripts, which are connected to the immune synapse in the circulating immune system. The contact-dependent communication channel known as the immune synapse connects T and B cells on the one hand, and a range of antigen-presenting and immunomodulating cells on the other. One of the genes with the greatest differential expression is fibromodulin (FMOD), which is upregulated 2–8 times in CAD. A number of additional regulated transcripts encode proteins associated with the immunological synapse's structure and operation. Nebulette, the transcript with the greatest down-regulation (2.4-fold), is a crucial "cytolinker" that joins actin and desmin to promote vesicular motion and cytoskeletal function. Changes in tubulin, a crucial microtubule protein, and fidgetin, an enzyme that severs tubulin and is a GWAS marker for cardiovascular risk, further regulate the endocytic pathway. Changes in the ubiquitin ligase MARCHF10 and the proteasomal regulator SIAH3 would regulate protein recycling (Figure 1.1).

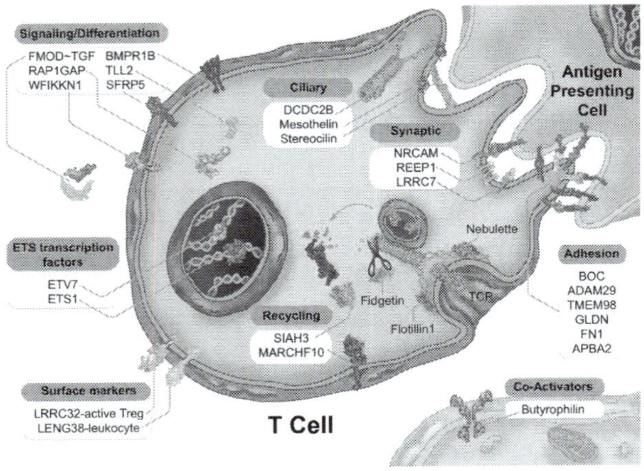

Figure 1.1. *Schematic representation of Treg-related TRACs identified by RNAseq. The differentially expressed genes (DEGs) identified by RNAseq were curated by automated and manual analysis to identify the molecular pathways involved. The resulting pattern points to changes in the 'immune synapse,' which involves both endocytic pathways of T cell receptor (TCR)-containing vesicles, as well as ciliary protrusions that couple to intracellular signaling pathways.*

Source: *https://upload.wikimedia.org/wikipedia/commons/thumb/9/91/Schematic_representation_of_Treg-related_TRACs_identified_by_RNAseq.jpg/800px-Schematic_representation_of_Treg-related_TRACs_identified_by_RNAseq.jpg.*

Many of the altered transcripts on the ciliary side of the immune synapse are connected to the length and function of the cilia. Mutations in Steriocilin (STRC), which is primarily found in outer sensory hair cells, cause deafness. Mesothelin (MSN), a related super-helical protein whose transcript is also altered in CAD, is a partner of stromatocilin. Similarly, DCDC2, a double-cortin protein, is recognized for its ability to regulate ciliary length. Many transcripts directly related to T cell function and differentiation regulation were found in the immune synapse's signaling pathways. One well-known co-regulator for T cell activation is butyrophilin (BTN1A1). Tre cell differentiation is primarily determined by the TGF-beta signaling pathway, which is modulated by the well-known protein fibromodulin. Concurrent alterations in the BMP receptor 1B RNA (BMPR1B) indicate additional influence on the TGF-beta pathway. This is because bone morphogenic proteins influence Treg differentiation and are members of the TGF-beta superfamily. As mentioned, TMEM98, NRCAM, SFRP5, SHISA2, and other transcripts are known components of the Wnt signaling pathway, a key factor in Treg differentiation.

1.2.4.4. Other

- Endometriosis in females under the age of 40.
- Depression and hostility appear to be risks.
- The number of categories of adverse childhood experiences (psychological, physical, or sexual abuse; violence against mother; or living with household members who used substances, mentally ill, suicidal, or incarcerated) showed a graded correlation with the presence of adult diseases including coronary artery (ischemic heart) disease.
- Hemostatic factors: High levels of fibrinogen and coagulation factor VII are associated with an increased risk of CAD.
- Low hemoglobin.
- In the Asian population, the b fibrinogen gene G-455A polymorphism was associated with the risk of CAD.
- Patient-specific vessel ageing or remodeling determines endothelial cell behavior and thus disease growth and progression. Such 'hemodynamic markers' are thus patient-specific risk surrogates.

1.2.5. Pathophysiology

The muscle cells of the heart experience ischemia, or cell starvation due to a lack of oxygen, when blood flow is restricted. A myocardial infarction, also known as a heart attack, occurs when the heart's muscle cells run out of oxygen. Without heart muscle cell regeneration, it causes damage, death, and ultimately scarring of the heart muscle. A dangerous heart rhythm known as ventricular fibrillation, which frequently results in death, can be induced by transient ischemia caused by chronic high-grade coronary artery narrowing. Ventricular fibrillation is a subtype of ventricular arrhythmia (Figure 1.2).

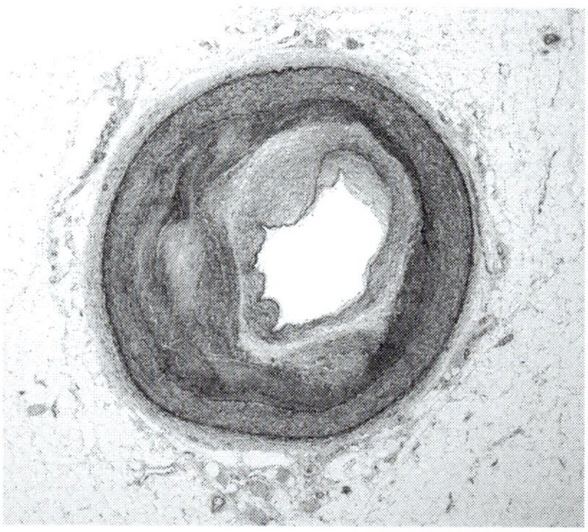

Figure 1.2. *Micrograph of a coronary artery with the most common form of coronary artery disease (atherosclerosis) and marked luminal narrowing. Masson's trichrome.*

Source: *https://upload.wikimedia.org/wikipedia/commons/thumb/f/f2/RCA_atherosclerosis.jpg/800px-RCA_atherosclerosis.jpg.*

Coronary artery disease is typically caused by the development of atherosclerosis in the smooth, elastic lining of the coronary arteries, which supply blood to the heart muscle. Atherosclerosis leads to the hardening and accumulation of calcium, fatty lipids, and abnormal cells in the artery lining, forming a plaque. Calcium deposits in the blood vessels appear to play a role in stiffening the arteries and initiating coronary arteriosclerosis. This process can be seen in the metastatic mechanism of calciphylaxis in individuals with chronic kidney disease. Despite kidney dysfunction, nearly half of these individuals die as a result of coronary artery disease. Plaques in the arteries can cause partial obstruction to blood flow, resembling large pimples in the artery channel. Some people with coronary artery disease may have one or two plaques, while others may have multiple plaques distributed throughout their coronary arteries. In more severe cases, chronic total occlusion occurs when a coronary artery is completely blocked for an extended period of more than 3 months (Figure 1.3).

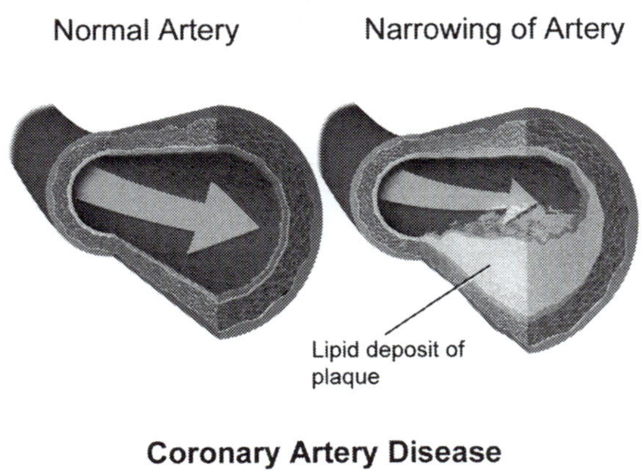

Figure 1.3. *Illustration depicting coronary artery disease.*

Source: https://upload.wikimedia.org/wikipedia/commons/thumb/6/6d/Blausen_0259_CoronaryArteryDisease_02.png/800px-Blausen_0259_CoronaryArteryDisease_02.png.

When an angiography (coronary angiogram) is being conducted, patients with microvascular angina, a form of angina pectoris, experience chest pain and discomfort without exhibiting any symptoms of blockages in their hearts' larger coronary arteries. It is unknown what specifically causes microvascular angina. Microvascular dysfunction and epicardial atherosclerosis are two possible explanations. Females are more likely than males to have it for unknown reasons, though hormones and other specific risk factors that are specific to women may be involved.

1.2.6. Diagnosis

The type of symptoms is a major factor in determining the diagnosis of CAD. When CAD is suspected, an electrocardiogram (ECG/EKG) is performed to rule out acute coronary syndrome as well as stable angina. Blood tests, resting echocardiography, and a chest X-ray are carried out. Depending on the pre-assessment of the risk profile, there are some non-invasive tests to diagnose CAD in patients who are symptomatic but stable. Non-invasive imaging techniques include stress echocardiography, single-photon emission computed tomography (SPECT), nuclear stress testing, myocardial scintigraphy, and computed tomography angiography (CTA), which is anatomical imaging and the best test to rule out CAD in patients with low-risk profiles. The three latter techniques can be summed up as functional non-invasive methods and are usually better to rule in. Because there is a chance of both false negative and false positive test results, exercise ECG and stress testing are not as reliable as non-invasive imaging techniques. If a person is asymptomatic and otherwise at low risk of developing coronary disease, then non-invasive imaging is not recommended. When non-invasive testing is unsatisfactory or indicates a high event risk, invasive testing using coronary angiography (ICA) may be used (Figure 1.4).

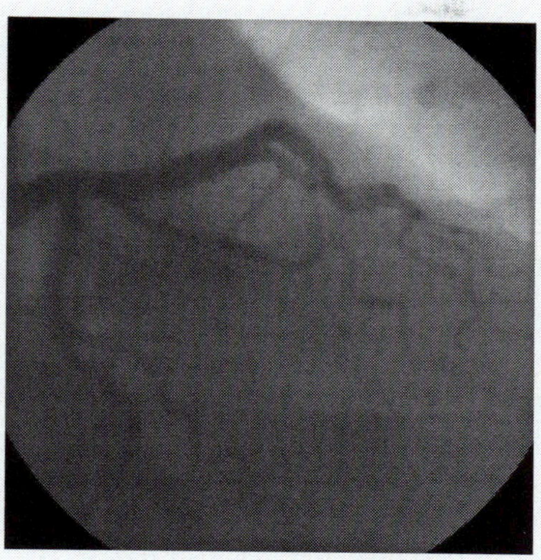

Figure 1.4. *Coronary angiogram of a male.*

Source: *https://upload.wikimedia.org/wikipedia/en/d/d2/Coro_Man.jpg.*

The diagnosis of microvascular angina (previously known as *cardiac syndrome X* – the rare coronary artery disease that is more common in females, as mentioned, is a diagnosis of exclusion. Therefore, usually, the same tests are used in any person suspected of having coronary artery disease:

- Intravascular ultrasound
- Magnetic resonance imaging (MRI)

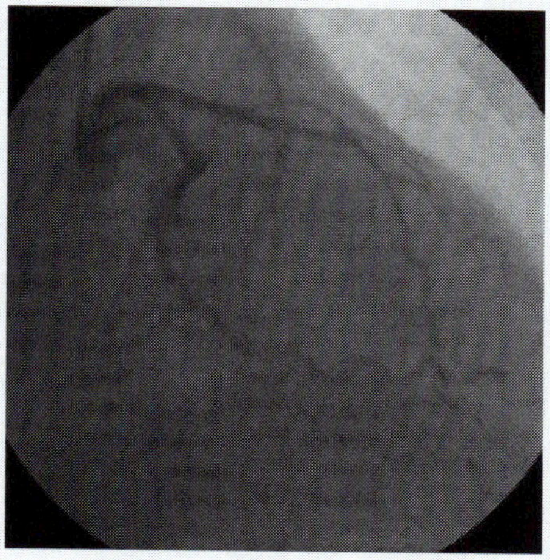

Figure 1.5. *Coronary angiogram of a female.*

Source: *https://upload.wikimedia.org/wikipedia/en/c/cf/Coro_Woman.jpg.*

1.2.6.1. Stable Angina

The most prevalent type of ischemic heart disease, stable angina, is linked to a lower quality of life and a higher death rate. It is brought on by epicardial coronary stenosis, which lowers the myocardium's blood flow and oxygen supply. Short-term chest pain during physical exertion that results from an imbalance between the oxygen supply and demand in the heart is known as stable angina. Cardiac stress tests can be designed to produce symptoms and identify alterations through electrocardiography (ECG), echocardiography (heart ultrasound), or scintigraphy (heart muscle uptake of radionuclide). In cases where there appears to be an inadequate blood supply to a portion of the heart, coronary angiography can be utilized to diagnose coronary artery stenosis and determine if an angioplasty or bypass surgery is appropriate.

Nitroglycerine can be used in mild to moderate cases to treat the acute symptoms of stable angina or can be used right before physical activity to stop angina from occurring. Most patients with refractory and recurrent angina use sublingual nitroglycerine to complement anti-anginal treatments and to quickly relieve acute angina attacks. Nitroglycerine produces free radical nitric oxide, or NO, in the bloodstream. This activates guanylate cyclase, which in turn triggers the release of cyclic GMP. This molecular signaling promotes smooth muscle relaxation, which in turn causes vasodilation and better blood flow to the parts of the heart where atherosclerotic plaque is present. Another common name for stable coronary artery disease (SCAD) is stable ischemic heart disease (SIHD).

Increased troponin T (above 14 pg/mL) was found to be associated with an increased 5-year event rate of ischemic cardiac events (myocardial infarction, percutaneous coronary intervention, or coronary artery bypass surgery) in patients with non-severe asymptomatic aortic valve stenosis and no overt coronary artery disease (Mozaffarian et al., 2016; Benjamin et al., 2019).

1.2.6.2. Acute Coronary Syndrome

Acute coronary syndrome is typically diagnosed in the emergency room, where successive ECG readings may be taken to spot changing abnormalities (signaling continuous myocardial damage). When an ECG reveals elevation of the ST segment, it is highly suggestive of an acute myocardial infarction (MI). This condition is known as a ST segment-elevation myocardial infarction (STEMI) and is treated as an emergency with either thrombolysis using medications to break up clots or urgent coronary angiography and percutaneous coronary intervention (angioplasty with or without stent insertion). The diagnosis is evident in this case. Blood tests that identify damage to the heart muscle are known as cardiac markers. These are used to detect heart damage in the absence of ST-segment elevation. These include Troponin I and Troponin C, Lactate Dehydrogenase, Creatinine Kinase, Myoglobin, and Copeptin. The chest pain is linked to a non-ST elevation MI (NSTEMI) if there is evidence of damage (infarction). The term "unstable angina" is used in the absence of any damage. To monitor for potential complications (like cardiac arrhythmias, or irregularities in the heart rate), this procedure typically requires hospital admission and close observation in a coronary care unit. Patients who have experienced an NSTEMI or unstable angina may be treated for coronary artery disease using angiography or stress testing, depending on the results of the risk assessment.

1.2.6.3. Risk Assessment

Different risk assessment systems exist to ascertain the likelihood of coronary artery disease, with varying degrees of emphasis placed on the variables mentioned above. One prominent instance is the Framingham Heart Study, which employed the Framingham Score. It is primarily determined by systolic blood pressure, age, gender, diabetes, total cholesterol, HDL cholesterol, and tobacco use. This estimates the risk of an individual in developing a myocardial infarction within 10 years. In terms of risk prediction for younger adults (18–39 years old), the Framingham Risk Score is consistently below 10–12% across all baseline-predicted risk deciles. An additional method of assessing risk is the polygenic score. In a particular study, individuals with high genetic risk had a 91% higher relative risk of incident coronary events compared to those with low genetic risk.

1.2.7. Prevention

If known risk factors are avoided, up to 90% of cardiovascular disease cases may be avoided. Adequate physical activity, reducing obesity, managing high blood pressure, maintaining a nutritious diet, lowering cholesterol, and quitting smoking are all components of prevention. Exercise and medication work about equally well. An estimated 25% lower risk of coronary artery disease is associated with high levels of physical activity. According to the American Heart Association, there are eight essential steps to improve and sustain cardiovascular health. These are called Life's Essential 8. In 2022, AHA included sleep as a factor affecting heart health. The majority of guidelines advise combining these preventative measures. There is some evidence, according to a 2015 Cochrane Review, that counseling and education aimed at changing behavior may be beneficial for high-risk populations. Nevertheless, there wasn't enough data to demonstrate a difference in mortality or real cardiovascular events. Although there is little evidence that very strict blood sugar control reduces the risk of heart attacks in people with diabetes mellitus, better blood sugar control does seem to reduce the risk of other complications like kidney failure and blindness.

1.2.7.1. Diet

Consuming a lot of fruits and vegetables lowers the risk of heart disease and death. It is possible that vegetarians' higher fruit and vegetable consumption lowers their risk of heart disease. Additionally, data point to a decreased risk associated with a high-fiber and Mediterranean diet. It has been demonstrated that consuming trans fat, which is frequently present in hydrogenated products like margarine, increases the risk of coronary artery disease and causes a precursor to atherosclerosis. There is insufficient evidence to suggest that taking supplements of omega-3 fatty acids can help prevent cardiovascular disease, which includes myocardial infarction and sudden cardiac death. Menaquinone (Vitamin K2) intake, but not phylloquinone (Vitamin K1), may lower the risk of CAD mortality, according to preliminary research.

1.2.7.2. Secondary Prevention

Secondary prevention is preventing further sequelae of already established disease. Effective lifestyle changes include:

- Weight control
- Smoking cessation
- Avoiding the consumption of trans fats (in partially hydrogenated oils)
- Decreasing psychosocial stress
- Exercise

Walking, running, or swimming are examples of aerobic exercise that can lower the risk of coronary artery disease-related death. Over time, aerobic exercise can assist in lowering blood pressure and low-density lipoprotein (LDL) levels in the blood.

Moreover, it raises HDL cholesterol. Based on a non-systematic review, the American Heart Association advises physicians to give patients exercise advice.

People with CHD frequently experience psychological symptoms, and although numerous psychological interventions may be suggested after cardiac events, there is no proof that these interventions affect mortality, the likelihood of revascularization procedures, or the frequency of non-fatal myocardial infarction.

1.2.7.2.1. Antibiotics for Secondary Prevention of Coronary Heart Disease

Patients with coronary disease may be able to lower their risk of heart attacks and strokes by taking antibiotics. Recent data, however, points to the dangers of using antibiotics as a secondary preventive measure for coronary heart disease, including an increased risk of stroke and death. Therefore, there is currently no evidence to support the use of antibiotics to prevent secondary coronary heart disease.

1.2.7.3. Neuropsychological Assessment

A comprehensive systematic review revealed that there is a connection between female CHD patients and brain dysfunction. Therefore, people with cardiovascular diseases, such as congestive heart failure (CHD), should undergo neuropsychological evaluations because research indicates that these conditions can act as a risk factor for dementia, such as Alzheimer's disease.

1.2.8. Treatment

There are some treatment options for coronary artery disease:

- Lifestyle changes
- Medical treatment – commonly prescribed drugs (e.g., cholesterol-lowering medications, beta-blockers, nitroglycerin, calcium channel blockers, etc.);

- Coronary interventions such as angioplasty and coronary stent;
- Coronary artery bypass grafting (CABG)

1.2.8.1. Medications

- Statins, which reduce cholesterol, reduce the risk of coronary artery disease
- Nitroglycerin
- Calcium channel blockers and/or beta-blockers
- Antiplatelet drugs such as aspirin

It is recommended that blood pressure be reduced to less than 140/90 mmHg. The diastolic blood pressure however should not be lower than 60 mmHg. Beta-blockers are recommended as first line for this use.

- *Aspirin:* Aspirin lowers the risk of a myocardial infarction but does not alter the overall risk of death in people without a history of heart disease. Therefore, the only adults who should take aspirin therapy to prevent heart disease are those who are at an increased risk for cardiovascular events. These individuals may include males over 40, postmenopausal women, and younger people who have coronary heart disease risk factors such as high blood pressure, diabetes, or a family history of the condition. People at high risk for a cardiovascular event—high risk is defined as having at least a 3% chance over a five-year period—benefits outweigh the risks most favorably, but those at lower risk may still find the potential benefits outweigh the risks.
- *Anti-platelet therapy:* In patients with a STEMI, clopidogrel plus aspirin (dual anti-platelet therapy) reduces cardiovascular events more than aspirin alone. The evidence is weak for those who are at high risk but have not experienced an acute event. It has no effect on this group's risk of dying. More than a year of clopidogrel plus aspirin does not change the risk of death in patients who have had a stent.
- *Surgery:* Revascularization reduces mortality in cases of acute coronary syndrome. For stable ischemic heart disease, percutaneous revascularization does not seem to be any better than medication therapy alone. Percutaneous coronary interventions seem to be less effective than coronary artery bypass grafts in patients with multiple artery disease. Revascularization procedures for the an aortic or no-touch off-pump coronary arteries have demonstrated lower postoperative stroke rates than percutaneous coronary intervention. Although it is more expensive, hybrid coronary revascularization has also been demonstrated to be a safe and practical procedure that may have some benefits over traditional CABG.

1.3. Arrhythmias

Heart rhythm abnormalities, such as an abnormally fast or slow heartbeat, are referred to as arrhythmias. Adults with resting heart rates exceeding 100 beats per minute, are said to have tachycardia, and those with resting heart rates falling below 60 beats per minute, are said to have bradycardia. Certain arrhythmias don't show any symptoms at all. When symptoms arise, one could feel a pause in between heartbeats or palpitations. In more severe situations, symptoms like dizziness, fainting, dyspnea, chest pain, or an altered state of consciousness could occur. Although the majority of arrhythmia cases are not dangerous, some put a person at risk for consequences like heart failure or stroke. Others might cause unexpected death. Extra beats, supraventricular tachycardias, ventricular arrhythmias, and bradyarrhythmias are the four main categories into which arrhythmias are commonly divided. Premature contractions of the atrial, ventricular, and junctional regions are examples of extra beats. Atrial fibrillation, atrial flutter, and paroxysmal supraventricular tachycardia are examples of supraventricular tachycardias. Ventricular tachycardia and fibrillation are examples of ventricular arrhythmias. Atrioventricular conduction abnormalities or dysfunction of the sinus node are the causes of bradyarrhythmias. Arrhythmias result from issues with the heart's electrical conduction system. A Holter monitor and an electrocardiogram (ECG) are two tests that can aid in the diagnosis. An echocardiogram is also ordered to find any underlying structural defects.

Treatments for many arrhythmias are effective. Medication, surgery, and medical procedures like pacemaker implantation are examples of possible treatments. Beta-blockers and antiarrhythmic drugs like procainamide, which work to normalize the heart rhythm, are two types of medications that can be used to treat an elevated heart rate. The latter group might experience more severe adverse effects, particularly if used repeatedly. Slow heart rates such as atrioventricular blocks may be treated with pacemakers. Blood thinners are used to lower the risk of complications in atrial fibrillation.

Those who are medically unstable or exhibit severe symptoms such as in supraventricular tachycardias may require immediate treatment with cardioversion or defibrillation, which involves a controlled electric shock. Arrhythmias impact millions of individuals. As of 2014, 2–3% of people in Europe and North America suffered from atrial fibrillation. From 29,000 in 1990 to 112,000 in 2013, atrial fibrillation and atrial flutter were responsible for 29,000 deaths. Furthermore, due to the infection's capacity to cause myocardial injury, cardiac arrhythmias are frequently developed and linked to high morbidity and mortality among hospitalized COVID-19 infection patients in the majority of recent SARS-CoV-2 pandemic cases. About 15% of all deaths worldwide and roughly half of deaths from cardiovascular disease are caused by sudden cardiac death. Ventricular arrhythmias account for about 80% of cases of sudden cardiac death. While arrhythmias can happen to anyone at any age, they are more common in the elderly. Children can also experience arrhythmias, but the normal range for heart rate changes with age.

1.3.1. Causes

When the electrical impulses that coordinate heartbeats are interfered with, an abnormal heart rhythm results, causing irregular or erratic heartbeats. The complexity and diversity of arrhythmias can be attributed to a variety of intrinsic and extrinsic factors that can cause these disruptions. Underlying cardiac disorders, such as coronary artery disease, heart failure, cardiomyopathy, or congenital heart defects, can interfere with the electrical activity of the heart. These conditions are one of the main causes of arrhythmias. Arrhythmias can also result from disruptions in the normal conduction of electrical impulses caused by scarring from prior cardiac surgeries or damage to the heart muscle from myocardial infarction. Furthermore, structural irregularities in the heart, like thicker walls, enlarged chambers, or aberrant heart valves, can change the electrical characteristics of the heart or obstruct the transmission of electrical signals, which can lead to the formation of substrates for arrhythmias. Electrolyte imbalances, such as abnormal potassium, calcium, or magnesium, can also cause disturbances in the electrical system of the heart. Changes in these electrolyte levels impact the excitability of cardiac cells and interfere with the production and transmission of electrical impulses. Similarly, hormonal imbalances can affect heart rhythm by changing the sensitivity of cardiac cells to electrical signals or by modifying the activity of ion channels involved in cardiac conduction. Examples of these imbalances include thyroid conditions and dysfunctional adrenal glands.

Arrhythmias can also be brought on by outside causes or lifestyle decisions that worsen underlying predispositions. Stimulants like nicotine, caffeine, or some medications (e.g., bronchodilators, decongestants, or some antidepressants) can change the characteristics of cardiac conduction or raise heart rate, which can cause or exacerbate arrhythmias. Similar consequences can arise from excessive alcohol intake, especially in those with underlying cardiac conditions. Arrhythmias can also be brought on by emotional stress or anxiety, as this can trigger the sympathetic nervous system, which causes the heart to beat more rapidly and irregularly. Certain arrhythmias, such as familial forms of atrial fibrillation, long QT syndrome, or Brugada syndrome, which are brought on by inherited mutations affecting ion channels or proteins involved in cardiac electrical signaling, are significantly influenced by genetic predisposition. Particularly in young people without obvious structural heart disease, these genetic abnormalities can impair the normal function of cardiac cells, resulting in abnormal rhythms and an elevated risk of sudden cardiac death. Arrhythmias can also be brought on by infections or inflammations that affect the heart, such as myocarditis or endocarditis, which can interfere with the electrical function of the heart. The electrical characteristics of the heart can be indirectly impacted by inflammatory conditions elsewhere in the body, such as autoimmune diseases or systemic infections, through cytokine-mediated mechanisms or dysregulation of the autonomic nervous system.

1.3.2. Signs and Symptoms

The most typical sign of an arrhythmia is palpitations, or the awareness of an irregular heartbeat. They could occur regularly, sporadically, or continuously. While some of these arrhythmias are benign (although they can be annoying for patients), others put patients at risk for negative consequences. Breathlessness and chest pain are additional symptoms of arrhythmias. Certain arrhythmias are asymptomatic and do not raise the risk of death. Nonetheless, a few asymptomatic arrhythmias are linked to unfavorable outcomes. Examples include an increased chance of blood clotting inside the heart and an increased risk of inadequate blood flow to the heart as a result of a weak heartbeat. Heart failure, sudden cardiac death, embolization, and stroke are additional increased risks. Lower blood pressure may be the first sign of an arrhythmia. Other symptoms include bradycardia, tachycardia, lightheadedness, dizziness, syncope, loss of consciousness, coma, persistent vegetative state, or brain death from a lack of blood and oxygen reaching the brain. Sudden death, or cardiac arrest, is a result of certain arrhythmias.

1.3.3. Types of Supraventricular Arrhythmias

Types of supraventricular arrhythmias include:

- Premature atrial contractions (PACs): Early, extra heartbeats that originate in the atria.
- Paroxysmal supraventricular tachycardia (PSVT): A rapid

but regular heart rhythm that comes from the atria. This type of arrhythmia begins and ends suddenly.

- Accessory pathway tachycardias (such as Wolff- Parkinson-White syndrome): An additional, aberrant electrical pathway or connection between the ventricles and atria that results in a rapid heartbeat. In addition to the regular path, the impulses also pass through the additional pathways. The heart beats abnormally fast as a result of the impulses being able to move around the heart more quickly.
- AV nodal re-entrant tachycardia (AVNRT): A fast heart rhythm caused by the presence of more than one pathway through the atrioventricular (AV) node.
- Atrial tachycardia: A rapid heart rhythm that originates in the atria.
- Atrial fibrillation: A fairly typical irregular cardiac rhythm. Numerous impulses start in the atria and spread out, vying for passage through the AV node. The ensuing rhythm is erratic, fast, and disjointed. The loss of coordinated atrial contraction is caused by the disorderly impulses moving through the atria.
- Atrial flutter: An atrial arrhythmia caused by one or more rapid circuits in the atrium. Atrial flutter is usually more organized and regular than atrial fibrillation.

1.3.4. Physiotherapy

A wealth of research suggests that regular, moderate exercise is advantageous for people with cardiovascular disease as well as healthy individuals. However, people with arrhythmias should avoid vigorous or demanding exercise. They might have negative consequences, such as provoking arrhythmias or making them worse, which could put lives in danger. Depending on what caused the arrhythmia and whether there are other heart disease types, there will be differences in the kind and quantity of exercise that is permitted.

To determine how much activity the heart can withstand and guide the exercise schedule, a stress ECG test, an electrocardiogram (ECG), and a physical examination are performed. An exercise program typically includes three main components: strength training (e.g., lifting light weights), aerobic exercise, and stretching. Make sure that the patient is aware of their symptoms. If they experience palpitations, chest pain, or lightheadedness or dizziness, they should cease their exercise and take some time off.

1.3.5. Risk Factors

Unusual cardiac rhythms, or arrhythmias, can result from a mix of internal and external causes, and some risk factors can contribute to their onset and recurrence. Underlying heart disease, which includes ailments like coronary artery disease, heart failure, cardiomyopathy, congenital heart defects, or structural anomalies in the heart's chambers or valves, is one of the main intrinsic risk factors. These disorders may interfere with the electrical function of the heart, change the way electrical impulses conduct, or provide reentrant circuit substrates, making people more susceptible to arrhythmias. Furthermore, due to ongoing cardiac remodeling or scarring, a history of prior arrhythmias or cardiac procedures, such as atrial fibrillation ablation or implantable cardioverter-defibrillator (ICD) placement, may increase the risk of recurrent arrhythmias. The excitability of cardiac cells and normal electrical signaling can be disrupted by metabolic imbalances, including low potassium, calcium, or magnesium levels. This increases the risk of arrhythmias. Similar to this, changes in the activity of ion channels involved in cardiac conduction or changes in the sensitivity of cardiac cells to electrical impulses are two ways that hormonal fluctuations, such as hyperthyroidism or hypothyroidism, or dysfunction of the adrenal glands, can affect heart rhythm.

Arrhythmia risk is significantly influenced by both external factors and lifestyle choices. Stimulants like nicotine, caffeine, or some medications (e.g., bronchodilators, decongestants, or certain antidepressants) can change the characteristics of cardiac conduction or raise heart rate, which can cause or worsen arrhythmias. Similar to this, excessive alcohol intake can cause arrhythmias, especially in vulnerable people or those with underlying cardiac conditions. Anxiety or emotional stress can stimulate the sympathetic nervous system, which can result in elevated cardiac excitability and sympathetic tone, both of which can cause arrhythmias. The prevalence of some arrhythmias, like atrial fibrillation, rises with age because of changes in the structure and function of the heart that come with aging as well as the cumulative effects of long-term exposure to cardiovascular risk factors. Age is an unmodifiable risk factor for arrhythmias. Arrhythmia risk is also significantly influenced by genetic predisposition and family history, especially in the case of inherited arrhythmia syndromes like familial forms of atrial fibrillation, Brugada syndrome, and long QT syndrome. The underlying cause of these disorders is genetic mutations that impact ion channels or proteins involved in electrical signaling in the heart, making people more vulnerable to arrhythmias and sudden cardiac death.

People with diabetes, hypertension, chronic kidney disease, obstructive sleep apnea, or autoimmune disorders may also be at risk for arrhythmias due to endothelial dysfunction, dysregulation of the autonomic nervous system, inflammation, or fibrosis, among other potential causes. Furthermore, proarrhythmic effects may be caused by some medications, such as antiarrhythmics, antipsychotics, or chemotherapeutic agents, which raises the risk of arrhythmias in those who are vulnerable.

1.3.6. Treatments for Arrhythmias

There are distinct treatment options for every kind of arrhythmia, or irregular heartbeat. Maintaining control over certain arrhythmias may also depend on managing any underlying underlying causes, such as hypertension or coronary heart disease. Treatments of the following kinds could be taken into consideration:

- **Medication.** The medication used will depend on the type of arrhythmia.
- **Catheter destruction (ablation) treatment.** A wire is inserted into the femoral vein to enter the heart chambers. A tiny piece of heart tissue that serves as the origin or trigger for aberrant electrical impulses may be removed by the wire or catheter tip.
- **Cardioversion.** This may be an option for some types of tachycardia. Whilst under an anesthetic, you are given an electrical shock over the heart to restore a normal regular heartbeat. This may revert the abnormal rhythm back to normal.
- **Artificial pacemakers.** These are employed in cases of total heart block. A tiny device called an artificial pacemaker is placed just beneath the skin on the upper chest. At that point, the pacemaker can

continue to pump blood through the heart to keep it beating normally.

- **Implantable cardioverter defibrillators (ICDs).** These are tiny, under-the-skin devices that are placed in the upper chest and resemble pacemakers. The heartbeat is tracked by the gadget. The gadget can shock the heart briefly with electricity if it notices a shift in an irregular heartbeat.

1.3.7. Stages of Heart Arrhythmias

Heart arrhythmias are often categorized into four groups:

- **Extra beats (ectopy)**. The extra beats throw off the heart's regular rhythm, giving rise to feelings of heart palpitations or skipped beats. These are usually benign.
- The atria, the heart's upper chambers, are affected by supraventricular tachycardias, which are rapid heartbeats. An excessively rapid heartbeat impairs the heart's ability to circulate blood throughout the body. Although they rarely result in cardiac arrest or fainting, supraventricular tachycardias are generally not life-threatening.
- **Ventricular arrhythmia** are irregular heart rhythms that affect the lower chambers of the heart, known as ventricles. The ventricles may beat excessively fast, produce extra beats, or twitch instead of completely contracting and relaxing as a result of ventricular arrhythmias. When the ventricles don't work properly, it can seriously affect the body because they are essential for pumping blood from the heart to other parts of the body.
- **Bradyarrhythmias**, occur when the heart rate is abnormally slow and has an irregular rhythm. Sometimes, bradyarrhythmias produce no symptoms. However, since they can reduce the amount of blood flow to the brain and other body parts, they can lead to fainting, dizziness, shortness of breath, or other symptoms.

1.4. Heart Valve Disease

One or more of the four heart valves can be impacted by heart valve disease. The valves function to maintain proper blood flow by opening and closing in response to each heartbeat. Heart valve issues can arise from regurgitation, stenosis, or atresia, which are conditions where the valves are too narrow, leak, or have an improper opening, respectively. Any of several disorders that impair the proper functioning of one or more of your heart's valves is referred to as heart valve disease. If left untreated, this makes the heart work harder, lowering one's quality of life. Heart valves can often be replaced or repaired by minimally invasive surgery.

The valves make sure blood flows in only one direction through your heart. These are:

- **Tricuspid valve.** Located between the right atrium and the right ventricle
- **Pulmonary valve.** Located between the right ventricle and the pulmonary artery
- **Mitral valve.** Located between the left atrium and the left ventricle
- **Aortic valve.** Located between the left ventricle and the aorta

Heart valves are made up of tiny tissue flaps known as leaflets that open during the second half of a heartbeat to let blood pass through the organ. To stop blood from flowing backward, these leaflets close. The tricuspic, pulmonic, and aortic valves have three leaflets. The mitral valve only has two.

The chordae tendineae, which connect the valve leaflets to the papillary muscles inside the ventricles, are strong, fibrous strands of tissue found the tricuspid and mitral valves. The papillary muscles and chordae tendineae maintain the leaflets stable against any blood flow backward.

After circulating through the body, oxygen-poor blood enters the right atrium, passes through the tricuspid valve, and enters the right ventricle. To obtain oxygen from the lungs, it then passes through the pulmonary artery and pulmonary valve. The left atrium receives blood that has been oxygenated through the pulmonary veins. Blood flows from the left atrium to the left ventricle by passing through the mitral valve. After that, blood rich in oxygen leaves the heart through the aorta and passes through the aortic valve.

1.4.1. Heart Valves Function

As the heart muscle contracts and relaxes, the valves open and close, letting blood flow into the ventricles and out to the body at alternate times. The following is a step-by-step explanation of blood flow through the heart.

- The left and right atrium contract once they are filled with blood. This pushes open the mitral and tricuspid valves. Blood is then pumped into the ventricles.
- The left and right ventricles contact. This closes the mitral and tricuspid valves preventing back blood flow. At the same time, the aortic and pulmonic valves open to let blood be pumped out of the heart.
- The left and right ventricles relax. The aortic and pulmonic valves close preventing backward blood flow into the heart. The mitral and tricuspid valves then open to allow forward blood flow within the heart to fill the ventricles again.

1.4.2. Types of Heart Valve Disease

There are different types of heart valve disease, and more than one valve can be affected.

- **Valvular stenosis.** The tissues that make up the valve leaflets stiffen in valvular stenosis, which narrows the valve opening and lowers the volume of blood that can pass through it.
- **Valvular insufficiency.** The tissues that make up the valve leaflets stiffen in valvular stenosis, which narrows the valve opening and lowers the volume of blood that can pass through it.
- **Valvular atresia.** Valvular atresia happens when a heart valve does not form correctly before birth. This is usually diagnosed very early in infancy.

1.4.3. Causes

Numerous intrinsic and extrinsic factors that impact the structure and function of the heart valves can cause damage to the valves, impairing their opening or closure and interfering with the heart's blood flow.

- **Aging**. Degenerative alterations brought on by aging are a major contributor to heart valve damage. These alterations occur when the valves progressively deteriorate over time, thickening, stiffening, or calcifying valve leaflets or annular structures. The aging process can lead to alterations in the flexibility and mobility of the valves, which can affect their capacity to fully open (stenosis) or close completely (regurgitation). This can cause disturbances in normal blood flow and raise the possibility of valve malfunction.

- **Infectious endocarditis**. This is an infection of the heart's inner lining and valves. Pathogens that are bacterial, fungal, or, in rare cases, viral, can infiltrate the bloodstream and settle on the heart valves, resulting in tissue damage, inflammation, and the development of vegetations (clumps of infected tissue and blood cells) on the valve surfaces. This can cause scarring, perforation, thickening, or destruction of the valve, affecting its functionality and making people more susceptible to regurgitation or stenosis. People who have a history of invasive dental procedures, surgeries, intravenous drug use, or congenital heart defects are more likely to develop infectious endocarditis.
- **Rheumatic fever**. A major contributor to heart valve damage is rheumatic fever, a systemic inflammatory disease brought on by untreated or insufficiently treated streptococcal infections. This condition is more common in developing nations with poor access to healthcare. When the body's immune reaction to streptococcal antigens cross-reacts with host tissues, including the heart valves, it can result in rheumatic fever and rheumatic heart disease, which is characterized by inflammation, scarring, and fibrosis. This may cause the valve leaflets to thicken, fuse, or calcify, which could result in aortic valve regurgitation or mitral valve stenosis. In areas where rheumatic fever is still prevalent, rheumatic heart disease is a leading cause of acquired heart valve disease in children and young adults.
- **Congenital heart defects.** Due to their impact on the development, alignment, or functionality of the heart valves during fetal development, congenital heart defects—structural abnormalities present at birth—can also put a person at risk for heart valve damage. Abnormal valve morphology, leaflet motion, or annular dimensions can result from malformations like bicuspid aortic valve, mitral valve prolapse, or atrioventricular septal defects. These conditions raise the risk of valve dysfunction in later life.
- **Genetic syndromes** like Ehlers-Danlos syndrome, Marfan syndrome, or familial thoracic aortic aneurysms and dissections can also be linked to connective tissue disorders that impair the strength and integrity of heart valves, potentially resulting in prolapse or degeneration of the valves.
- **Systemic illnesses** like hypertension, atherosclerosis, or autoimmune disorders can also

cause damage to the heart valve by encouraging thickening, calcification, or inflammation of the valve via a variety of pathways, such as fibrosis, valvular calcification, or carcinoid heart disease, chronic kidney disease, radiation therapy, or specific drugs, such as ergot alkaloids or fenfluramine derivatives, may also raise the risk of valve damage.

- **Lifestyle choices** like obesity, smoking, or being sedentary can aggravate underlying risk factors for valve disease like atherosclerosis or hypertension, which over time raises the chance of valve damage.

1.4.4. Symptoms

There are individuals who may not exhibit any symptoms but still require medical attention for a valve issue. Some people get very obvious symptoms all of a sudden.

If valve disease is severe, symptoms may also appear very quickly. Other diseases advance very slowly, and the heart can eventually make up for it, making the symptoms hardly noticeable. For patients who may be at risk, education and knowledge regarding the potential reasons for a gradual onset of symptoms is crucial because the risk and damage could still be substantial.

Some physical signs of heart valve disease can include:

- Chest pain or palpitations (rapid rhythms or skips)
- Shortness of breath, difficulty catching your breath, fatigue, weakness, or inability to maintain regular activity level
- Lightheadedness or fainting
- Swollen ankles, feet or abdomen

Symptoms don't necessarily determine the seriousness of the valve problems in a patient.

A valve problem can be severe with no symptoms. A valve problem also can be insignificant in terms of leakage, but problematic because of the uncomfortable symptoms.

1.4.5. Diagnosis

1.4.5.1. Tests

Tests to diagnose heart valve disease may include:

- **Echocardiogram.** This test creates images of the beating heart using sound waves. It displays the condition of the heart valves and the flow of blood through the heart.
- **Electrocardiogram (ECG or EKG).** The electrical signals in the heart are recorded during this brief test. It displays the heart's rhythm. Electrodes, which are sensors, are affixed to the chest and occasionally the legs. The sensors are wired to a computer, which prints or displays the data.
- **Chest X-ray.** A chest X-ray shows the heart and lungs. The test can tell if the heart is larger than usual or if there is fluid around the lungs. Fluid could be due to some types of heart valve disease.
- **Cardiac MRI.** A cardiac MRI uses magnetic fields and radio waves to create detailed images of the heart. It can help determine the severity of heart valve disease.
- **Exercise tests or stress tests.** These examinations entail using a stationary bike or treadmill while the heart is monitored. Exercise

testing reveals the heart's response to physical exertion and whether symptoms of valve disease appear during exercise. If a patient is unable to exercise (i.e., due to paralysis or shortness of breath) medications that induce the heart-related effects of exercise are given while the heart is monitored.

- **Cardiac catheterization.** Heart valve disease is not frequently diagnosed with this test. However, if no other test can identify a heart valve issue, it might be done. Alternatively, it may be used to assess the severity of heart valve disease. A catheter is a long, thin, flexible tube that is inserted into a blood vessel, usually in the wrist or groin. It finds its way to the heart. The catheter allows the dye to enter the heart's arteries. The dye enhances the visibility of the arteries in video and X-ray images.

1.4.5.2. Heart Valve Disease Stages

The staging process aids in choosing the best course of action. Numerous factors, such as the disease's severity, the valve structure, and blood flow through the heart and lungs, determine the stage of heart valve disease.

Heart valve disease is staged into four basic groups:

- Stage A: At risk. Risk factors for heart valve disease are present.
- Stage B: Progressive. Valve disease is mild or moderate. There are no heart valve symptoms.
- Stage C: Asymptomatic severe. There are no heart valve symptoms but the valve disease is severe.
- Stage D: Symptomatic severe. Heart valve disease is severe and is causing symptoms.

1.4.6. Heart Valve Repair

The heart is a pump made of muscle tissue. It has four pumping chambers: two upper chambers, called atria, and two lower chambers, called ventricles. Valves between each of the heart's pumping chambers keep blood flowing forward through the heart.

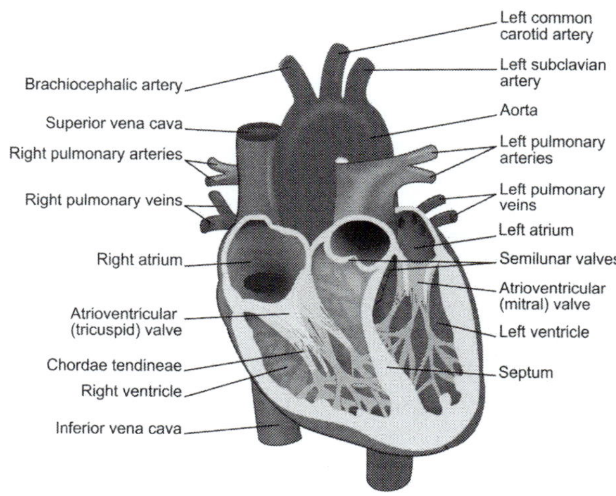

Figure 1.6. *Valves of the heart.*

Source: *By ZooFari – Own workSupporting references ↑ [1] (cache) ↑ [2] (cache), CC BY-SA 3.0, https://commons.wikimedia.org/w/index.php?curid=9841860.*

- **Tricuspid valve.** Located between the right atrium and the right ventricle
- **Pulmonary valve.** Located between the right ventricle and the pulmonary artery
- **Mitral valve.** Located between the left atrium and the left ventricle
- **Aortic valve.** Located between the left ventricle and the aorta

When valves are damaged or diseased and do not work the way they should they may need to be repaired or replaced. Conditions that may cause heart valve dysfunction are valve stenosis (stiffness) and valve regurgitation (leaky valve).

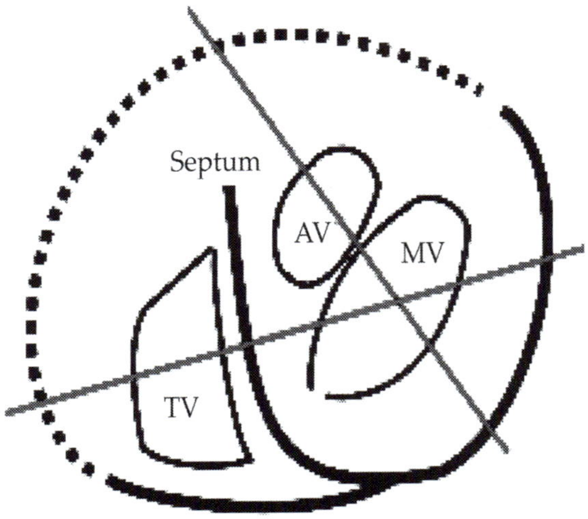

Figure 1.7. *Heart valves.*

Source: *By Kjetil Lenes – Own work, CC BY-SA 3.0, https://commons.wikimedia.org/w/index.php?curid=3705979.*

Note: MV: Mitral valve, TV: Tricuspid valve, AV: Aortic valve, Septum: Interventricular septum. Continuous lines demarcate septum and free wall seen in echocardiogram, dotted line is a suggestion of where the free wall of the right ventricle should be. The red line represents where the upper left loop in the echocardiogram transects the 3D-loop, the blue line represents the lower loop.

The heart must work harder to pump blood through stenotic (stiff) valves, which can affect one or more valves. Aging and infections (like staph or rheumatic fever) can cause valves to narrow and stiffen. Leaky valves cause blood to leak backward, which reduces the amount of blood pumped in the proper direction.

Heart valve replacement or repair is typically accomplished through open heart surgery. To repair or replace the valve(s), a large incision is made in the chest, and the patient's heart is temporarily stopped. Heart valve replacement or repair can now be accomplished with less intrusive, more advanced procedures. Smaller incisions are made during minimally invasive procedures, which also result in less pain following and shorter hospital stays. A ring to support the damaged valve can be used to repair the diseased valve or the damaged valve may be removed and replaced with an artificial valve. Artificial valves can be made from tissue (derived from donated human or animal valves) or carbon-coated plastic.

1.4.6.1. Why One Might Need Heart Valve Repair or Replacement Surgery?

Valve repair or replacement surgery is done to correct the problems caused by one or more diseased heart valves.

If your heart valve(s) becomes damaged or diseased, you may have the following symptoms:

- Dizziness
- Chest pain
- Breathing difficulties
- Palpitations
- Edema (swelling) of the feet, ankles, or abdomen (belly)
- Rapid weight gain due to fluid retention

1.4.6.2. What Are the Risks of Heart Valve Repair or Replacement Surgery?

Possible risks of heart valve repair or replacement surgery include:

- Bleeding during or after the surgery

- Blood clots that can cause heart attack, stroke, or lung problems
- Infection
- Pneumonia
- Pancreatitis
- Breathing problems
- Arrhythmias (abnormal heart rhythms)
- The repaired or replaced valve doesn't work correctly
- Death

There may be other risks depending on the patient's specific medical condition.

A Closer Look

Symptoms of Heart Failure

Heart failure is a complex clinical syndrome characterized by the heart's inability to pump blood effectively to meet the body's metabolic demands. The symptoms of heart failure can vary widely depending on the severity of the condition, the underlying cause, and individual factors such as age, comorbidities, and overall health status. Common symptoms of heart failure include shortness of breath (dyspnea), which may occur during physical exertion or at rest and worsen when lying flat (orthopnea) or during sleep (paroxysmal nocturnal dyspnea). Dyspnea in heart failure results from pulmonary congestion and fluid accumulation in the lungs due to impaired cardiac function, leading to reduced oxygen exchange and increased respiratory effort. Another hallmark symptom is fatigue or weakness, which can result from reduced cardiac output and inadequate tissue perfusion, leading to diminished energy reserves and exercise intolerance. Individuals with heart failure may experience reduced exercise tolerance, with symptoms such as decreased exercise capacity, early onset of fatigue, or difficulty performing routine activities of daily living. Swelling of the legs, ankles, feet, or abdomen (edema) is also common in heart failure, reflecting fluid retention due to impaired circulation and increased venous pressure. Edema may be present bilaterally or asymmetrically and can worsen with prolonged standing or sitting. Additionally, individuals with heart failure may experience weight gain due to fluid retention, despite reduced appetite or dietary intake. Other symptoms of heart failure may include persistent coughing or wheezing, especially when lying down, due to fluid accumulation in the lungs (pulmonary edema), as well as palpitations, chest pain, or a feeling of fullness or bloating in the abdomen due to fluid buildup in the liver or gastrointestinal tract. In advanced stages of heart failure, symptoms may progress to include confusion, dizziness, or lightheadedness, reflecting reduced cerebral perfusion and impaired cognitive function. It is important to note that the symptoms of heart failure can fluctuate over time and may be influenced by factors such as medication adherence, dietary intake, fluid balance, and exacerbating factors such as infections or other medical conditions. Prompt recognition and management of symptoms are essential for optimizing heart failure outcomes, preventing complications, and improving the quality of life for individuals living with this chronic condition (Mozaffarian et al., 2016; Benjamin et al., 2019).

Summary

- Heart disease includes many diseases that affect your heart, but coronary artery disease (CAD) is the most common and familiar one. CAD can create a waxy buildup in your heart's arteries that can cause a heart attack.
- Heart disease refers to a range of conditions that affect the heart's structure and function, leading to various complications. It is a broad term encompassing conditions such as coronary artery disease, heart rhythm problems (arrhythmias), heart defects present at birth (congenital heart defects), and others.
- Heart disease symptoms depend on the type of heart disease. Coronary artery disease is a common heart condition that affects the major blood vessels that supply the heart muscle. Cholesterol deposits (plaques) in the heart arteries are usually the cause of coronary artery disease.
- Heart disease can stem from a multitude of factors, both modifiable and non-modifiable, contributing to its complexity and prevalence worldwide. Among the primary causes is atherosclerosis, a condition characterized by the buildup of plaque in the arteries, which can narrow or block blood flow to the heart.
- Heart arrhythmias, or irregular heartbeats, can manifest with a variety of symptoms, ranging from mild to severe, depending on the type and severity of the arrhythmia.
- Congenital heart defects are structural abnormalities present at birth, affecting the heart's chambers, valves, walls, or blood vessels. The symptoms of congenital heart defects vary widely depending on the type and severity of the defect.
- Cardiomyopathy refers to diseases of the heart muscle, where the heart becomes enlarged, thickened, or stiffened, impairing its ability to pump blood effectively. The symptoms of cardiomyopathy can vary depending on the type of cardiomyopathy, the underlying cause, and the severity of the condition.
- Valvular heart disease refers to conditions that affect the heart's valves, impairing their function and disrupting blood flow within the heart.
- The management and treatment of heart disease encompass a multifaceted approach aimed at addressing underlying risk factors, alleviating symptoms, preventing complications, and improving overall cardiovascular health.
- Cardiac rehabilitation programs play a vital role in the post-treatment phase, providing structured exercise training, education, counseling, and support to individuals recovering from heart disease or cardiac procedures.
- Coronary artery disease is a common heart condition. The major blood vessels that supply the heart (coronary arteries) struggle to send enough blood, oxygen and nutrients to the heart muscle. Cholesterol deposits (plaques) in the heart arteries and inflammation are usually the cause of coronary artery disease.
- Coronary artery disease is characterized by heart problems that result from atherosclerosis. Atherosclerosis is a type of arteriosclerosis that is the "chronic inflammation of the

arteries which causes them to harden and accumulate cholesterol plaques (atheromatous plaques) on the artery walls."

- Arrhythmias, also known as cardiac arrhythmias, are irregularities in the heartbeat, including when it is too fast or too slow. A resting heart rate that is too fast - above 100 beats per minute in adults - is called tachycardia, and a resting heart rate that is too slow - below 60 beats per minute - is called bradycardia.
- The term cardiac arrhythmia covers a very large number of very different conditions. The most common symptom of arrhythmia is an awareness of an abnormal heartbeat, called palpitations. These may be infrequent, frequent, or continuous.
- Heart valve diseases are problems affecting one or more of the four valves in the heart. Heart valves open and shut with each heartbeat to keep blood flowing in the right direction. Problems with heart valves can occur if the valves are leaky (a condition called regurgitation), too narrow (stenosis), or don't have a proper opening (atresia).
- Heart valve damage can result from various intrinsic and extrinsic factors that affect the structure and function of the heart valves, leading to impaired valve opening or closure and disrupting blood flow within the heart (Lloyd-Jones et al., 2010).

References

1. Benjamin, E. J., Muntner, P., Alonso, A., Bittencourt, M. S., Callaway, C. W., Carson, A. P., & Virani, S. S. (2019). Heart disease and stroke statistics—2019 update: A report from the American heart association. *Circulation, 139*(10), e56–e528.
2. Libby, P., Ridker, P. M., & Hansson, G. K. (2011). Progress and challenges in translating the biology of atherosclerosis. *Nature, 473*(7347), 317–325.
3. Lloyd-Jones, D. M., Hong, Y., Labarthe, D., Mozaffarian, D., Appel, L. J., Van Horn, L., & Greenlund, K. (2010). Defining and setting national goals for cardiovascular health promotion and disease reduction: The American heart association's strategic impact goal through 2020 and beyond. *Circulation, 121*(4), 586–613.
4. Mozaffarian, D., Benjamin, E. J., Go, A. S., Arnett, D. K., Blaha, M. J., Cushman, M., & Turner, M. B. (2016). Heart disease and stroke statistics—2016 update: A report from the American heart association. *Circulation, 133*(4), e38–e360.
5. Yusuf, S., Hawken, S., Ôunpuu, S., Dans, T., Avezum, A., Lanas, F., & Lisheng, L. (2004). Effect of potentially modifiable risk factors associated with myocardial infarction in 52 countries (the Interheart study): Case-control study. *The Lancet, 364*(9438), 937–952.

Chapter 2

SYMPTOMS OF BREAST DISEASE

Contents

Introduction

A variety of illnesses, including benign disorders and malignant cancers, can impact the breast tissue and are collectively referred to as breast diseases. For efficient treatment and early detection, it is essential to identify the symptoms. A lump or mass in the breast that can be felt by the patient or by a medical professional is the main indicator of breast disease. Even though not all lumps are cancerous, a medical examination is necessary for any lump that is new, persistent, or changing. Another typical symptom is mastalgia, or pain in the breasts. This pain can range in intensity from a minor, sporadic ache to a severe, ongoing soreness. Even though breast pain is frequently associated with hormonal fluctuations and may not be a sign of cancer, any persistent or unusual pain needs to be looked into.

Alterations in the breast's appearance may also indicate illness. These include skin dimpling or puckering, alterations to the breast's size or form, and redness or peau d'orange, a texture resembling orange peel. These signs could point to an infection like mastitis or an underlying problem like inflammatory breast cancer. Changes in the breasts are important markers of breast disease. Nipple inversion or retraction, discharge that is unrelated to nursing, particularly if it is clear or bloody, and scaling or flaking of the nipple skin are among the symptoms. Such alterations may indicate Paget's disease or ductal carcinoma in situ (DCIS) of the breast.

Even in the absence of a noticeable lump, breast swelling may indicate breast disease. The lymph nodes under the armpit and those surrounding the collarbone may also swell. Expanded lymph nodes may be a sign of an infection or the progression of breast cancer. Breast conditions can also manifest as skin irritation or changes, such as continuous itching or the emergence of a rash. Even though these symptoms are frequently linked to dermatological problems, if they persist, they should not be disregarded.

Lastly, systemic symptoms such as fatigue, bone pain, or unexplained weight loss may be signs of advanced breast cancer. Although these symptoms are not specific to breast disease, their co-occurrence with other symptoms related to breast health should encourage additional medical research. To effectively manage breast disease, early detection through awareness of these symptoms, regular self-examinations, and routine screenings are essential. It is important to consult a healthcare professional as soon as you notice any unusual changes in your breasts to rule out serious conditions and guarantee prompt treatment (Guray & Sahin, 2006; Collins & Schnitt, 2014; Esteva & Gutiérrez, 2014; Overmoyer & Pierce, 2014; Sabel, 2021).

Orientation and Directional Terms

Terms	Definition	Illustration
Breast diseases	Breast diseases make up a number of conditions. The most common symptoms are a breast mass, breast pain, and nipple discharge.	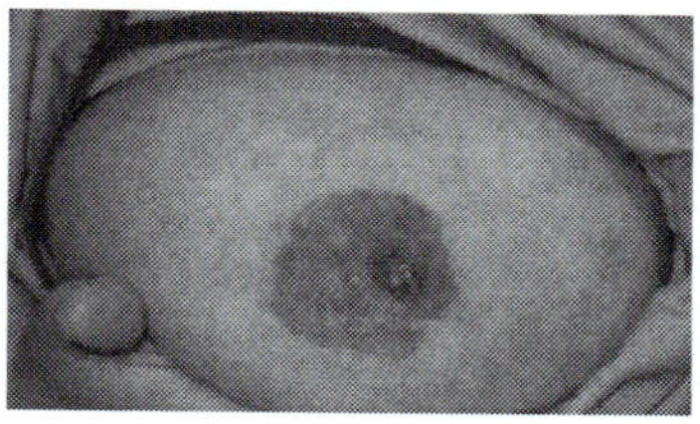
Mammography	Mammography is the process of using low-energy X-rays to examine the human breast for diagnosis and screening.	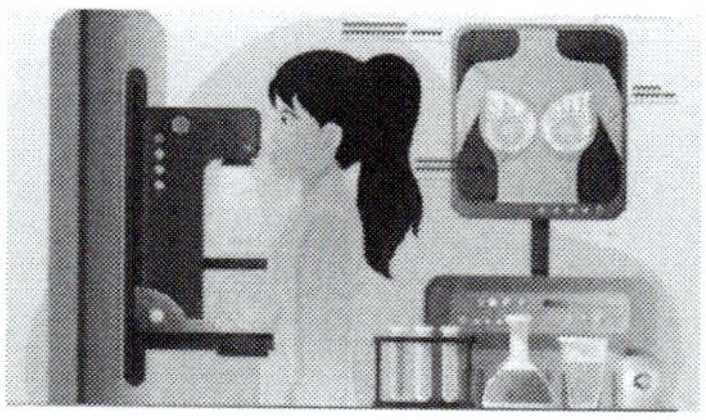
Fibrocystic breasts	Fibrocystic breasts are painful, lumpy breasts. Formerly called fibrocystic breast disease, this common condition is, in fact, not a disease.	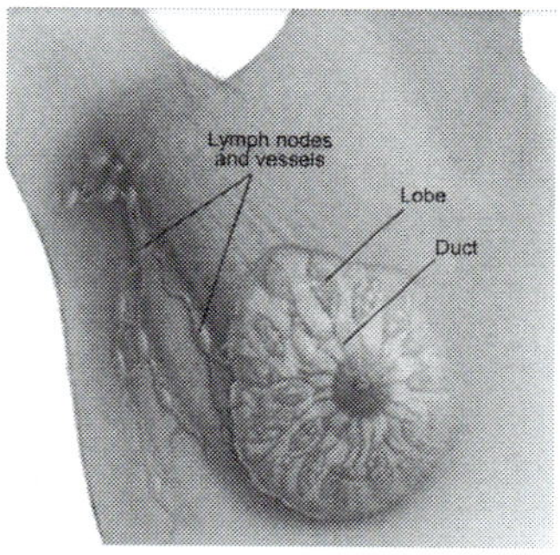
Gynecomastia	Gynecomastia is an increase in the amount of breast gland tissue in boys or men. An imbalance of the hormones estrogen and testosterone causes it.	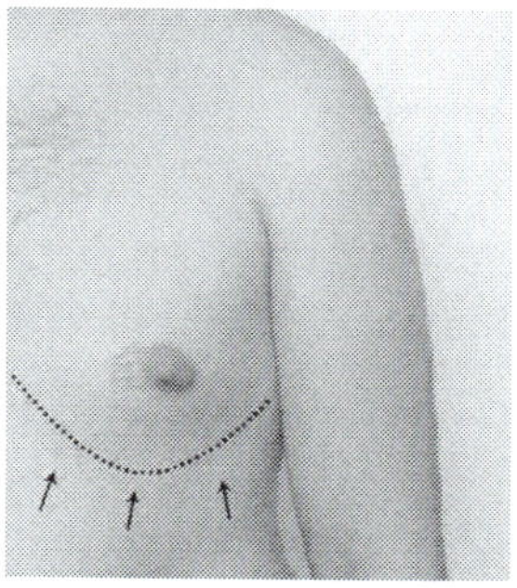
Polymastia	Polymastia, or accessory breasts, is a rare, congenital (present at birth) condition in which a child is born with an additional breast or breast tissue.	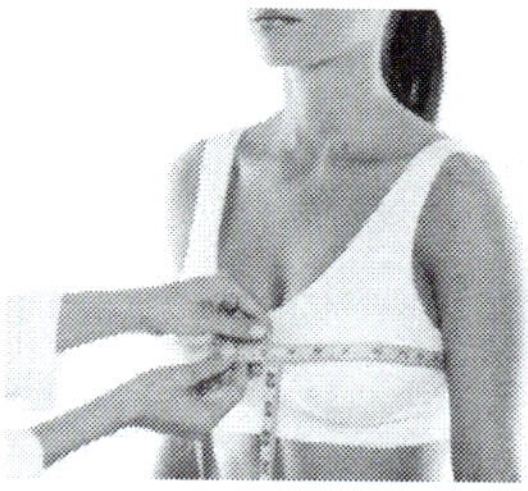

2.1. Overview of Symptoms of Breast Disease

Breast disorders can be classified as benign (non-cancerous) or malignant (cancerous). The majority are not fatal and are not cancerous. They frequently don't need to be treated. On the other hand, treatment for breast cancer is necessary and may include surgery or other intensive cancer treatments.

Potential problems can often be detected early by the following:

- Regular breast examinations with a healthcare professional;
- Mammograms as recommended;
- Early detection of breast cancer can be essential to successful treatment.

Women ought to know what their natural breast and nipple appearance and sensation are. A woman might wish to perform a breast self-examination if she detects a change. Women should notify a healthcare provider of any changes as soon as possible. The majority of medical associations no longer advise regular breast self-examinations on a monthly or weekly basis to screen for cancer. For women who get screening mammograms regularly, doing these exams when there is no lump or other change does not aid in the early detection of breast cancer.

2.1.1. Symptoms of Breast Disorders

Symptoms related to the breast are common, leading to millions of visits to the doctor each year. These symptoms include

- Breast pain
- Breast lumps
- A discharge from the nipple
- Changes in the breast skin (e.g., the breast skin may become pitted, puckered, red, thickened, or dimpled)

Breast symptoms do not always indicate breast cancer or another serious illness in women. For instance, monthly breast tenderness associated with premenstrual hormonal changes does not necessarily signify a serious illness.

However, women should see their doctor if they observe any change in a breast, particularly any of the following:

- A lump or thickened area that feels distinctly different from other breast tissue
- A lump that is stuck to the skin or chest wall
- A lump that does not go away
- Swelling that does not go away
- Pitting, puckering, reddening, thickening, or dimpling in the skin of the breast
- Scaly skin around the nipple
- Changes in the shape of the breast
- Changes in the nipple, such as being pulled inward

- Discharge from the nipple, especially if it is bloody and/or occurs spontaneously (that is, without the nipple's being squeezed or stimulated by other means)

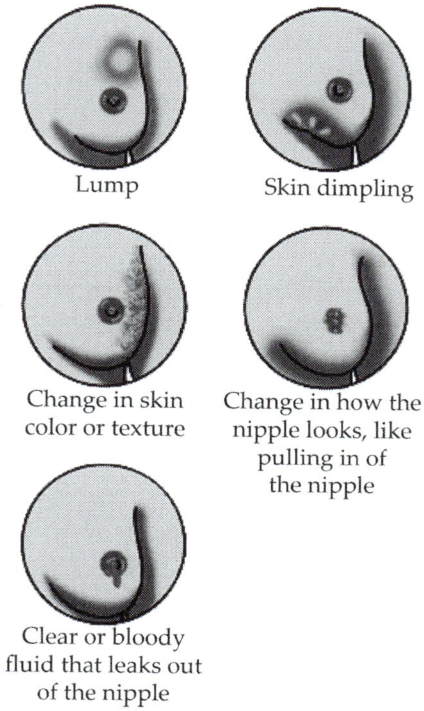

Figure 2.1. *An illustration of breast cancer.*

Source: *By Morning2k – http://www.4woman.gov/faq/cancer-illustrations-with-t.gif, Public Domain, https://commons.wikimedia.org/w/index.php?curid=37747125.*

2.1.2. Evaluation of Breast Disorders

Doctors ask a woman about the symptoms she is having and other information related to possible causes, including:

- What the symptoms are
- How long she has had the symptoms
- Whether the symptoms occur at certain times of the month (related to the menstrual cycle)
- Whether she has a discharge from the nipple, and if so, what it looks like and whether it was from one breast or both
- Whether she is pregnant
- What medications she is taking
- Whether she or a family member has had breast cancer
- When she had her last mammogram and what the results were

2.1.2.1. Breast Examination

The doctor examines each breast while the patient is lying down, and again while the patient is sitting. The physician first looks for skin over the breast that has tightened, thickened, dimpled, or reddened, then looks for nipple inversion (nipples that turn inward). The physician then feels for lumps and tenderness over the breast and axillary areas. Enlarged lymph nodes over the axilla or armpits are also noted. To observe a discharge, the doctor applies pressure around the nipples. The discharge is examined for consistency, color, and presence of blood.

A woman may be asked to stand or sit for the examination of her breasts and underarms. She might be asked to, for instance, put her palms together in front of her forehead while she is seated. The contraction of the chest muscles in this position draws attention to even the slightest changes in the breast.

2.1.2.2. Testing

Imaging tests are used to:

- Check for breast abnormalities before they are noticed by a woman or her doctor (called breast cancer screening)
- Evaluate abnormalities that have been identified, such as a breast

lump found during the doctor's examination

Mammography involves taking X-rays of both breasts to check for abnormalities. A low dose of radiation is used. Only about 10 to 15% of abnormalities detected by mammography result from cancer.

Experts agree that all women should be screened for breast cancer. However, experts disagree about

- When it should start
- How often it should be done
- When (or if) it should be stopped

Screening may include:

- Mammography
- A breast examination by a healthcare professional
- Magnetic resonance imaging (MRI) for high-risk patients

The typical age range to begin screening mammography is between 40 and 50. Next, a mammogram is performed every year or two. Different experts have different opinions on when to begin routine mammography. Since screening mammography is more accurate in women over 50, some experts advise beginning at that age. Depending on a woman's life expectancy and desire for ongoing screening, routine mammography may be discontinued at age 75. The ability of a mammography to identify an anomaly depends on the types of tissue present in the breast. The breast is made up of fatty tissue and fibroglandular tissue, which is made up of glands and fibrous tissue. Women's breast tissue composition changes with age, with more fatty tissue and less fibroglandular tissue present. With a mammography, abnormalities adjacent to fatty tissue are simpler to find. Because of this, mammogram accuracy increases beyond the age of 50.

Certain women have full breasts. Women with dense breasts have less fatty tissue and more fibroglandular tissue. On mammography, abnormalities in dense breasts are more difficult to spot. Additionally, there is a higher chance of breast cancer in women with dense breasts. As a result, these women might need to undergo additional testing, like magnetic resonance imaging (MRI), breast ultrasonography, or 3-dimensional mammography (tomosynthesis).

Mammography can be used to do the following:

- Provide images of any abnormalities (such as a tumor or an abscess) and the tissues around the abnormality
- Provide images of lymph nodes to check for abnormalities
- Help doctors place a biopsy needle into abnormal tissue
- After surgery, help doctors determine whether all the cancer was removed

Mammography may also be done if a woman or doctor finds a lump while examining the breasts or if a woman has breast pain or a discharge from the nipple.

Ultrasonography can be used to do the following:

- Provide the first image of abnormalities that were detected during a breast examination in women under 30 years old
- Provide more information about abnormalities detected by magnetic resonance imaging or mammography—for example, ultrasonography can show whether lumps are solid or filled with fluid (fluid-filled lumps—called cysts—are rarely cancerous)

- Help doctors place a biopsy needle into abnormal tissue
- Identify abnormal lymph nodes that may require biopsy
- Stage breast cancer

Magnetic resonance imaging (MRI) can be used to do the following:

- Evaluate abnormal findings on breast examination or other imaging studies
- After breast cancer is diagnosed, determine the size and number of the tumors, especially in women with dense breast tissue
- Identify abnormal lymph nodes and thus help stage breast cancer

2.1.3. Causes

Most breast cancers have an unknown exact cause. Certain factors have been found by researchers to raise the risk of breast cancer. These consist of environmental factors, lifestyle decisions, and hormones. However, the question of why some people with no risk factors develop cancer while others with risk factors never do remains unclear. Breast cancer most likely results from a complex interplay between environmental factors and your genetic makeup.

Medical professionals are aware that genetic alterations within breast tissue cells are the primary cause of breast cancer. The instructions that tell a cell what to do are encoded in its DNA. The DNA in healthy cells contains instructions on how to divide and grow at a specific rate. The cells are instructed to die at a predetermined time. Different instructions are given by the altered DNA in cancerous cells. The alterations instruct the cancer cells to proliferate rapidly. When healthy cells would die, cancer cells can survive. This results in an excess of cells. The cancer cells may aggregate into a mass known as a tumor. The tumor has the potential to spread and engulf healthy bodily tissue. Cancer cells can split off and travel to other areas of the body over time. Metastatic cancer is the term for cancer that spreads.

The cells lining the milk ducts are typically where the DNA alterations that cause breast cancer occur. The tubes in these ducts are meant to transport milk to the nipple. Invasive ductal carcinoma is the name given to breast cancer that begins in the ducts. Cells in the milk glands may also serve as the source of breast cancer. The purpose of these glands, known as lobules, is to produce breast milk. Invasive Lobular carcinoma is the name for cancer that develops in the lobules. Though it is uncommon, other breast cells have the potential to develop into cancerous ones.

2.1.4. Risk Factors

Factors that may increase the risk of breast cancer include:

- **A family History of Breast Cancer:** If a parent, sibling or child had breast cancer, the risk of breast cancer is increased. The risk is higher when the relative developed breast cancer at a young age. The risk also is higher when multiple family members have had breast cancer. Still, most people diagnosed with breast cancer don't have a family history of the disease.
- **A Personal History of Breast Cancer:** Cancer in one breast increases the risk of getting cancer in the other breast.
- **A Personal History of Breast Conditions:** Certain breast conditions are markers for a higher risk of breast cancer. These

conditions include lobular carcinoma in situ, also called LCIS, and atypical hyperplasia of the breast. The diagnosis of LCIS, typically through breast biopsy, increases the risk of breast cancer.

- **Menarche at a Younger Age:** Menstrual period before age 12 increases the risk of breast cancer.
- **Beginning Menopause at an Older Age:** Menopause after age 55 increases the risk of breast cancer.
- **Being Female:** Women are much more likely than men to get breast cancer. Everyone is born with some breast tissue, so anyone, male or female, can develop breast cancer.
- **Dense Breast Tissue:** Breast tissue is made up of fatty tissue and dense tissue. Dense tissue is made of milk glands, milk ducts and fibrous tissue. Denser breasts have more dense tissue than fatty tissue. Having dense breasts can make it harder to detect breast cancer on a mammogram. If a mammogram shows dense breasts, the risk of breast cancer is increased.
- **Drinking Alcohol:** Drinking alcohol increases the risk of breast cancer.
- **Having a first child at an older age:** Giving birth to their first child after age 30 may increase the risk of breast cancer.
- **Having Never Been Pregnant (Nulligravid):** Having been pregnant one or more times lowers the risk of breast cancer. Never having been pregnant increases the risk.
- **Increasing Age:** The risk of breast cancer goes up with age.
- **Inherited DNA Changes That Increase Cancer Risk:** Certain DNA changes that increase the risk of breast cancer can be passed from parents to children. The most well-known changes are called BRCA1 and BRCA2. These changes can greatly increase the risk of breast cancer and other cancers, but not everyone with these DNA changes gets cancer.
- **Menopausal Hormone Therapy.** Taking certain hormone therapy medicines to control the symptoms of menopause may increase the risk of breast cancer. The risk is linked to hormone therapy medicines that combine estrogen and progesterone. The risk goes down after discontinuing these medicines.
- **Obesity:** People with obesity have an increased risk of breast cancer.
- **Radiation Exposure:** Radiation treatments to the chest as a child or young adult, increases the risk of breast cancer.

2.1.5. Prevention

Making changes in your daily life may help lower your risk of breast cancer. Try to:

- **Ask About Breast Cancer Screening:** Talk with your doctor or other healthcare professional about when to begin breast cancer screening. Ask about the benefits and risks of screening. Together, you can decide what breast cancer screening tests are right for you.
- **Become Familiar With Your Breasts Through Breast Self-Exam for Breast Awareness:** You may

choose to become familiar with your breasts by occasionally inspecting them during a breast self-exam for breast awareness. If there is a new change, a lump or something not typical in your breasts, report it to a healthcare professional right away.

Breast awareness can't prevent breast cancer. But it may help you to better understand the look and feel of your breasts. This might make it more likely that you'll notice if something changes.

- **Drink Alcohol in Moderation, if at All:** Limit the amount of alcohol you drink to no more than one drink a day, if you choose to drink. For breast cancer prevention, there is no safe amount of alcohol. So, if you're very concerned about your breast cancer risk, you may choose to not drink alcohol.
- **Exercise Most Days of the Week:** Aim for at least 30 minutes of exercise on most days of the week. If you haven't been active lately, ask a healthcare professional whether it is OK and start slowly.
- **Limit Menopausal Hormone Therapy:** Combination hormone therapy may increase the risk of breast cancer. Talk with a healthcare professional about the benefits and risks of hormone therapy.

Some people have symptoms during menopause that cause discomfort. These people may decide that the risks of hormone therapy are acceptable to get relief. To reduce the risk of breast cancer, use the lowest dose of hormone therapy possible for the shortest amount of time.

- **Maintain a Healthy Weight:** If your weight is healthy, work to maintain that weight. If you need to lose weight, ask a healthcare professional about healthy ways to lower your weight. Eat fewer calories and slowly increase the amount of exercise.

2.1.5.1. Medicines and Operations for Those at a High Risk of Breast Cancer

You may want to look into other options if your risk of breast cancer is high. If breast cancer runs in your family, you may be at a higher risk. Additionally, if you have a history of precancerous cells in your breast tissue, your risk may be increased. Discuss your risk with your medical team.

Your team might have options for lowering your risk, such as:

- **Preventive Medicines:** Using estrogen-blocking medicines can lower the risk of breast cancer in those who have a high risk. Options include medicines called selective estrogen receptor modulators and aromatase inhibitors. These medicines also are used as hormone therapy treatment for breast cancer.

These medicines carry a risk of side effects. For this reason, they're only used in those who have a very high risk of breast cancer. Discuss the benefits and risks with your healthcare team.

- **Preventive Surgery:** If you have a very high risk of breast cancer, you may consider having surgery to lower the risk of breast cancer. One option might be surgery to remove the breasts, called prophylactic mastectomy. Another option is surgery to remove the ovaries, called prophylactic oophorectomy. This operation lowers the risk of breast cancer and ovarian cancer

(Guray & Sahin, 2006; Collins & Schnitt, 2014; Esteva & Gutiérrez, 2014; Overmoyer & Pierce, 2014; Sabel, 2021)

2.2. Benign Breast Disease

The term "benign breast disease" describes a group of common, non-cancerous conditions that affect the breast tissue. Because these conditions can mimic the symptoms of cancer, they can cause significant anxiety. Fibrocystic changes, fibroadenomas, intraductal papillomas, and mastitis are a few of the benign breast diseases that can occur. The most common benign breast change, known as fibrocystic breast changes, is characterized by lumpy, tender breasts, particularly before menstruation. Hormonal fluctuations are the cause of these changes, which can result in cysts, which are fluid-filled sacs that are generally benign and can vary in size.

Solid, benign tumors called fibroadenomas are most common in young women. When palpated, they are usually smooth, rubbery, and movable. Any new or growing lump should be evaluated to rule out malignancy even though they are not cancerous. Small, wart-like growths called intraductal papillomas form in the breast ducts close to the nipple. They may result in clear or bloody nipple discharge. Even though they are benign, they occasionally need to be removed because of the symptoms they cause and to make sure they aren't concealing more serious conditions.

Mastitis is a common infection in breastfeeding women that can lead to redness, swelling, pain, and sometimes a fever. Treatment typically involves antibiotics and continued breastfeeding or pumping to reduce engorgement. Other noncancerous conditions of the breast include duct ectasia, which may cause nipple discharge and retraction, and fat necrosis, resulting from breast trauma and causing firm, painless lumps. Recognizing benign breast diseases is important for easing concerns and receiving proper care. Regular self-exams and medical check-ups can help distinguish between benign and malignant conditions, providing peace of mind and maintaining good health. If you discover a lump in your breast, it is natural to worry about cancer. However, most breast lumps are not cancerous. Breasts are complex structures that can develop various benign conditions like cysts or tumors. While these conditions are generally not life-threatening, they may increase the risk of future breast cancer. To confirm the nature of a breast lump, it is best to contact a healthcare provider. Additionally, becoming familiar with the look and feel of your breasts can help you notice any changes early on.

2.2.1. Common Types of Benign Breast Disease

Benign breast disease comes in a variety of forms. Any lump, cyst, or other non-cancerous change in your breast tissue is referred to as a benign breast disorder.

Most of the following types don't increase your cancer risk and don't require treatment:

- **Breast Cysts:** Up to 25% of breast lumps are fluid-filled cysts. Breast cysts can be tender and lumpy, but they don't make you more prone to cancer. Cysts often go away without treatment.
- **Fibroadenomas:** These are the most common noncancerous solid breast tumors providers find in people with a vagina between the ages of 15 to 35. Fibroadenomas don't increase cancer risk and often go away on their own.

- **Fibrocystic Breast Changes:** Fluctuating hormone levels can make breasts feel lumpy, dense and tender, especially right before menstruation. People with a vagina between the ages of 30 to 50 are more likely to experience fibrocystic breast changes, which go away without treatment.
- **Hyperplasia:** This condition occurs from an overgrowth of cells that line your mammary ducts or glands. A condition called usual (typical) hyperplasia slightly increases breast cancer risk but doesn't require surgery. If you have atypical hyperplasia, your healthcare provider may recommend surgically removing the affected breast tissue because the condition may make you more prone to breast cancer.
- **Intraductal Papilloma:** These small, wart-like growths form inside your mammary duct near your nipple. Intraductal papilloma may cause nipple discharge. The condition most commonly affects people with a vagina between the ages of 30 to 50. Your risk of cancer goes up if you have five or more papillomas at one time. Surgery can remove these growths and reduce your cancer risk.
- **Mammary Duct Ectasia:** People who have reached menopause are more prone to mammary duct ectasia. It causes your milk ducts to swell, thicken and sometimes become blocked. Your nipple may turn inward or leak discharge. Also known as periductal mastitis, this condition doesn't increase cancer risk. You may need antibiotics if a bacterial infection causes inflammation and blockage. Otherwise, you don't need treatment.
- **Traumatic Fat Necrosis:** These breast lumps form when scar tissue replaces breast tissue that's been damaged by an injury, surgery or radiation therapy. Fat necrosis doesn't raise your cancer risk and doesn't need treatment.
- **Adenosis:** This is when the lobules (milk-producing part of your breast) in your breast grow larger and contain more glands than usual.

Benign breast lumps are a common occurrence for women and individuals assigned female at birth (AFAB). Approximately half of all women will experience fibrocystic changes that result in noncancerous breast lumps at some point in their lives. While men and individuals assigned male at birth (AMAB) can also develop benign breast disease, it is less prevalent.

2.2.2. Symptoms and Causes

2.2.2.1. What Are the Symptoms of Benign Breast Disease?

As you shower, put on clothes, or perform a breast self-examination, you might notice changes in your breasts or a lump. Your doctor may occasionally notice these changes when doing a mammography or clinical breast exam.

Besides a breast lump, other signs of benign breast disease include:

- Breast pain (mastalgia).
- Nipple discharge.
- Change in breast size, shape or contour.

- Inverted, creased or scaly nipple.
- Dimpled, puckered or scaly breasts.

2.2.2.2. What Causes Benign Breast Disease?

Common causes of noncancerous breast lumps include:

- Changes in breast tissue (fibrocystic breast changes).
- Breast infection (mastitis).
- Scar tissue from a breast injury.
- Hormone fluctuations, especially during menstruation, pregnancy or menopause.
- Medication use, such as hormonal contraceptives (birth control pills) and hormone replacement therapy.
- Consuming too much caffeine.

Men and people can develop enlarged, swollen breasts with lumps, a condition called gynecomastia. Gynecomastia happens due to hormone imbalance, obesity and certain diseases or medications.

2.2.2.3. What Are the Risk Factors for Benign Breast Disease?

Benign breast disease can affect anyone. Your risk for benign breast disease increases if you:

- Have a family history of breast cancer or benign breast disease.
- Use hormone replacement therapy.
- Have a hormonal imbalance.

2.2.2.4. What Are the Complications of This Condition?

Breast cancer risk is increased by certain benign breast diseases, such as atypical hyperplasia. Benign breast lumps can occasionally hurt or enlarge. Your doctor might advise surgery to remove large or uncomfortable lumps. Regretfully, following surgery, some fibroadenoma lumps recur.

2.2.3. Diagnosis and Tests

- **How Is Benign Breast Disease Diagnosed?**

If you feel a lump or notice breast changes, see your healthcare provider immediately. Your provider may order one or more of these tests:

- o Imaging scans, including mammogram, ultrasound or magnetic resonance imaging (MRI).
- o Image-guided core needle breast biopsy, fine-needle aspiration biopsy or excisional biopsy to test cells for cancer. An excisional (or surgical) biopsy involves removing a larger piece of tissue from your breast.

2.2.4. Management and Treatment

- **How Is Benign Breast Disease Managed or Treated:** The majority of benign breast diseases don't need to be treated. If you have atypical hyperplasia or another benign breast disease that raises your risk of breast cancer in the future, your doctor might suggest treatment. To lower your risk, this can entail surgical excision or specific medications.

If you experience pain or discomfort or have an increased cancer risk, these treatments can help:

- o Fine needle aspiration to drain fluid-filled cysts.
- o Surgery to remove lumps

- Oral antibiotics for infections like mastitis.
- **Can I Get Benign Breast Disease More Than Once?:** Benign breast lumps can happen frequently throughout your lifetime and are fairly common. When hormone levels fluctuate as a result of menstruation or menopause, your breasts may feel lumpy or sensitive. Anytime you detect a change in your breasts or feel a lump, you should get in touch with your healthcare provider.
- **How Does Pregnancy Affect Benign Breast Disease?:** Breast lumps, tenderness, and nipple discharge during pregnancy can be caused by changes in hormone levels. Additionally, while breastfeeding (chest feeding), you run the risk of developing a breast infection known as mastitis or experiencing benign breast changes. Rarely are changes to the breasts that occur during pregnancy or nursing malignant. Nevertheless, as soon as you notice any changes to your breasts, you should consult your healthcare provider.
- **Do Benign Breast Tumors Need to Be Removed?:** Sometimes. It depends on the results of any diagnostic tests, your risk for cancer and if the tumor is painful or large. Your healthcare provider can discuss removing a benign tumor with you.

2.2.5. Prevention

- **How Can I Prevent Benign Breast Disease?**

You may not be able to prevent benign breast disease, but you can take steps to reduce your risk. These steps may lower your risk of some benign breast disease:

- Decreasing caffeine intake (coffee, tea, soda or chocolate, for example).
- Wearing well-fitted bras and avoiding underwire bras.
- Not smoking or quitting smoking.
- Avoid drinking beverages containing alcohol.

These steps may lower cancer risk and help detect disease early when it is most treatable:

- Get regular mammogram screenings.
- Perform self-breast exams to be familiar with how your breasts look and feel.
- Maintain a weight that's healthy for you.
- Exercise regularly.
- Eat a nutritious diet.
- Drink alcoholic beverages in moderation or not at all.
- Quit smoking cigarettes or using other tobacco products.
- Reconsider the use of hormone replacement therapy.
- Switch to a non-hormonal birth control option.

2.2.6. Breast Anatomy

The structure of the mammary gland, an ectodermal organ common to mammals, reflects its unique purpose of producing milk for lactation. The human breast possesses an indisputable aesthetic value, having served as the inspiration for countless artistic creations over the ages. It also has an erotic significance because many cultures identify the breast with sensuality and sexuality. There is a wide range in women's breast size and shape. Some women have larger breasts and a lot of breast tissue. Some have less tissue and less fat in their breasts. Rarely are a woman's breasts the same size; instead, one is typically slightly bigger, smaller, higher, or shaped differently than the other.

The lobules (where milk is produced) that connect to the ducts that run out to the nipple comprise the epithelial components that make up the inner structure of the mammary gland. The background fibrous tissue and adipose tissue that make up the breast's main mass are home to these lobules and ducts. Except for the absence of specialized lobules in the male breast tissue due to the lack of a physiological requirement for milk production, the structure of the male and female breasts is nearly identical.

2.2.6.1. Development of the Breast (Embryology)

The development of human breast tissue starts in the fifth or sixth week of fetal life. It begins as a single ectodermal bud and develops into longitudinal bands of thickened ectoderm called "milk lines" that run from the axilla to the pelvis on the ventral side of the embryo. By the ninth week of pregnancy, only one pair of mammary glands forms in the pectoral region of the milk line in humans, in contrast to the majority of mammals that develop a series of paired glands along this ridge.

The nipple bud develops from a mass of proliferating basal cells in this area. By the 12th week, squamous cells from the surface start to invade the nipple bud. Meanwhile, mesenchymal cells differentiate into the smooth muscle of the nipple and areola, and epithelial cells grow downward as mammary ducts, terminating in lobular buds. By the 20th to 24th weeks of gestation, this specialized epithelium buds into 15–20 branches that initially consist of solid epithelial columns. Eventually, the branches canalize to form the lactiferous ducts. The placental sex hormones that enter the fetal circulation during the third trimester stimulate the canalization of these branched epithelial tissues.

Colostrum is a yellow, sticky, serous fluid that is contained in lobulo-alveolar structures, which are formed at the ends of these branches. This colostral milk, also known as "witch's milk," can be expressed for 4-5 days following birth in both male and female newborns and is triggered by placental hormones. 1,2 The mammary gland's mass steadily increases in the last few weeks of pregnancy, and the nipple-areola complex (NAC) grows and pigments. Following delivery, the withdrawal of placental hormones causes the breast to begin an involution and cease colostral secretion. The mesenchyme that invades and envelops the epithelium is the source of the connective tissue and fat that make up the breast's supporting structure.

Congenital anomalies of the breast may arise from the failure of some of these stages of breast development. Etiological breast tissue has been reported in 1-6% of cases. For instance, accessory nipples, or polythelia, are common along the milk line and are typically located on the chest wall beneath the breast (Figure 2.2). These develop as a result of the milk streak's regression failing. Additionally common are inverted nipples, which result from the small mammary pit's inability to evaginate at birth. Patients who have accessory mammary glands (polymastia), which are typically located in the axilla and cause pain or a mass in that area, typically do so because the milk line has failed to fully atrophy. A rare congenital anomaly known as absence of the breast (amastia) is caused by an arrested mammary ridge around the sixth week of pregnancy.

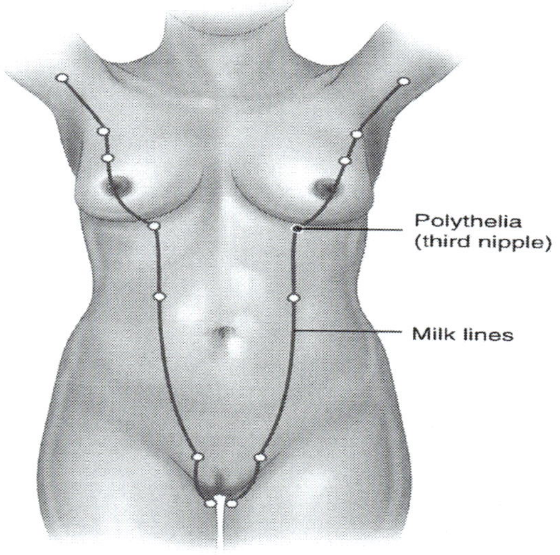

Figure 2.2. *The milk line extends from the axilla to the groin. Aberrant breast and/or vestigial nipple and areola development can occur anywhere along this line.*

Source: *By The Geneva Foundation for Medical Education and Research – http://www.gfmer.ch/genetic_diseases_v2/gendis_detail_list.php?cat3=1518, CC BY-SA 3.0, https://commons.wikimedia.org/w/index.php?curid=25931398.*

2.2.6.2. Development of the Breast from Birth until Puberty

There are no alveoli in the breast during this time; only lactiferous ducts exist. The circulating estrogen causes the stroma and ductal epithelium to grow as puberty progresses. These ducts start to arborize, forming terminal duct lobular units and collecting ducts. In the end, these develop into buds before additional breast lobules. Adipose tissue is replaced by connective tissue, which is more elastic and has increased in volume, surrounding the ducts and supporting the formation of ducts. One of the earliest indications of adolescence in girls is breast budding, which can start at any age between eight and thirteen.

2.2.6.3. Development of the Breast During Pregnancy

Pregnancy is when the breast reaches its full potential. Under the influence of prolactin, luteal and placental sex steroids, and other factors, secreting alveoli emerge and the ducts, lobules, and alveoli grow noticeably. In the initial weeks, ductal sprouting and lobular proliferation occur due to the influence of estrogen. By the second month, the breasts have significantly grown larger and have become more pigmented in the areolar and nipple areas. The secretory cells have now formed a lumen encircling the alveoli. Progesterone causes the lobular formation to outpace ductal sprouting during the second trimester of pregnancy, accompanied by a discernible increase in prolactin levels. The breast is still growing at this point, and colostrum is present in the alveoli. The breast begins to secrete colostrum in the final trimester, which is later replaced by real milk secretion, as the stroma surrounding the lobules shrinks to make room for the hypertrophied lobules. The glandular tissue goes back to resting when lactation stops.

2.2.6.4. Development of the Breast During Menopause

Menopause is characterized by a range of symptoms related to the loss of estrogen and progesterone, and it usually strikes women in their late 40s and early 50s. The breast's glandular tissue shrinks, the connective tissue loses some of its cellularity, and there is less collagen overall. The breast typically sags and gains volume as a result of the connective tissue losing its strength. These atrophic changes, however, differ and are not consistent from woman to woman (Guray & Sahin, 2006; Collins & Schnitt, 2014; Esteva & Gutiérrez, 2014; Overmoyer & Pierce, 2014; Sabel, 2021).

2.3. Breast Pathology

The breast can develop a broad variety of benign and malignant lesions.

2.3.1. Benign Breast Conditions

Most people think that breast cancer is related to breast abnormalities. But not every breast condition is cancerous. Numerous benign (non-cancerous) breast disorders exist. A benign breast condition is any non-cancerous lump, cyst, or nipple discharge (fluid) on the breast of a man or woman.

For women, the most common ones are:

- **Fibrocystic Breast Changes**: Fibrosis feels like scar tissue and can be rubbery and firm.
- **Cysts***:* These are sacs filled with fluid. They may enlarge and feel tender right before your period.
- **Fibroadenomas***:* These are the most common breast lumps in younger women and are usually small.
- **Mastitis***:* Your breast can become enlarged because of infection. This can happen to anyone but usually happens when breastfeeding.
- **Fat Necrosis***:* These lumps form when areas of fatty breast tissue are damaged.
- **Calcification***:* Small spots of calcium salts can show up anywhere in breast tissue. Usually, these are asymptomatic.
- **Nipple Discharge***:* Your nipples may leak fluid for a variety of reasons.
- **Hyperplasia, Adenosis, Intraductal Papilloma, and Lipoma***:* These are made up of mostly fat tissue.

Less common types of benign breast conditions include:

- **Atypical Hyperplasia***:* This is an abnormal increase in cell growth in the breast.
- **Adenosis***:* The lobules in your breasts can become enlarged and contain more glands than usual.
- **Intraductal Papillomas***:* Small tumors can form in your nipple's milk ducts.

2.3.1.1. Fibrocystic Changes in the Breast

Fibrocystic changes, collectively known as fibrosis and/or cysts, are non-cancerous (benign) alterations in fibrous tissue that frequently manifest as breast lumps. Previously known as "fibrocystic disease," these alterations are a common occurrence in many women. Although they can affect women at any age, fibrocystic changes are most common in women who are childbearing age.

- **Fibrosis:** Fibrosis refers to an area of fibrous tissue, the same tissue that ligaments and scar tissue are made of. Areas of fibrosis can feel rubbery or firm to the touch.
- **Cysts:** Cysts are round or oval sacs inside the breasts that are filled with fluid. They frequently feel like a movable, round lump or lumps that may be sensitive to touch. Although they can affect women at any age, they are most common in those in their 30s and 40s. Cysts frequently enlarge, become painful, and occasionally become more noticeable right before the menstrual period due to monthly hormone fluctuations. When fluid begins to accumulate inside the breast glands, cysts develop. They begin as extremely tiny cysts called

microcysts, which are too small to feel unless they are part of a cluster. Should fluid accumulation persist, these may transform into macrocysts, which are sizable cysts. These are frequently easily felt and can measure up to one or two inches in diameter.

- **Diagnosis of Fibrocystic Changes:** The majority of the time, symptoms such as breast lumps, swelling, and/or tenderness or pain are used to diagnose fibrocystic changes. These symptoms usually peak right before your menstrual period, and they may fluctuate depending on where you are in the menstrual cycle (e.g., lumps may grow or shrink). You might occasionally detect some nipple discharge.

If there is a concern about a lump possibly being cancer, a breast ultrasound typically is done to see if the lump is solid or if it has fluid in it (that is, if it is a cyst). There are different types of cysts:

- o A simple cyst is filled entirely with fluid. Simple cysts are not a cause for concern.
- o A complicated cyst is similar to a simple cyst, but it has what looks like 'debris' floating in the fluid. Complicated cysts are very unlikely to be cancer, but in some cases a doctor might advise a follow-up exam or a procedure to remove the fluid with a thin, hollow needle, just to be sure.
- o A complex cystic and solid mass has features such as a solid component or thick outer walls. These findings have a higher chance of being cancer, so a biopsy is usually needed to find out for sure.

- **How Do Fibrocystic Changes Affect Your Risk for Breast Cancer?:** Simple cysts and fibrosis do not raise your chance of acquiring breast cancer in the future. Depending on the results of a biopsy, there is a slight possibility that complex cysts, solid masses, and cystic cysts may contain cancer or increase your chance of developing breast cancer in the future.
- **Treatment of Fibrocystic Changes:** As fibrocystic alterations in the breast are believed to be natural, treatment is typically not required unless they become uncomfortable. A thin, hollow needle can be used to drain painful cysts, and this procedure may be performed to confirm the diagnosis. Pressure and pain may temporarily subside after the fluid is removed. If removed, the fluid may reappear later, but cysts may eventually disappear as well. Cysts that recur and cause symptoms may need to be surgically removed. Treatment is not necessary for the majority of women with fibrocystic changes who do not have any bothersome symptoms, but the doctor may advise close observation of the changes. If your discomfort is moderate, wearing supportive bras that fit well, heating up your body, or taking over-the-counter painkillers could help.

Some women claim that if they stay away from coffee, tea, chocolate, and many soft drinks that contain caffeine and other stimulants, their breast symptoms get better. Although research has not conclusively linked these stimulants to breast symptoms, many women believe it is worthwhile to try abstaining from these foods and beverages for a few months.

Some physicians advise taking over-the-counter painkillers like acetaminophen or ibuprofen, as well as other medications because breast swelling during the end of the menstrual cycle can be uncomfortable for certain women. Although some vitamin or herbal supplements have been proposed as potential symptom relievers, none have been shown to be effective to date, and some may cause negative effects if taken in excess. Certain physicians prescribe hormones, including androgens, tamoxifen, and oral contraceptives (birth control pills). However, because they may have harmful side effects, these are typically only prescribed to women who have severe symptoms. If you have breast symptoms that aren't improving or are getting worse, it is important to see your doctor for further evaluation.

2.3.1.2. Hyperplasia of the Breast

The overgrowth of cells lining the lobules (milk-producing glands) or ducts (small tubes) inside the breast is known as hyperplasia. Certain forms of hyperplasia are associated with an increased risk of breast cancer, but they are not the same as cancer.

Hyperplasia can be described as either typical or atypical, based on how the cells look under a microscope.

- In usual ductal hyperplasia (UDH), there is an overgrowth of cells lining the ducts in the breast, but the cells look very close to normal.
- In atypical hyperplasia (or hyperplasia with atypia), the cells look more distorted and abnormal. This can be either atypical ductal hyperplasia (ADH) or atypical lobular hyperplasia (ALH).

- **Diagnosis of Hyperplasia:** Although hyperplasia rarely results in a palpable lump, it can occasionally cause abnormalities that show up on a mammography. A biopsy is used to diagnose it, removing a sample of the abnormal breast tissue for testing using a hollow needle or surgery.
- **How Does Hyperplasia Affect Your Risk for Breast Cancer?:** Hyperplasia can affect your risk for breast cancer, but how much depends on what type it is:
    - **Usual Ductal Hyperplasia (Also Known as Moderate or Florid Hyperplasia of the Usual Type, Without Atypia):** The risk of breast cancer is about 1½ to 2 times higher than that of a woman with no breast abnormalities.
    - **Atypical Hyperplasia (Either ADH or ALH):** The risk of breast cancer is about 4 to 5 times higher than that of a woman with no breast abnormalities.
- **Treatment of Hyperplasia:** Treatment is not necessary for usual ductal hyperplasia in the breast since it is regarded as a normal finding. In the event that a needle biopsy sample reveals the presence of ADH, additional breast tissue removal may be advised. This is to ensure that nothing more dangerous, like cancer, is present in the area.

2.3.1.3. Lobular Carcinoma in Situ (LCIS)

A breast biopsy may occasionally reveal lobular carcinoma in situ (LCIS), a form of breast alteration. The lining of the breast's milk-producing glands, or lobules, is home to cells that resemble cancer cells in LCIS, but they do not break through the lobules' walls. If left untreated, LCIS is not classified as cancer and usually does not spread to the surrounding tissue, meaning it does not progress to become invasive breast cancer.

However, having LCIS raises your chances of subsequently getting invasive breast cancer in either breast. Lobular neoplasia includes LCIS and another type of breast change known as atypical lobular hyperplasia, or ALH. Both of these benign (non-cancerous) conditions raise your chance of developing breast cancer.

The different types of LCIS are:

i. **Classic LCIS:** The cells lining the lobules of the breast are smaller and are about the same size.

ii. **Pleomorphic LCIS:** The cells lining the lobules of the breast are larger and look more abnormal.

iii. **Florid LCIS:** The cells lining the lobules have grown into a large enough group that they have formed a mass, typically with an area of dead cells in the middle (called central necrosis).

- **Diagnosis of LCIS:** Although pleomorphic and florid LCIS can occasionally be detected in this manner, classic LCIS typically does not result in a palpable lump or changes that can be seen on a mammography. LCIS is typically discovered during a breast biopsy performed for a related issue. Tiny bits of breast tissue are taken out and examined in a lab during a biopsy.
- **How Does LCIS Affect Breast Cancer Risk?:** The risk of developing invasive breast cancer in either breast is approximately 7–12 times higher for women with LCIS. Because of this, medical professionals usually advise women with LCIS to undergo routine screening for breast cancer and to follow up with a physician for the remainder of their lives.
- **Treatment for LCIS:** Having LCIS does increase your risk of developing invasive breast cancer later on. However, since LCIS is not a true cancer or pre-cancer, often no treatment is needed after the biopsy. In certain cases, if a needle biopsy reveals LCIS, the physician may advise its total removal (through excisional biopsy or another kind of breast-conserving surgery) to ensure that LCIS was the only anomaly discovered. This is particularly true if the LCIS is characterized as florid or pleomorphic, which may increase its likelihood of growing quickly. If pleomorphic or florid LCIS is discovered even after an excisional biopsy, some physicians may suggest a second, more involved procedure to ensure that it has been completely removed.

2.3.1.4. Adenosis of the Breast

Adenosis is a benign (non-cancerous) breast condition characterized by enlarged lobules (milk-producing glands) and an increased number of glands relative to normal. Women with fibrocystic changes in their breasts frequently have adenosis in their biopsy samples. This condition is also known by several other names, such as aggregate adenosis, tumoral adenosis, or adenosis tumor. Adenosis is not breast cancer, even though it is referred to as a tumor in some of these terms. Sclerosing adenosis is a unique kind of adenosis where scar-like tissue distorts the enlarged lobules. This kind could result in breast pain.

- **Diagnosis of Breast Adenosis:** Enlarged lobules may be large enough to be felt as a breast lump if they are located close to one another. A breast exam might not be sufficient in these circumstances to determine whether the lump is an adenosis or something else (like breast cancer). Both breast cancers and adenosis, including sclerosing adenosis, can develop calcifications (mineral deposits). Mammograms may reveal these, which can make it challenging to distinguish between the two conditions. Due to these uncertainties, determining whether the breast change is due to cancer or adenosis usually requires a breast biopsy. (Tiny bits of breast tissue are removed during a biopsy and examined under a microscope.).
- **Treatment of Adenosis:** Adenosis does not usually need to be treated, unless it is causing bothersome symptoms.
- **How Does Adenosis Affect Your Risk for Breast Cancer?:** Most types of adenosis are not thought to increase breast cancer risk, although some studies have found that women with sclerosing adenosis have a slightly higher risk of breast cancer.

2.3.1.5. Fibroadenomas of the Breast

Fibroadenomas are frequently occurring, non-cancerous growths in the breast that consist of glandular and stromal tissues. They are most prevalent in women between the ages of 20 and 30 but can be found in women of all ages. Typically, fibroadenomas decrease in size after menopause.

2.3.1.5.1. Diagnosis of Fibroadenomas

While some fibroadenomas are too tiny to feel, others can measure up to several inches in diameter. One or more fibroadenomas can occur in a woman. It is common for fibroadenomas to feel like a marble inside the breast. They usually have distinct borders and are spherical or oval in shape. Although they are not sensitive, they are typically firm or rubbery and moveable under the skin. A mammogram or ultrasound are two examples of imaging tests that are necessary to detect certain fibroadenomas. To determine with certainty whether a breast mass is a fibroadenoma (or some other condition), a breast biopsy (removing some breast tissue to check it in the lab) may be required.

Under a microscope, the majority of fibroadenomas have an identical appearance. We refer to these as simple fibroadenomas. Complex fibroadenomas, on the other hand, are fibroadenomas that also exhibit additional changes. Patients who have complex fibroadenomas typically age and have larger tumors.

2.3.1.5.2. How Do Fibroadenomas Affect Your Risk for Breast Cancer?

Simple fibroadenomas do not seem to increase breast cancer risk by much, if at all. Complex fibroadenomas seem to increase the risk slightly more than simple fibroadenomas.

2.3.1.5.3. Treatment of fibroadenomas

Most fibroadenomas don't require medical attention. However, in certain situations, particularly if they continue to grow or alter the breast's shape, doctors may advise their removal. Fibroadenomas can occasionally stop growing or even shrink on their own without any medical intervention. The masses can frequently be left in place and monitored to make sure they don't grow provided the doctor is certain that they are fibroadenomas rather than breast cancer. For women who have numerous non-growing fibroadenomas, this method can be helpful. In these situations, excising them could involve removing a significant portion of the surrounding normal breast tissue, leaving scars and altering the breast's texture and shape.

Women who have fibroadenomas must undergo routine imaging tests or breast exams to ensure that the tumors are not getting bigger. Following the removal of one fibroadenoma, one or more may occasionally develop. This typically indicates the formation of a new fibroadenoma rather than the return of the previous one.

2.3.1.6. Phyllodes Tumors of the Breast

Phyllodes tumors are uncommon breast tumors originating in the connective tissue of the breast, rather than the ducts or glands where most breast cancers develop. The majority of phyllodes tumors are noncancerous, with only a small percentage being malignant. These tumors typically affect women in their 40s, although they can occur at any age. Individuals with Li-Fraumeni syndrome, a rare hereditary genetic disorder, are at a higher risk for developing phyllodes tumors.

Phyllodes tumors are often divided into 3 groups, based on how they look under a microscope:

- Benign (non-cancerous) tumors account for more than half of all phyllodes tumors. These tumors are the least likely to grow quickly or to spread.
- Borderline tumors have features in between benign and malignant (cancerous) tumors.
- Malignant (cancerous) tumors account for about 1 in 4 phyllodes tumors. These tend to grow the fastest and are the most likely to spread or to come back after treatment.

2.3.1.6.1. Diagnosis of Phyllodes Tumors

Although some may hurt, phyllodes tumors are typically felt as a firm, painless breast lump. They frequently stretch the skin and tend to grow larger rather quickly. When these tumors are initially detected by imaging tests (such as mammograms or ultrasounds), it can be challenging to distinguish them from fibroadenomas. A core needle biopsy is frequently sufficient to make the diagnosis; however, in certain cases, an excisional biopsy is required to confirm the diagnosis and determine whether the tumor is malignant or not.

2.3.1.7. How Do Phyllodes Tumors Affect Your Risk for Breast Cancer?

The presence of a benign phyllodes tumor has no effect on the risk of breast cancer. Having a malignant phyllodes tumor has no bearing on the likelihood of developing other forms of breast cancer. Even so, since phyllodes tumors can recur after surgery, you might still be under closer observation and undergo routine imaging tests.

2.3.1.7.1. Treatment of Phyllodes Tumors

Surgery is usually required to completely remove phyllodes tumors. As long as the tumor is completely removed, an excisional biopsy may be sufficient if the tumor turns out to be benign. A larger margin—the region of normal tissue surrounding the tumor—usually needs to be removed as well if the tumor is malignant or borderline. Breast-conserving surgery (lumpectomy or partial mastectomy) may be used to accomplish this, in which a portion of the breast is removed. Alternatively, a mastectomy may be necessary to remove the entire breast, particularly if breast-conserving surgery is unable to remove a margin of healthy breast tissue. After surgery, radiation therapy may be administered to the affected area, particularly if it is unclear whether the entire tumor was removed.

Phyllodes tumors that are malignant differ from the more prevalent forms of breast cancer. They are also less likely to react to some of the standard treatments for breast cancer, like hormone therapy or the drugs used in chemotherapy. When a phyllodes tumor spreads to other body parts, it is typically treated more like a soft-tissue cancer, or sarcoma, than it is like a breast cancer. Tumors of the phyllodes sometimes recur in the same location. As a result, after treatment, frequent imaging tests and close follow-up are typically advised.

2.3.1.8. Intraductal Papillomas of the Breast

Benign (non-cancerous) wart-like tumors called intraductal papillomas develop inside the breast's milk ducts. They consist of fibrous tissue, blood vessels, and gland tissue (also referred to as fibrovascular tissue). Single tumors known as solitary papillomas (also called solitary intraductal papillomas) frequently develop in the sizable milk ducts close to the nipple. They are frequently the source of bloody or clear nipple discharge, particularly if it originates from a single breast. They could feel like a little lump behind or beside the nipple. They may cause pain at times. Small ducts in parts of the breast that are farther away from the nipple may also contain papillomas. Several growths (multiple papillomas) are frequently present. Nipple discharge is less likely to result from these. Small patches of cell growth within the ducts are present in papillomatosis, but they are not as noticeable as they are in papillomas.

2.3.1.8.1. Diagnosis of Breast Papillomas

Papillomas can lead to symptoms like clear or bloody discharge from the nipple, a lump in the breast, or an abnormal finding on a mammogram or breast ultrasound. A ductogram, involving the injection of dye into the nipple duct followed by an X-ray, may be used to locate the papilloma. If there is cause for concern, a breast biopsy may be performed to confirm the diagnosis. In certain situations, surgery (duct excision) may be necessary to further evaluate the affected area.

2.3.1.8.2. How Do Intraductal Papillomas Affect Your risk for Breast Cancer?

Having a single (solitary) papilloma does not raise breast cancer risk unless it contains other breast changes, such as atypical hyperplasia. However, having multiple papillomas increases breast cancer risk slightly.

2.3.1.8.3. Treatment of Breast Papillomas

The size, presence of multiple, and presence of symptoms of papillomas all influence whether or not treatment is required. Surgery to remove papillomas and the portion of the duct they are in may be advised by doctors due to the possibility that they are associated with other, more serious breast abnormalities.

2.3.1.9. Fat Necrosis and Oil Cysts in the Breast

An injury to a fatty breast tissue area may result in fat necrosis, a benign (non-cancerous) breast condition. It may also appear following radiation therapy or breast surgery. Different stages of fat necrosis exist. When fat cells degrade, their contents leak out, creating an oil cyst—a sac-shaped collection of greasy fluid. Mammograms frequently show calcifications, or tiny calcium deposits, surrounding the cyst's walls over time. Denser scar tissue typically replaces the damaged breast tissue as the body repairs it.

2.3.1.9.1. Diagnosis of Fat Necrosis and Oil Cysts

Although they usually don't hurt, oil cysts and areas of fat necrosis can form a lump that can be felt. The skin surrounding the lump may appear redder, thicker, or bruised. Sometimes, on a breast exam or even a mammography, it can be difficult to distinguish these changes from cancers. If this is the case, determining whether the lump contains cancer cells may require a breast biopsy, which involves removing all or a portion of the lump to examine the tissue under a microscope. Oil cysts are typically identifiable by their appearance on mammograms or breast ultrasonography images. However, if there's a chance it could be something else, a fine needle aspiration or core needle biopsy could be performed.

2.3.1.9.2. How Do Fat Necrosis and Oil Cysts Affect Breast Cancer Risk?

These breast changes do not affect your risk for breast cancer.

2.3.1.9.3. Treatment of Fat Necrosis and Oil Cysts

Fat necrosis and oil cysts typically don't require treatment as long as medical professionals are certain of the diagnosis. Fat necrosis can occasionally disappear on its own. A needle biopsy can be used as treatment if it is performed to extract the fluid from an oil cyst. However, surgery may be required to remove the lump if it grows larger or starts to bother you.

2.3.1.10. Mastitis

Breast inflammation, or swelling, is known as mastitis and is typically brought on by an infection. While it can occur at other times, breastfeeding is the most common time for it to occur. An infection may result from a blocked milk duct that prevents milk from completely draining from the breast or from breaks in the nipple's skin. This results in the release of chemicals by the body's white blood cells to combat the infection, which may cause swelling and an increase in blood flow. The breast area that is infected may swell, hurt, turn red, and feel warm to the touch. In addition, fever, headaches, and other flu-like symptoms can be caused by mastitis.

- **Diagnosis of Mastitis:** Mastitis can often be diagnosed based on symptoms and the results of a breast exam. It usually affects only one breast.
- **How Does Mastitis Affect Your Risk of Breast Cancer?:** Having mastitis does not raise your risk of developing breast cancer.
- **Treatment of Mastitis:** Antibiotics and breast milk emptying are the usual treatments for mastitis. A breast abscess, or collection of pus, may occur occasionally. Antibiotics are used after aspiration—a thin, hollow needle used under ultrasound guidance—or surgery to remove pus from an abscess. The symptoms of inflammatory

breast cancer can be mistaken for an infection because they closely resemble those of mastitis. If a week or so after receiving an antibiotic diagnosis for mastitis, you may require a skin biopsy to rule out cancer. If your symptoms persist after receiving antibiotic treatment, don't wait to see a doctor again because inflammatory breast cancer can spread quickly.

2.3.1.11. Duct Ectasia

When a milk duct in the breast widens and its walls thicken, a benign (non-cancerous) breast condition known as duct ectasia, also called mammary duct ectasia, results. This may result in a blockage in the duct and a build-up of fluid. Women who are approaching menopause are more likely to experience it. However, it can also occur at other ages.

- **Diagnosis of Duct Ectasia:** This disorder frequently goes undiagnosed until a biopsy—the removal of tiny samples of breast tissue for microscopic examination—is performed to treat another breast issue. A thick, sticky nipple discharge is a less common side effect of duct ectasia. The nipple may be pulled inward, and the surrounding breast tissue may be red and tender. Occasionally, the hard lump that develops around the abnormal duct can be mistaken for cancer due to scar tissue. To find out more information about the altered area of your breast, you might have a mammography or breast ultrasound.
- **How Does Duct Ectasia Affect Your Breast Cancer Risk?:** Duct ectasia does not increase your risk for breast cancer.
- **Treatment of Duct Ectasia:** Duct ectasia that is causing symptoms sometimes gets better without treatment. Warm compresses and antibiotics may be used in some cases. If the symptoms don't go away, the abnormal duct might need to be surgically removed.

2.3.1.12. Radial Scars and Some Other Non-Cancerous Breast Conditions

These are some of the less common types of benign (non-cancerous) tumors and conditions that can be found in the breast.

- **Radial Scars:** Another name for radial scars is complex sclerosing lesions. Most frequently, they are discovered during a breast biopsy performed for another reason. Radial scars can occasionally be seen on mammograms as a distortion of the normal breast tissue.

Radial scars are not really scars, but they look like scars when seen with a microscope. They don't usually cause symptoms, but they are important because:

- o If they are large enough, they may look like cancer on an imaging test such as a mammogram, or even on a biopsy.
- o They seem to be linked to a slight increase in a woman's risk of developing breast cancer.

Doctors often recommend surgery to remove radial scars, but in some cases they can use imaging tests instead to watch for any concerning changes.

- **Other Breast Changes That Are Not Cancer:** Other types of benign masses and other changes can also be found in the breast. Many of these are described on other Non-cancerous Breast Conditions pages.

Some types of benign breast changes that are not covered on those pages are listed below. None of these conditions raise breast cancer risk, but they may need to be biopsied or removed to know what they are and to be sure they don't have any cancer cells in them.

   - o **Lipoma:** a fatty tumor that can appear almost anywhere in the body, including the breast. It is usually not painful.
   - o **Hamartoma:** a smooth, painless lump formed by the overgrowth of mature breast cells, which can be made up of fatty, fibrous, and/or gland tissues
   - o **Hemangioma:** a rare tumor made up of blood vessels
   - o **Hematoma:** a collection of blood within the breast caused by internal bleeding
   - o **Adenomyoepithelioma:** a very rare tumor formed by certain cells in the milk duct walls
   - o **Neurofibroma:** a tumor that's an overgrowth of nerve cells
   - o **Granular Cell Tumor:** a tumor that starts in early forms of Schwann cells, which normally surround and help insulate nerve cells. These tumors rarely start in the breast.

2.3.2. The Symptoms of Breast Cancer

Different people have different symptoms of breast cancer. Some people do not have any signs or symptoms at all.

Some warning signs of breast cancer are:

- New lump in the breast or underarm (armpit).
- Thickening or swelling of part of the breast.
- Irritation or dimpling of breast skin.
- Redness or flaky skin in the nipple area or the breast.
- Pulling in of the nipple or pain in the nipple area.
- Nipple discharge other than breast milk, including blood.
- Any change in the size or the shape of the breast.
- Pain in any area of the breast.

Keep in mind that these symptoms can happen with other conditions that are not cancer.

Other signs and symptoms of breast cancer may include:

- A breast lump or thickened area of skin that feels different from the surrounding tissue.
- A nipple that looks flattened or turns inward.
- Changes in the color of the breast skin. In people with white skin, the breast skin may look pink or red. In people with brown and Black skin, the breast skin may look darker than the other skin on the chest or it may look red or purple.
- Change in the size, shape or appearance of a breast.
- Changes to the skin over the breast, such as skin that looks dimpled or looks like an orange peel.

- Peeling, scaling, crusting or flaking of the skin on the breast.

2.3.3. Incidence of Breast Cancer

Worldwide, breast cancer is the most common cancer to affect women. With a higher incidence rate among women than men, it is the most prevalent cancer in the UK. The lifetime risk of breast cancer for a British woman born after 1960 is estimated to be 1 in 7, while the risk for a British man born after 1960 is approximately 1 in 870. 15% of female cancer deaths are attributable to this disease. In England and Wales, 15,000 women lose their lives to breast cancer annually. These statistics attest to the significance of breast cancer as a health issue, and research indicates that inviting women between the ages of 50 and 70 once every three years helps to avert about 1300 breast cancer-related deaths annually.

2.3.3.1. Screening with Mammography

Every randomized controlled trial that has demonstrated a statistically significant reduction in the population's death rate from breast cancer has used mammography as its screening modality. It is still acknowledged as the preferred method for screening the general public for breast cancer. It is available to women in the UK between the ages of 50 and 70, with the option for older women to self-refer. Although it can be completed quickly and interpreted fairly quickly, producing mammograms of the highest quality requires a mammographer to possess exceptional skill. Technically speaking, this can be difficult, and some women find the process uncomfortable. The prevalent screen is the initial screening exam given to women; subsequent screenings are referred to as incident screens. Women who are more likely to be recalled for evaluation are those whose prior mammograms are not available for comparison.

By comparing the number of cancers that occur between routine screening exams, or intervals, with the incidence of breast cancer in an age-matched non-screened population, one can estimate the sensitivity of screening mammography. According to these calculations, the number of cases of breast cancer with symptoms drops by 76% in the first year after a negative screen. This decreases to 21% and 21% in the following years following a negative screen.

2.3.3.2. Radiation Dose

Since mammography uses ionizing radiation, breast cancer could theoretically be caused by it. A woman undergoing full-field digital mammography (two views) through the National Health Service Breast Screening Program (NHSBSP) has a one in 49,000 to one in 98,000 chance of developing a radiation-induced cancer each visit. For every cancer that is induced, the NHSBSP is estimated to detect 400–800 cancers; additionally, the mortality benefit of screening outweighs the damage caused by radiation by a ratio of approximately 150:1 to 300:1.

2.3.3.3. Number of Views

At the beginning of the screening program, only mediolateral oblique (MLO) mammograms were performed. As a result of further research, all mammography screening exams now include craniocaudal (CC) views of each breast, contributing to the evolution of practice. Studies revealed that the second perspective lowered the recall rate by 15% and raised breast cancer detection by 24%. It was especially significant when it came to the identification of invasive cancer smaller than 10 mm. These are the tumors that are most likely to result in the screening-associated mortality benefit. Although the cost was undoubtedly higher than with single-view mammography, the addition of two views was determined to be cost-effective due to the enhanced screening performance.

2.3.3.4. Digital Mammography

The use of mammography has been considerably more flexible since the transition from X-ray film screening to full-field digital imaging, which has high-resolution and reconstructive algorithms. For digital breast tomosynthesis (DBT), a series of low-dose mammography images taken across the breast at various angles are used. To achieve sharp focus on any plane of the breast and blurry appearance on other structures outside of it, the resulting digital images are reconstructed into a series of high-resolution 1-mm slices (or thicker slabs).

The advantages of DBT are:

- Increased invasive cancer detection rate and in most studies decrease the false positive recall rate.
- Unexpected multifocal disease can be demonstrated.
- It increases sensitivity in the dense breast.
- It may help to localize lesions that are seen initially on a single projection only.
- It has the potential to reduce the biopsy rate of normal/benign densities present in full-field digital mammography which subsequently resolve on DBT.

Disadvantages are:

- It currently has no significant effect on calcification (ductal carcinoma in situ [DCIS]) detection although the performance of newer machines in this area is improving.
- The examination and interpretation time are typically longer than for a standard set of images.
- DBT images are larger data file sizes than standard mammographic images, which can present IT challenges and associated cost implications.

Research is ongoing, and these aspects of its use need to be addressed before it can be taken into consideration for population screening. DBT is currently authorized for use with the symptomatic population as well as in the assessment clinic. When it comes to abnormalities only detected by DBT and not by two-dimensional mammography or ultrasound (US), departments that use DBT should take into consideration the availability of DBT-guided biopsy. Digital mammography also makes it possible to perform Contrast-enhanced spectral mammography (CESM). Just before the digital mammography scan, contrast media is injected, much like it would be for a computed tomography scan. This provides information on the extra blood supply linked to the development of cancer as well as the typical shape and size changes observed on mammography that may be indicative of cancer. Because it is more affordable, accessible in the breast unit, and well-liked by most patients, this method is showing promise as a substitute for magnetic resonance imaging (MRI) in certain contexts, where it can enhance cancer detection. However, it is currently limited to use in the symptomatic population and is not appropriate as a mass population screening technique.

2.3.3.5. What Are the Reasons for a Mammogram?

Mammography can be used for diagnosis or for screening. If a woman has any of the following symptoms—a palpable lump, thickening or indentation of the breast skin, discharge or retraction of the nipple, erosive sore of the nipple, or breast pain—she should have a diagnostic mammography performed before turning 30. Breast pain may be assessed with a mammogram if the results of a physical examination and history are inconclusive. Mammography screening may be used for women whose breasts are dense, lumpy, or very large, as physical examination may be challenging in these cases. Mammograms may be performed on women who have a history of breast cancer or who are at high risk for the disease. Your healthcare provider might recommend a mammography for additional reasons.

2.3.3.6. Who Should Get a Screening Mammogram?

Different health experts have different recommendations for mammography.

The following screening guidelines are for early detection of cancer in women who have no symptoms:

- The American College of Radiology (ACR) and the Society of Breast Imaging (SBI) recommend that women get yearly mammograms starting at age 40.
- The National Cancer Institute guidelines state that women in their 40s and older should have a screening mammogram regularly, every 1 to 2 years.
- The American Cancer Society recommends that women with an average risk of breast cancer should have regular screening mammograms starting at age 45. Mammograms should be done every year for all women ages 45 to 54. Then you can switch to mammograms every 2 years. Or you have the choice to continue annual mammograms.
- Currently, the U.S. Preventive Services Task Force (USPSTF) recommends screening every 2 years for women ages 50 to 74.
- Women who are at an increased risk (family history, genetic tendency, past breast cancer) should talk with their healthcare providers about the benefits and limitations of starting mammography screening earlier, having additional tests (breast ultrasound, MRI), or having more frequent exams.

2.3.3.7. What Are the Risks of a Mammogram?

It might be a good idea to inquire with your healthcare provider about the risks associated with the procedure and the amount of radiation used. To let your healthcare provider know about any prior radiation exposure, such as scans or other X-rays, it is a good idea to maintain a record of them. Radiation exposure risks may be correlated with the total number of X-ray exams and/or treatments received over an extended period of time.

You should let your healthcare provider know if you are pregnant or think you might be. Radiation exposure during pregnancy may lead to birth defects. Should mammography be required, extra care will be taken to reduce the radiation exposure to the developing fetus. Some discomfort may be felt as the breast is compressed against the X-ray plate during the procedure. Nonetheless, the breast won't be harmed by this compression. There may be other risks depending on your specific medical condition. Before the procedure, make sure to discuss any concerns you may have with your healthcare provider. Certain factors or conditions may interfere with a mammogram. These include, but are not limited to, the following:

- Talcum powder, deodorant, creams, or lotions applied under the arms or on the breasts
- Breast implants, as they may prevent complete visualization of the breast. If you have breast implants, be sure to tell your mammography facility that you have them when you make your appointment. You will need an X-ray technologist who is trained in working with patients with implants. This is important because breast implants can hide some breast tissue, which could make it difficult for the radiologist to see breast cancer when looking at your mammogram images.
- Previous breast surgery
- Hormonal breast changes (Guray & Sahin, 2006; Collins & Schnitt, 2014; Esteva & Gutiérrez, 2014; Overmoyer & Pierce, 2014; Sabel, 2021).

A Closer Look

Breast Lumps

The majority of breast lumps are benign because they are not cancerous. Finding a breast lump may surprise you, but it is crucial to keep in mind that it might not have a long-term impact on your health. A breast lump, however, may indicate cancer. It is a good idea to get any lumps or swelling on your breasts evaluated by a doctor. Men and women both have breast tissue, even though breasts are typically associated with women. This tissue is affected by your hormones. Lomas can develop and, in certain situations, go away on their own due to hormonal fluctuations. Breast lumps can appear at any age.

Because babies receive estrogen from their mothers during birth, some of them end up with breast lumps. Usually, these go away when the estrogen leaves their bodies. Prepubescent girls may develop tender breast lumps from time to time. Puberty usually causes these to disappear on their own. During puberty, adolescent boys may also develop breast lumps. These are also transient, usually going away after a few months.

- **Causes of Breast Lumps**

There are many possible causes for a lump in your breast, including:

- breast cysts, which are soft, fluid-filled sacs
- milk cysts, referring to sacs filled with milk
- that can occur during breast-feeding
- fibrocystic breasts, a condition in which breast
- tissue feels lumpy in texture and is sometimes accompanied by pain
- fibroadenoma, meaning noncancerous rubbery lumps
- that move easily within the breast tissue and rarely become cancerous
- hamartoma, which is a benign, tumorlike growth
- intraductal papilloma, referring to a small,
- non-cancerous tumor in a milk duct
- lipoma, which is a slow-growing, noncancerous,
- fatty lump
- mastitis, or an infection of the breast
- injury
- breast cancer
- **Treatment for Breast Lumps**

Before developing a treatment plan, your doctor needs to ascertain the cause of your breast lump. Not every breast lump requires medical attention. Your doctor will likely prescribe antibiotics to treat your breast infection. Your cyst may be emptied of fluid if you have one. Cysts typically disappear after they are drained. Cysts may go away on their own in certain situations and not require medical attention.

If the lump is found to be breast cancer, treatment can include:

- lumpectomy, or removing the lump
- mastectomy, which refers to removing your breast
- tissue
- chemotherapy, which uses drugs to fight or
- destroy the cancer
- radiation, a treatment that uses radioactive
- rays or materials to fight the cancer

The kind of breast cancer you have, the size and location of the tumor, and whether the cancer has spread outside of your breast will all affect your course of treatment.

There are various reasons for breast lumps that may not necessitate treatment. If your breast lump is a result of an injury, your doctor may suggest giving it time to heal naturally. Some types of breast lumps, like fibroadenoma, often do not require removal or treatment. It is crucial not to jump to conclusions if you discover a breast lump. Consulting with your doctor will help determine if additional testing is necessary and if any treatment is recommended (Guray & Sahin, 2006; Collins & Schnitt, 2014; Esteva & Gutiérrez, 2014; Overmoyer & Pierce, 2014; Sabel, 2021).

Summary

- Breast disease encompasses a range of conditions that can affect the breast tissue, including benign disorders and malignant cancers. Recognizing the symptoms is crucial for early detection and effective treatment.
- Breast disorders may be noncancerous (benign) or cancerous (malignant). Most are noncancerous and not life-threatening.
- Breast symptoms do not necessarily mean that a woman has breast cancer or another serious disorder. For example, monthly breast tenderness that is related to hormonal changes before a menstrual period does not indicate a serious disorder.
- Benign breast disease refers to non-cancerous conditions that affect the breast tissue, which are common and often cause considerable anxiety due to their potential mimicry of cancerous symptoms.
- The mammary gland is an organ of ectodermal origin, typical of mammalians, whose structure reflects its special function: the production of milk for lactation.
- Most people associate breast abnormalities with breast cancer. However, not all breast disorders are cancerous.

References

1. Dixon, J. M., & Pariser, K. M. (2021). Nonlocational mastitis in adults. *UpToDate*. Retrieved from: https://www.uptodate.com/contents/nonlactational-mastitis-in-adults (accessed on 16 July 2024).
2. Golshan, M. (2021). Breast pain. *UpToDate*. Retrieved from: https://www.uptodate.com/contents/breast-pain (accessed on 16 July 2024).
3. Guray, M., & Sahin, A. A. (2006). Benign breast diseases: Classification, diagnosis, and management. *Oncologist, 11*, 435–449.
4. Hartmann, L. C., Sellers, T. A., Frost, M. H., et al. (2005). Benign breast disease and the risk of breast cancer. *New England Journal of Medicine, 353*, 229–237.
5. Orr, B., & Kelley, J. L. (2016). Benign breast diseases: Evaluation and management. *Clinical Obstetrics and Gynecology, 59*(4), 710–726.
6. Sabel, M. S. (2021). Clinical manifestations, differential diagnosis, and clinical evaluation of a palpable breast mass. *UpToDate*. Retrieved from: https://www.uptodate.com/contents/clinical-manifestations-differential-diagnosis-and-clinical-evaluation-of-a-palpable-breast-mass (accessed on 16 July 2024).

Chapter 3

SYMPTOMS OF LUNG DISEASE

Contents

Introduction

Lung diseases encompass a diverse array of conditions that affect the respiratory system, ranging from acute infections to chronic disorders. These diseases can involve the airways, lung tissue, blood vessels, or a combination of these components, leading to a wide spectrum of symptoms and complications. Understanding lung disease is crucial given the pivotal role the lungs play in respiration and overall health.

The lungs are essential organs responsible for oxygenating the blood and expelling carbon dioxide, facilitating the exchange of gases vital for cellular function. However, they are also vulnerable to various insults, including infections, environmental toxins, genetic predispositions, and autoimmune processes, all of which can disrupt their normal function and structure.

Symptoms of lung disease can vary widely depending on the specific condition, its severity, and the individual patient. However, there are several common symptoms that may indicate the presence of a lung disorder.

One of the most prevalent symptoms of lung disease is dyspnea or shortness of breath. Dyspnea can manifest as difficulty breathing, a sensation of breathlessness, or an inability to get enough air. It may occur at rest or during physical activity and can range from mild to severe, depending on the underlying cause.

Orientation and Directional Terms

Term	Definition	Illustration
Pulmonary Embolism	A pulmonary embolism is a sudden blockage in your pulmonary arteries, the blood vessels that send blood to your lungs. It usually happens when a blood clot in the deep veins in your leg breaks off and travels to your lungs.	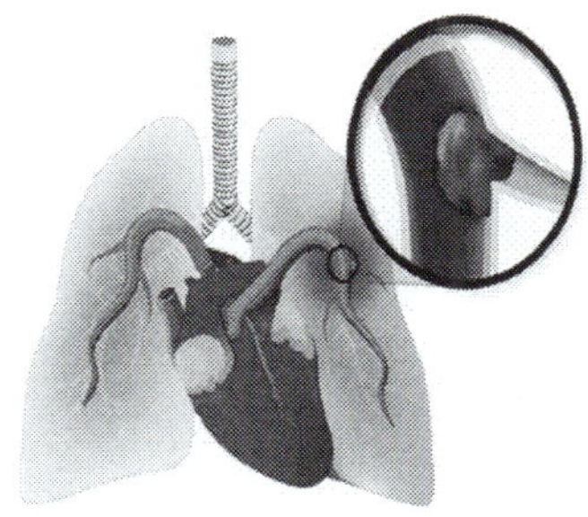
Airway Hyperresponsiveness	Airway hyperresponsiveness is a characteristic feature of asthma and consists of an increased sensitivity of the airways to an inhaled constrictor agonist, a steeper slope of the dose-response curve, and a greater maximal response to the agonist	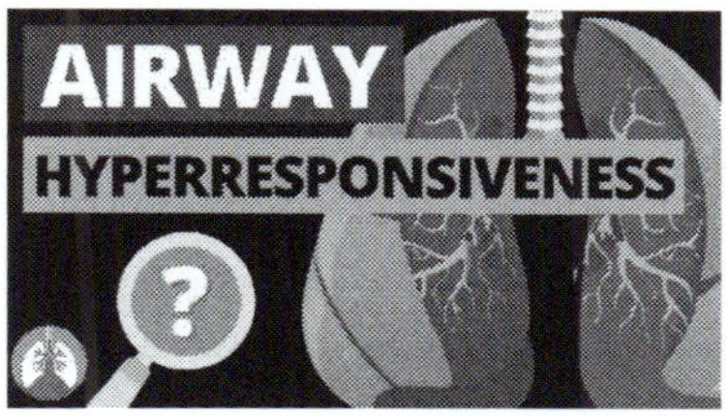
Emphysema	Emphysema is a lung disease that damages the alveoli in your lungs. The primary symptom of emphysema is shortness of breath.	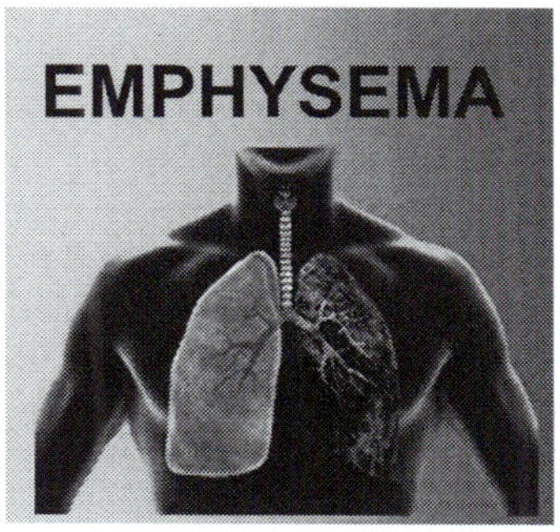
Forced Vital Capacity	Forced vital capacity: the maximum amount of air you can forcibly exhale from your lungs after fully inhaling. It is about 80% of total capacity, or 4.8 liters, because some air remains in your lungs after you exhale.	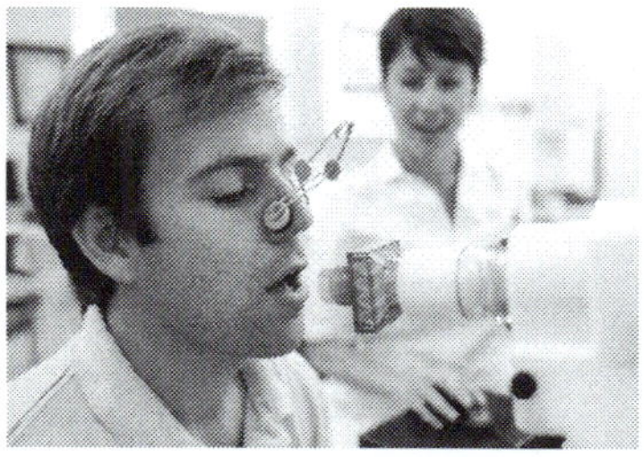
Cystic Fibrosis (CF)	Cystic fibrosis (CF) is an inherited disorder that causes severe damage to the lungs, digestive system and other organs in the body.	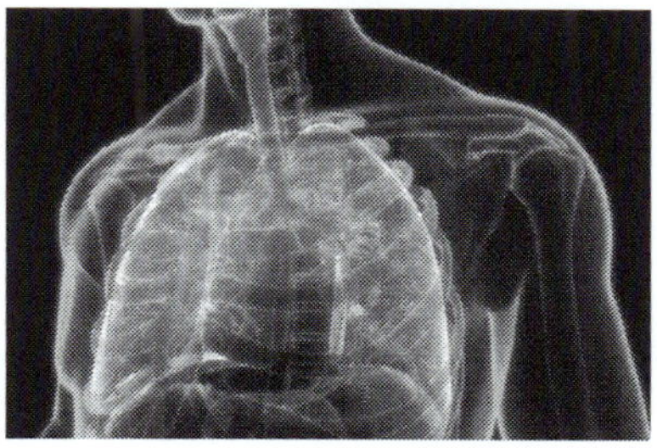

3.1. Overview of Lung Disease

Any issue that hinders the lungs' normal function is referred to as a lung disease. Lung disease can be of three main types:

1. **Airway Diseases:** The tubes, or airways, that carry gases other than oxygen into and out of the lungs are impacted by these diseases. Usually, they result in an obstruction or narrowing of the airways. Asthma, bronchiolitis, chronic obstructive pulmonary disease (COPD), and bronchiectasis—which is also the primary condition affecting people with cystic fibrosis—are examples of airway diseases. Individuals suffering from respiratory disorders frequently describe feeling as though they are exhaling through a straw.
2. **Lung Tissue Diseases:** Lung tissue's structural integrity is impacted by these illnesses. The lungs can't enlarge to their full potential due to tissue inflammation or scarring (restrictive lung disease). The lungs find it difficult to exhale carbon dioxide and take in oxygen as a result. People who have this kind of lung disease frequently describe feeling as though they are wearing a vest or sweater that is too tight. They are unable to breathe deeply as a result. Lung tissue diseases include sarcoidosis and pulmonary fibrosis.
3. **Lung Circulation Diseases:** The lungs' blood vessels are impacted by these illnesses. They are brought on by blood vessel inflammation, scarring, or clotting. They have an impact on the lungs' capacity to absorb oxygen and expel carbon dioxide. Heart function may also be impacted by these conditions. Pulmonary hypertension is a disease of the lung circulation. When they exert themselves, people with these conditions frequently experience severe dyspnea (Figure 3.1).

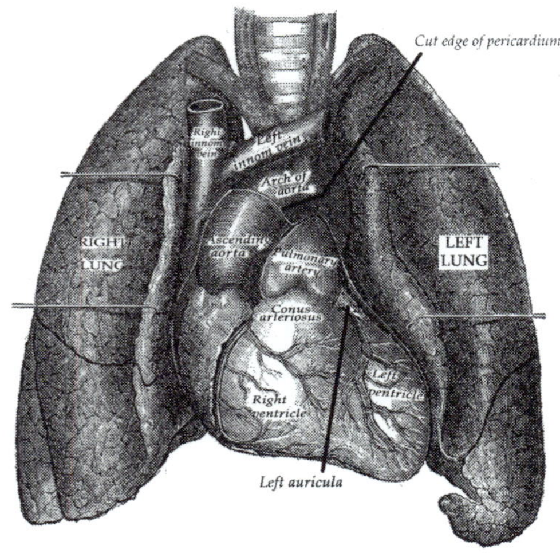

Figure 3.1. *Lungs.*

Source: By Gray's Anatomy – Gray's Anatomy at http://www.bartleby.com/107/138.html, Public Domain, https://commons.wikimedia.org/w/index.php?curid=141450.

The most common lung diseases include:

- Asthma
- Collapse of part or all of the lung (pneumothorax or atelectasis)
- Swelling and inflammation in the main passages (bronchial tubes) that carry air to the lungs (bronchitis)
- COPD
- Lung cancer
- Lung infection (pneumonia)
- Abnormal buildup of fluid in the lungs (pulmonary edema)
- Blocked lung artery (pulmonary embolus)

3.2. Airway Diseases

Airway diseases primarily affect the tubes that carry air in and out of your lungs. These conditions can restrict airflow, making it difficult to breathe. Here are some common airway diseases:

1. **Asthma:** Asthma is a chronic inflammatory disorder of the airways that causes recurrent episodes of wheezing, breathlessness, chest tightness, and coughing, particularly at night or in the early morning. These episodes are often triggered by exposure to allergens, irritants, or exercise. Asthma affects people of all ages, but it most commonly begins in childhood. According to the World Health Organization (WHO), an estimated 235 million people worldwide suffer from asthma, making it a significant public health concern (Boulet & Godbout, 2020; Cloutier et al., 2020) (Figure 3.1).

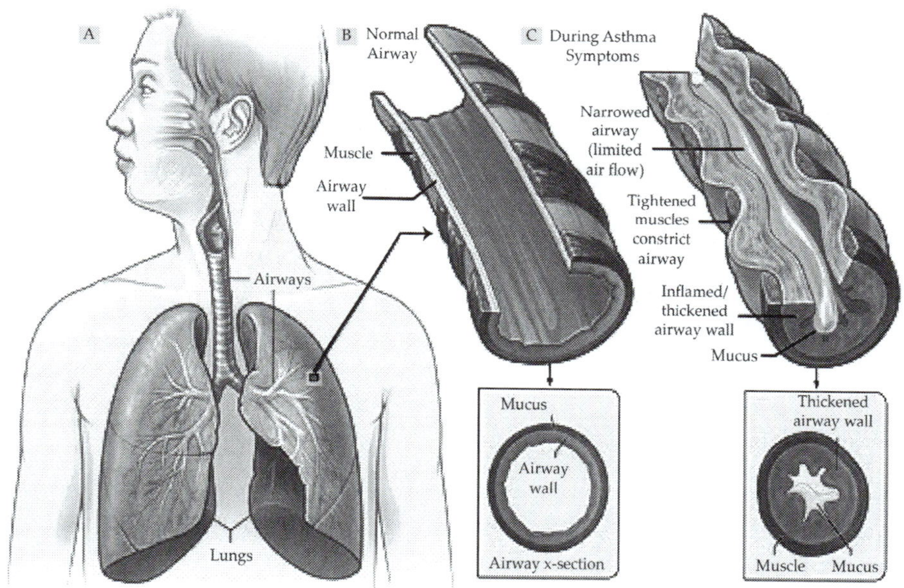

Figure 3.2. *Asthma causes bronchospasms, inflammation, thick mucus and constriction in the airways.*

Source: *By United States-National Institute of Health: National Heart, Lung, Blood Institute – http://www.nhlbi.nih.gov/health/health-topics/topics/asthma/, Public Domain, https://commons.wikimedia.org/w/index.php?curid=24760677.*

2. **Pathophysiology:** The pathophysiology of asthma involves a complex interplay of genetic, environmental, and immunological factors. In susceptible individuals, exposure to allergens or irritants triggers an inflammatory response in the airways. This inflammation leads to airway hyperresponsiveness (AHR), causing the airways to constrict and become narrow, making it difficult to breathe. Chronic inflammation can also lead to airway remodeling, characterized by structural changes such as thickening of the airway walls and increased mucus production.

3. **Causes and Risk Factors**

   i. **Genetic Factors:** Genetic predisposition plays a significant role in the development of asthma. Individuals with a family history of asthma or allergic conditions are at a higher risk of developing the disease. Several genes have been implicated in asthma susceptibility, including those involved in immune regulation, airway inflammation, and response to environmental triggers.

   ii. **Environmental Factors:** Exposure to environmental factors such as allergens, air pollution, tobacco smoke, and respiratory infections can increase the risk of developing asthma and trigger asthma symptoms in susceptible individuals. Common allergens that can trigger asthma include pollen, dust mites, pet dander, mold, and certain foods. Occupational exposure to allergens or irritants in the workplace can also contribute to the development of occupational asthma.

4. **Clinical Presentation**

   i. **Symptoms:** The symptoms of asthma can vary in severity and frequency from person to person. Common symptoms include:

   a. **Wheezing:** A whistling or squeaky sound when breathing, particularly during exhalation.

   b. **Shortness of Breath:** Difficulty breathing or feeling out of breath.

   c. **Chest Tightness:** A sensation of pressure or constriction in the chest.

   d. **Coughing:** A persistent cough, especially at night or in the early morning.

Symptoms may worsen during asthma attacks, which can be triggered by factors such as allergen exposure, respiratory infections, exercise, cold air, or emotional stress.

   ii. **Asthma Exacerbations:** Asthma exacerbations, also known as asthma attacks, are episodes of worsening symptoms that require prompt medical intervention. During an exacerbation, airway inflammation and bronchoconstriction lead to a sudden worsening of symptoms, often accompanied by coughing, wheezing, shortness of breath, and chest tightness. Severe exacerbations can be life-threatening and may require emergency medical treatment, including the administration of bronchodilators, corticosteroids, and oxygen therapy.

5. **Diagnosis**

   i. **Clinical Evaluation:** Diagnosing asthma begins with a thorough clinical evaluation, including a detailed medical history and physical examination. The healthcare provider will ask about the patient's symptoms, triggers, family history of asthma or allergies, and exposure to environmental factors.

ii. Pulmonary Function Tests

Pulmonary function tests, such as spirometry and peak flow measurement, are essential for diagnosing and monitoring asthma. Spirometry measures lung function by assessing airflow obstruction and bronchodilator responsiveness. Peak flow measurement measures the maximum airflow rate during forced expiration and can help assess the severity of airflow limitation.

iii. **Other Diagnostic Tests:** Additional tests may be performed to support the diagnosis of asthma and identify potential triggers. These tests may include:

a. **Allergy Testing:** Skin prick tests or blood tests to identify specific allergens that may trigger asthma symptoms.

b. **Exhaled Nitric Oxide Measurement:** A non-invasive test that measures the level of nitric oxide in exhaled breath, which is elevated in patients with allergic asthma.

c. **Chest X-Ray or CT Scan:** Imaging studies may be performed to rule out other respiratory conditions that can mimic asthma, such as pneumonia or chronic obstructive pulmonary disease (COPD) (Boulet & Godbout, 2020; Cloutier et al., 2020).

6. **Classification and Severity**

i. **Classification of Asthma:** Asthma is classified into different subtypes based on its severity and control. The classification system helps guide treatment decisions and management strategies. The two main classifications of asthma severity are intermittent and persistent, with persistent asthma further categorized into mild, moderate, and severe subtypes based on symptom severity and lung function impairment.

ii. **Assessment of Asthma Control:** Assessing asthma control is essential for determining treatment effectiveness and adjusting therapy as needed. The level of asthma control is assessed based on the frequency and severity of symptoms, as well as the use of rescue medications and pulmonary function tests. The goal of asthma management is to achieve and maintain optimal asthma control, minimizing symptoms and the risk of exacerbations.

7. **Treatment**

i. **Pharmacological Therapy:** Pharmacological therapy is the cornerstone of asthma management and aims to reduce airway inflammation, relieve bronchoconstriction, and control asthma symptoms. The main classes of asthma medications include:

a. **Inhaled Corticosteroids (ICS):** These anti-inflammatory medications are the most effective long-term control therapy for asthma and are recommended as first-line treatment for most patients with persistent asthma.

b. **Long-Acting Beta2-Agonists (LABAs):** These bronchodilators are often used in combination with ICS to provide additional bronchodilation and improve symptom control.

c. **Short-Acting Beta2-Agonists (SABAs):** These quick-relief medications provide rapid relief of asthma symptoms and are used as rescue therapy during asthma exacerbations.

d. **Leukotriene Modifiers:** These medications block the action of leukotrienes, inflammatory mediators that contribute to airway inflammation and bronchoconstriction.

e. **Mast Cell Stabilizers:** These medications help prevent the release of inflammatory mediators from mast cells, reducing airway inflammation and hypersensitivity.

f. **Biologic Agents:** These targeted therapies are used for severe asthma that is not well-controlled with standard medications and target specific pathways involved in asthma inflammation, such as IgE or interleukin-5 (IL-5).

ii. **Non-pharmacological Therapy:** In addition to pharmacological therapy, non-pharmacological interventions play a crucial role in asthma management. These interventions include:

a. **Allergen Avoidance:** Identifying and avoiding triggers such as allergens, irritants, and pollutants can help reduce asthma symptoms and exacerbations.

b. **Smoking Cessation:** Tobacco smoke is a potent asthma trigger and can worsen asthma symptoms. Quitting smoking is essential for improving asthma control and reducing the risk of complications.

c. **Education and Self-Management:** Patient education programs help empower individuals with asthma to better understand their condition, recognize early warning signs of worsening symptoms, use medications correctly, and adhere to treatment recommendations. Asthma action plans guide how to adjust medication doses and seek medical help during exacerbations.

D. **Regular Monitoring:** Regular monitoring of asthma symptoms, peak flow measurements, and lung function tests is essential for assessing asthma control, identifying triggers, and adjusting treatment as needed (Boulet & Godbout, 2020; Cloutier et al., 2020)

8. **Prevention:** While there's no way to prevent asthma, you and your doctor can design a step-by-step plan for living with your condition and preventing asthma attacks.

- Follow your asthma action plan. With your doctor and healthcare team, write a detailed plan for taking medications and managing an asthma attack. Then be sure to follow your plan.

Asthma is an ongoing condition that needs regular monitoring and treatment. Taking control of your treatment can make you feel more in control of your life.

- Get vaccinated for influenza and pneumonia. Staying current with vaccinations can prevent flu and pneumonia from triggering asthma flare-ups.

- Identify and avoid asthma triggers. Many outdoor allergens and irritants — ranging from pollen and mold to cold air and air pollution — can trigger asthma attacks. Find out what causes or worsens your asthma, and take steps to avoid those triggers.
- Monitor your breathing. You may learn to recognize warning signs of an impending attack, such as slight coughing, wheezing or shortness of breath.

But because your lung function may decrease before you notice any signs or symptoms, regularly measure and record your peak airflow with a home peak flow meter. A peak flow meter measures how hard you can breathe out. Your doctor can show you how to monitor your peak flow at home.

- Identify and treat attacks early. If you act quickly, you're less likely to have a severe attack. You also won't need as much medication to control your symptoms.

When your peak flow measurements decrease and alert you to an oncoming attack, take your medication as instructed. Also, immediately stop any activity that may have triggered the attack. If your symptoms don't improve, get medical help as directed in your action plan.

- Take your medication as prescribed. Don't change your medications without first talking to your doctor, even if your asthma seems to be improving. It is a good idea to bring your medications with you to each doctor's visit. Your doctor can make sure you're using your medications correctly and taking the right dose.
- Pay attention to increasing quick-relief inhaler use. If you find yourself relying on your quick-relief inhaler, such as albuterol, your asthma isn't under control. See your doctor about adjusting your treatment (Boulet & Godbout, 2020; Cloutier et al., 2020).

3.2.1. Chronic Obstructive Pulmonary Disease (COPD)

Chronic Obstructive Pulmonary Disease (COPD) is a common and preventable respiratory condition characterized by persistent airflow limitation that is not fully reversible. The airflow limitation is usually progressive and associated with an abnormal inflammatory response of the lungs to harmful particles or gases, primarily caused by cigarette smoking. COPD encompasses several respiratory conditions, including chronic bronchitis and emphysema, which commonly coexist and contribute to the overall disease burden.

COPD is a major global health concern, with an estimated 384 million people affected worldwide. It is a leading cause of morbidity and mortality, responsible for over 3 million deaths annually. The prevalence of COPD is higher in low- and middle-income countries, where exposure to indoor air pollution from biomass fuel combustion is a significant risk factor (Figure 3.3).

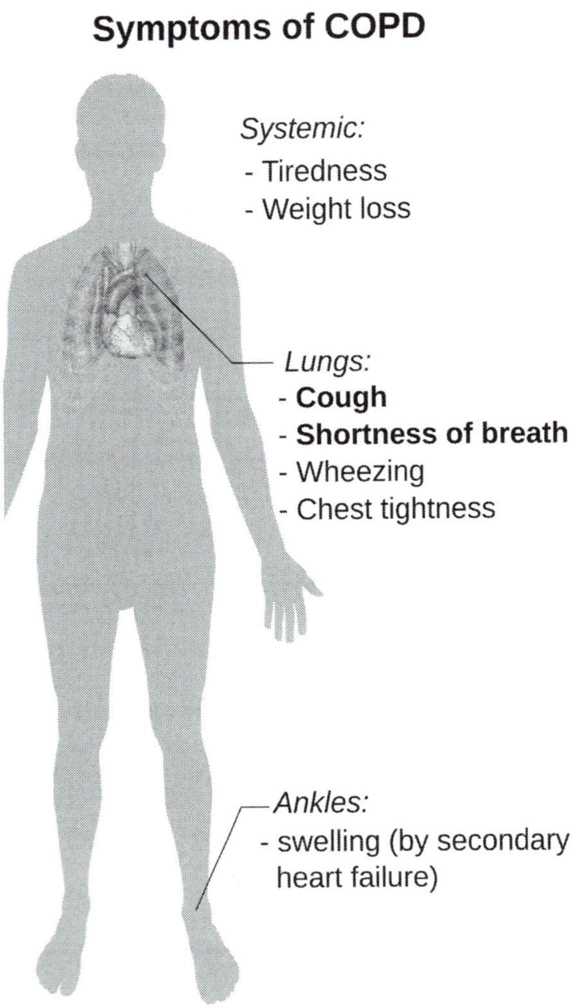

Figure 3.3. *Chronic obstructive pulmonary disease (COPD).*

Source: *By Mikael Häggström – All used images are in public domain., Public Domain, https://commons.wikimedia.org/w/index.php?curid=27469766.*

3.2.1.1. Pathophysiology

The pathophysiology of COPD involves complex interactions between genetic predisposition, environmental exposures, and inflammatory processes in the lungs. Cigarette smoking is the primary risk factor for COPD, accounting for up to 90% of cases. Other risk factors include exposure to indoor and outdoor air pollution, occupational dust and chemicals, biomass fuel smoke, and genetic factors such as alpha-1 antitrypsin deficiency.

Chronic inflammation in the airways and lung parenchyma leads to structural changes, including airway narrowing, mucous gland hyperplasia, and destruction of alveolar walls (emphysema). These structural changes result in airflow limitation, air trapping, and impaired gas exchange, leading to respiratory symptoms such as dyspnea, cough, and sputum production.

3.2.1.2. Causes and Risk Factors

- **Smoking:** Cigarette smoking is the single most significant risk factor for COPD. Smoking causes inflammation and damage to the airways and lung tissue, leading to the development and progression of COPD. Long-term exposure to tobacco smoke increases the risk of developing COPD, with approximately 20-30% of smokers developing the disease.
- **Environmental Exposures:** Exposure to indoor and outdoor air pollution, including biomass fuel smoke, industrial pollutants, and vehicle emissions, is a significant risk factor for COPD. Indoor air pollution from biomass fuel combustion is particularly common in low- and middle-income countries and affects millions of people worldwide.
- **Occupational Exposures:** Occupational exposure to dust, chemicals, and fumes can contribute to the development of COPD, particularly in industries such as mining, construction, agriculture, and manufacturing. Workers exposed

to these occupational hazards are at an increased risk of developing COPD, especially if they smoke cigarettes.

- **Genetic Factors:** Genetic factors also play a role in the development of COPD. Alpha-1 antitrypsin deficiency (AATD) is a genetic condition characterized by a deficiency of the alpha-1 antitrypsin protein, which protects the lungs from damage by neutrophil elastase. Individuals with AATD are at an increased risk of developing COPD, particularly if they smoke cigarettes.

3.2.1.3. Clinical Presentation

- **Symptoms:** The symptoms of COPD vary in severity and may include:
  - o Dyspnea (shortness of breath), which is often progressive and worsens with exertion.
  - o Chronic cough, which may be productive of sputum (mucus) and worsen in the morning.
  - o Wheezing, chest tightness, and recurrent respiratory infections may also occur, particularly during exacerbations.

Symptoms typically develop gradually and worsen over time, leading to a significant impact on quality of life and functional status.

- **Exacerbations:** COPD exacerbations are acute episodes of worsening respiratory symptoms that require additional treatment beyond routine therapy. Exacerbations are often triggered by respiratory infections, air pollution, or other factors that increase inflammation or airway irritation. Symptoms of a COPD exacerbation may include increased dyspnea, cough, sputum production, and changes in sputum color or volume. Severe exacerbations may require hospitalization and can be life-threatening, particularly in patients with advanced COPD.

3.2.1.4. Diagnosis

- **Clinical Evaluation:** Diagnosing COPD begins with a comprehensive clinical evaluation, including a detailed medical history, physical examination, and assessment of respiratory symptoms. The healthcare provider will inquire about the patient's smoking history, occupational exposures, environmental factors, and family history of COPD or other respiratory conditions.
- **Pulmonary Function Tests:** Pulmonary function tests (PFTs) are essential for diagnosing and monitoring COPD. Spirometry is the most commonly used PFT for assessing airflow limitation and is necessary to establish the diagnosis of COPD. Spirometry measures forced expiratory volume in one second (FEV1) and forced vital capacity (FVC), which are used to calculate the FEV1/FVC ratio. A post-bronchodilator FEV1/FVC ratio <0.70 confirms the presence of airflow limitation consistent with COPD.
- **Other Diagnostic Tests:** Additional tests may be performed to evaluate the severity of COPD, assess for complications, and rule out other respiratory conditions. These tests may include:

- o **Chest X-Ray or CT Scan:** Imaging studies may be performed to assess lung anatomy, detect signs of emphysema or other structural abnormalities, and rule out alternative diagnoses.
- o **Arterial Blood Gas (ABG) Analysis:** ABG analysis measures oxygen and carbon dioxide levels in the blood and helps assess the severity of hypoxemia and respiratory acidosis in patients with advanced COPD.

3.2.1.5. Classification and Severity

- **Staging of COPD:** COPD severity is classified based on the Global Initiative for Chronic Obstructive Lung Disease (GOLD) criteria, which take into account symptoms, spirometry results, and exacerbation history. The GOLD classification system divides COPD into four stages:
  - o **Stage I (mild):** FEV1 ≥80% predicted
  - o **Stage II (moderate):** FEV1 50-79% predicted
  - o **Stage III (severe):** FEV1 30-49% predicted
  - o **Stage IV (Very Severe):** FEV1 <30% predicted or <50% predicted with chronic respiratory failure

In addition to spirometry results, the GOLD classification system considers symptoms and exacerbation history to categorize patients as having either a low or high risk of exacerbations and hospitalizations.

3.2.1.6. Treatment

- **Pharmacological Therapy:** Pharmacological therapy is a cornerstone of COPD management and aims to reduce symptoms, improve lung function, and prevent exacerbations. The main classes of medications used to treat COPD include:
  - o **Bronchodilators:** Bronchodilators are medications that relax the muscles around the airways, improving airflow and relieving symptoms such as dyspnea and wheezing. Bronchodilators are classified as short-acting or long-acting and include beta2-agonists and anticholinergics.
  - o **Inhaled Corticosteroids (ICS):** Inhaled corticosteroids reduce airway inflammation and may be used in combination with long-acting bronchodilators in patients with moderate to severe COPD and a history of exacerbations.
  - o **Phosphodiesterase-4 (PDE4) Inhibitors:** PDE4 inhibitors are oral medications that reduce inflammation in the lungs and may be used in patients with severe COPD and chronic bronchitis who continue to experience exacerbations despite other treatments.
  - o **Antibiotics:** Antibiotics may be prescribed to treat exacerbations of COPD caused by bacterial infections, particularly in patients with

increased sputum purulence and worsening symptoms.

- **Non-Pharmacological Therapy:** In addition to pharmacological therapy, non-pharmacological interventions play a crucial role in COPD management. These interventions include:
  - o **Smoking Cessation:** Smoking cessation is the most effective intervention for slowing the progression of COPD and reducing symptoms. Healthcare providers should offer smoking cessation counseling and support to all patients with COPD who smoke.
  - o **Pulmonary Rehabilitation:** Pulmonary rehabilitation is a comprehensive program that includes exercise training, education, and support to improve symptoms, exercise capacity, and quality of life in patients with COPD.
  - o **Oxygen Therapy:** Long-term oxygen therapy (LTOT) is recommended for patients with severe COPD and chronic respiratory failure to improve survival and relieve symptoms of hypoxemia.
  - o **Nutritional Support:** Nutritional supplementation and dietary counseling may be beneficial for patients with COPD who are malnourished or at risk of weight loss.

3.2.1.7. Management of Exacerbations

The management of COPD exacerbations involves prompt assessment, treatment, and follow-up to minimize the impact on lung function and quality of life. The goals of treatment are to relieve symptoms, improve gas exchange, and prevent complications. Treatment of exacerbations may include:

- **Bronchodilators:** Short-acting bronchodilators are the cornerstone of treatment for COPD exacerbations and should be administered promptly to relieve airflow limitation and dyspnea.
- **Systemic Corticosteroids:** Oral corticosteroids reduce airway inflammation and improve symptoms in patients with COPD exacerbations. A short course of oral corticosteroids is recommended for patients with moderate to severe exacerbations.
- **Antibiotics:** Antibiotics are indicated for exacerbations associated with bacterial infections, particularly in patients with increased sputum purulence, worsening symptoms, or signs of systemic inflammation.
- **Oxygen Therapy:** Oxygen therapy should be initiated in patients with severe exacerbations and hypoxemia to maintain adequate oxygenation and prevent complications such as respiratory failure.

3.2.1.8. Complications and Prognosis

- **Complications:** COPD can lead to a range of complications that impact quality of life and prognosis. Common complications of COPD include:
  - o **Respiratory Infections:** Patients with COPD are at increased risk of developing

respiratory infections, including pneumonia, bronchitis, and influenza.

- **Respiratory Failure:** Advanced COPD can lead to respiratory failure, characterized by severe hypoxemia and hypercapnia, requiring supplemental oxygen therapy and mechanical ventilation.
- **Pulmonary Hypertension:** Chronic hypoxemia and pulmonary vascular remodeling can lead to pulmonary hypertension, which increases the risk of right heart failure and death.

- **Prognosis:** The prognosis of COPD varies depending on factors such as disease severity, comorbidities, and response to treatment. COPD is a progressive condition, and the prognosis tends to worsen over time, particularly in patients with severe airflow limitation and frequent exacerbations. Early diagnosis, comprehensive treatment, and adherence to management strategies can help improve symptoms, slow disease progression, and enhance quality of life in patients with COPD (Judson et al., 2022; Vohra & Nowak, 2023).

3.2.2. Bronchiectasis

Bronchiectasis is a chronic lung condition characterized by abnormal and irreversible widening of the bronchi, the large airways in the lungs.

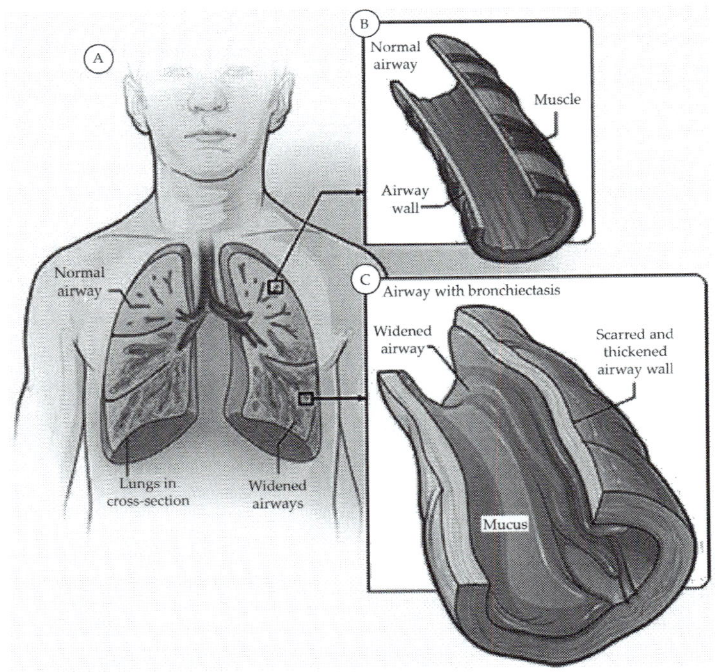

Figure 3.4. *The illustration shows the lungs with normal airways and with widened airways with bronchiectasis.*

Source: *By National Heart Lung and Blood Institute – National Heart Lung and Blood Institute, Public Domain, https://commons.wikimedia.org/w/index.php?curid=29583169*

This widening results from damage to the bronchial walls, leading to inflammation, scarring, and impaired clearance of mucus. Bronchiectasis can affect one or both lungs and can be focal or diffuse.

Bronchiectasis is considered an uncommon condition, but its prevalence varies widely depending on geographic location and underlying risk factors. In developed countries, the incidence of bronchiectasis has been increasing, particularly among older adults and individuals with predisposing conditions such as cystic fibrosis (CF) or primary ciliary dyskinesia (PCD) (Figure 3.4).

3.2.2.1. Pathophysiology

The pathophysiology of bronchiectasis involves a vicious cycle of airway inflammation, infection, and structural damage. The initial insult to the airway, such as infection, aspiration, or inflammation, leads to bronchial wall damage and impaired mucociliary clearance. This results in the accumulation of mucus and bacteria in the dilated bronchi, creating an environment conducive to recurrent respiratory infections and further inflammation. Over time, chronic inflammation and repeated infections lead to progressive bronchial dilation and remodeling, perpetuating the cycle of bronchiectasis.

3.2.2.2. Causes and Risk Factors

- **Underlying Conditions:** Bronchiectasis can occur as a primary condition or secondary to underlying respiratory or systemic disorders. Common underlying conditions associated with bronchiectasis include:
  - **Cystic Fibrosis (CF):** CF is a genetic disorder characterized by abnormal production of thick, sticky mucus that affects multiple organ systems, including the lungs.
  - **Primary Ciliary Dyskinesia (PCD):** PCD is a genetic disorder characterized by defects in the structure or function of cilia, hair-like structures that line the respiratory tract and help clear mucus and debris.
  - **Immunodeficiency Disorders:** Conditions that impair the immune system, such as human immunodeficiency virus (HIV) infection, immunoglobulin deficiency, or autoimmune disorders, can increase the risk of recurrent respiratory infections and bronchiectasis.
  - **Chronic Respiratory Infections:** Severe or recurrent respiratory infections, such as tuberculosis (TB), pneumonia, or severe viral infections, can lead to bronchiectasis, particularly if left untreated or inadequately treated.
  - **Obstructive Lung Diseases:** Conditions that cause airway obstruction, such as chronic obstructive pulmonary disease (COPD), asthma, or bronchiolitis obliterans, can predispose to bronchiectasis due to impaired clearance of mucus and debris from the airways.
- **Environmental Exposures:** Exposure to environmental pollutants, irritants, or toxins can contribute to the development or exacerbation of bronchiectasis. Common environmental risk factors for bronchiectasis include:

- **Air Pollution:** Exposure to indoor or outdoor air pollution, including particulate matter, vehicle emissions, and industrial pollutants, can irritate the airways and contribute to bronchial inflammation and structural damage.
- **Occupational Exposures:** Workers exposed to dust, chemicals, fumes, or other occupational hazards are at increased risk of developing bronchiectasis, particularly if proper protective measures are not implemented.
- **Tobacco Smoke:** Cigarette smoking is a significant risk factor for bronchiectasis and can exacerbate existing bronchial inflammation and structural damage.

3.2.2.3. Clinical Presentation

- **Symptoms:** The clinical presentation of bronchiectasis can vary widely depending on the extent and severity of bronchial dilation and associated respiratory complications. Common symptoms of bronchiectasis include:
  - **Chronic Cough:** A persistent cough that may be productive of large amounts of sputum, which can be foul-smelling or blood-tinged.
  - **Dyspnea:** Shortness of breath, particularly during physical activity or exacerbations.
  - Recurrent respiratory infections: Frequent episodes of acute bronchitis, pneumonia, or exacerbations of bronchiectasis.
  - **Hemoptysis:** Coughing up blood or blood-streaked sputum, which may occur during exacerbations or due to bronchial irritation.
  - **Fatigue, Malaise, and Weight Loss:** Symptoms of systemic illness may occur in severe or advanced cases of bronchiectasis.
- **Exacerbations:** Bronchiectasis exacerbations are acute episodes of worsening respiratory symptoms that require additional treatment beyond routine therapy. Exacerbations are often triggered by respiratory infections, air pollution, or other factors that increase inflammation or airway irritation. Symptoms of a bronchiectasis exacerbation may include increased cough, sputum production, dyspnea, and changes in sputum color or volume. Severe exacerbations may require hospitalization and can be life-threatening, particularly in patients with advanced bronchiectasis.

3.2.2.4. Diagnosis

- **Clinical Evaluation:** Diagnosing bronchiectasis begins with a thorough clinical evaluation, including a detailed medical history, physical examination, and assessment of respiratory symptoms. The healthcare provider will inquire about the onset, duration, and characteristics of symptoms, as well as any predisposing conditions or risk factors for bronchiectasis.

- **Imaging Studies:** Imaging studies are essential for confirming the diagnosis of bronchiectasis and assessing the extent and severity of bronchial dilation. The most commonly used imaging modalities for diagnosing bronchiectasis include:
  - **High-Resolution Computed Tomography (HRCT):** HRCT is the gold standard imaging modality for diagnosing bronchiectasis and provides detailed images of the lungs, airways, and surrounding structures.
  - **Chest X-Ray:** Chest X-ray may show characteristic findings of bronchiectasis, such as tram-track or ring-like opacities, but HRCT is more sensitive and specific for detecting bronchial dilation.
- **Pulmonary Function Tests:** Pulmonary function tests (PFTs) may be performed to assess lung function and identify any associated respiratory abnormalities, such as airflow limitation or gas exchange abnormalities. Spirometry, lung volume measurements, and diffusion capacity testing may be useful in evaluating the severity and impact of bronchiectasis on lung function.

3.2.2.5. Classification and Severity

- **Classification of Bronchiectasis:** Bronchiectasis can be classified based on etiology, anatomical distribution, and severity. Etiological classification distinguishes between primary (idiopathic) and secondary bronchiectasis, based on the presence or absence of underlying predisposing conditions. An anatomical classification describes the distribution of bronchial dilation within the lungs, such as focal, segmental, or lobar bronchiectasis. Severity classification assesses the extent and impact of bronchiectasis on lung function and quality of life, based on symptoms, exacerbation frequency, and imaging findings.

3.2.2.7. Treatment

- **Pharmacological Therapy:** Pharmacological therapy is a cornerstone of bronchiectasis management and aims to reduce symptoms, prevent exacerbations, and improve quality of life. The main classes of medications used to treat bronchiectasis include:
  - **Bronchodilators:** Bronchodilators such as beta2-agonists and anticholinergics may be used to relieve symptoms of bronchial obstruction and improve airflow in patients with bronchiectasis.
  - **Mucolytics:** Mucolytic agents such as hypertonic saline or dornase alfa may be used to thin and loosen mucus in the airways, making it easier to clear and reducing the risk of respiratory infections.
  - **Antibiotics:** Antibiotics are often prescribed to treat acute exacerbations of bronchiectasis caused by bacterial infections. Long-term or intermittent antibiotic therapy may also be considered for patients with

frequent exacerbations or chronic bacterial colonization.

- **Anti-Inflammatory Agents:** Corticosteroids or other anti-inflammatory medications may be used to reduce airway inflammation and suppress the immune response in patients with bronchiectasis.

3.2.2.8. Airway Clearance Techniques

Airway clearance techniques are an essential component of bronchiectasis management and help remove excess mucus from the airways, reduce the risk of respiratory infections, and improve lung function. Common airway clearance techniques include:

- **Chest Physiotherapy:** Chest physiotherapy techniques such as percussion, postural drainage, and vibration are used to loosen and mobilize mucus in the airways, making it easier to cough up and clear.
- **Active Cycle of Breathing Techniques (ACBT):** ACBT involves a combination of breathing exercises, deep breathing, and huffing or forced expiratory techniques to mobilize and clear mucus from the airways.
- **Oscillating Positive Expiratory Pressure (OPEP) Devices:** OPEP devices generate oscillating airflow during expiration, helping to mobilize mucus and improve airway clearance in patients with bronchiectasis.

3.2.3.9. Pulmonary Rehabilitation

Pulmonary rehabilitation programs are comprehensive interventions that combine exercise training, education, and support to improve symptoms, exercise capacity, and quality of life in patients with bronchiectasis. Pulmonary rehabilitation may include:

- **Exercise Training:** Aerobic exercise, strength training, and endurance exercises help improve cardiovascular fitness, muscle strength, and exercise tolerance in patients with bronchiectasis.
- **Education and Self-Management:** Patient education programs provide information on bronchiectasis, airway clearance techniques, medication management, nutrition, and coping strategies for managing symptoms and exacerbations.
- **Psychosocial Support:** Psychosocial support services such as counseling, support groups, and peer mentoring can help patients cope with the emotional and psychological impact of living with bronchiectasis.

3.2.2.10. Surgical Intervention

Surgical intervention may be considered in select cases of bronchiectasis with localized or severe bronchial dilation that is refractory to medical therapy. Surgical options for bronchiectasis include:

- **Lung Resection:** Lung resection involves the removal of diseased or damaged lung tissue to improve lung function and reduce the risk of recurrent infections. Lobectomy or segmentectomy may be performed in patients with localized bronchiectasis affecting one or more lung lobes.
- **Lung Transplantation:** Lung transplantation may be

considered in patients with end-stage bronchiectasis and severe respiratory compromise who are refractory to medical therapy and other interventions.

3.2.2.11. Management of Exacerbations

The management of bronchiectasis exacerbations involves prompt assessment, treatment, and follow-up to minimize the impact on lung function and quality of life. The goals of treatment are to relieve symptoms, control infection, and prevent complications. Treatment of exacerbations may include:

- **Antibiotics**: Antibiotics are the mainstay of treatment for bronchiectasis exacerbations caused by bacterial infections. Empiric antibiotic therapy should be initiated promptly based on the severity of symptoms, previous sputum culture results, and local antibiotic resistance patterns.
- **Bronchodilators:** Bronchodilators such as beta2-agonists and anticholinergics may be used to relieve bronchial obstruction and improve airflow in patients with exacerbations.
- **Corticosteroids:** Oral corticosteroids may be prescribed to reduce airway inflammation and suppress the immune response in patients with severe exacerbations or systemic symptoms.
- **Oxygen Therapy:** Oxygen therapy should be initiated in patients with severe exacerbations and hypoxemia to maintain adequate oxygenation and prevent complications such as respiratory failure.

3.2.2.12. Complications and Prognosis

- **Complications:** Bronchiectasis can lead to a range of complications that impact quality of life and prognosis. Common complications of bronchiectasis include:
    - o **Respiratory Infections:** Patients with bronchiectasis are at increased risk of developing respiratory infections, including acute bronchitis, pneumonia, and exacerbations of bronchiectasis, which can lead to hospitalization and respiratory failure.
    - o **Chronic Respiratory Failure:** Advanced bronchiectasis can lead to chronic respiratory failure, characterized by severe hypoxemia and hypercapnia, requiring supplemental oxygen therapy and mechanical ventilation.
    - o **Bronchiectasis-Related Complications:** Complications such as hemoptysis (coughing up blood), bronchial obstruction, lung abscess, and pleural effusion may occur in patients with severe or advanced bronchiectasis and can lead to significant morbidity and mortality.
- **Prognosis:** The prognosis of bronchiectasis varies depending on factors such as disease severity, underlying conditions, and response to treatment. Bronchiectasis is a chronic and progressive condition, and the prognosis tends to worsen over time, particularly in patients

with advanced bronchiectasis and frequent exacerbations. Early diagnosis, comprehensive treatment, and adherence to management strategies can help improve symptoms, slow disease progression, and enhance quality of life in patients with bronchiectasis (Judson et al., 2022; Vohra & Nowak, 2023).

3.2.3. Bronchiolitis

Bronchiolitis is an acute viral respiratory infection that primarily affects infants and young children under the age of two. It is one of the most common reasons for hospitalization in this age group, especially during the winter months. Bronchiolitis is typically caused by viral pathogens, with respiratory syncytial virus (RSV) being the most common etiological agent.

Bronchiolitis is characterized by inflammation, swelling, and mucus buildup in the bronchioles, leading to airway obstruction and respiratory symptoms. While most cases of bronchiolitis are mild and self-limiting, severe cases can result in respiratory distress, hypoxemia, and respiratory failure, particularly in infants with underlying health conditions or prematurity.

3.2.3.1. Causes and Risk Factors

- **Viral Pathogens:** Bronchiolitis is primarily caused by viral pathogens, with RSV being the most common culprit. RSV is highly contagious and spreads through respiratory droplets when an infected person coughs or sneezes. Other viruses that can cause bronchiolitis include human rhinovirus, adenovirus, influenza virus, and parainfluenza virus.
- **Age and Immune Status:** Infants and young children under the age of two are at the highest risk of developing bronchiolitis due to their immature immune systems and smaller airways. Premature infants, infants with underlying health conditions, and those who have not received adequate immunizations are also at increased risk of developing severe bronchiolitis.
- **Environmental Factors:** Environmental factors such as overcrowding, exposure to tobacco smoke, and poor air quality can increase the risk of bronchiolitis. Infants and children who attend daycare or have siblings are more likely to be exposed to viral pathogens and may have a higher risk of developing bronchiolitis.

3.2.3.2. Clinical Presentation

- **Symptoms:** The clinical presentation of bronchiolitis can vary depending on the severity of the illness and the age of the child. Common symptoms of bronchiolitis include:
  - **Runny or Stuffy Nose:** Nasal congestion and discharge are often the first symptoms of bronchiolitis.
  - **Cough:** A dry or wet cough may develop as the illness progresses, often worsening at night.
  - **Wheezing:** Wheezing, a high-pitched whistling sound heard during breathing, is common in children with bronchiolitis and indicates airway obstruction.

- o **Difficulty Breathing:** Rapid or labored breathing, retractions (visible inward movement of the chest wall), and nasal flaring may occur in infants with severe bronchiolitis.
- o **Fever:** Fever is common in infants with bronchiolitis, but its presence does not necessarily indicate the severity of the illness.

- **Clinical Course:** The clinical course of bronchiolitis typically follows a predictable pattern, with symptoms worsening over the first few days and gradually improving throughout one to two weeks. Infants with mild bronchiolitis may only experience mild respiratory symptoms, while those with severe bronchiolitis may develop respiratory distress, dehydration, and other complications requiring hospitalization.

3.2.3.3. Diagnosis

- **Clinical Evaluation:** Diagnosing bronchiolitis is primarily based on clinical evaluation, including a detailed medical history and physical examination. The healthcare provider will inquire about the child's symptoms, onset, duration, and severity of illness, as well as any underlying health conditions or risk factors for severe disease.
- **Laboratory and Imaging Studies:** Laboratory tests such as nasal swabs or throat swabs may be performed to identify the viral pathogen responsible for bronchiolitis, but these tests are not routinely recommended for diagnosis. Chest X-ray may be obtained in severe or complicated cases of bronchiolitis to assess for signs of pneumonia or other respiratory complications, but imaging studies are not typically necessary for diagnosis.

3.2.3.4. Treatment

- **Supportive Care:** The mainstay of treatment for bronchiolitis is supportive care, which aims to alleviate symptoms, maintain hydration, and ensure adequate oxygenation. Supportive care measures for bronchiolitis include:
  - o **Nasal Suctioning:** Gentle nasal suctioning with a bulb syringe or nasal aspirator can help remove mucus and improve nasal congestion in infants with bronchiolitis.
  - o **Humidified Air:** Humidified air or saline nasal drops may be used to moisturize the nasal passages and loosen mucus in infants with bronchiolitis.
  - o **Fluids:** Adequate hydration is essential for infants with bronchiolitis to prevent dehydration, particularly if they have feeding difficulties due to nasal congestion or respiratory distress.
  - o **Oxygen Therapy:** Oxygen therapy may be necessary for infants with severe bronchiolitis and hypoxemia to maintain adequate oxygenation and prevent complications such as respiratory failure.
- **Pharmacological Therapy:** Pharmacological therapy for

bronchiolitis is limited, as antibiotics are ineffective against viral infections, and bronchodilators have not been shown to provide significant benefit in most cases. However, in select cases of bronchiolitis with severe respiratory distress or wheezing, the following medications may be considered:

- o **Bronchodilators:** Short-acting bronchodilators such as albuterol may be used on a trial basis in infants with bronchiolitis and evidence of reversible airway obstruction or significant wheezing.
- o **Corticosteroids:** Oral or intravenous corticosteroids are not routinely recommended for the treatment of bronchiolitis but may be considered in infants with severe bronchiolitis and evidence of airway inflammation or wheezing refractory to bronchodilator therapy.

- **Respiratory Support:** In severe cases of bronchiolitis with respiratory distress, hypoxemia, or respiratory failure, respiratory support may be necessary to maintain adequate oxygenation and ventilation. Respiratory support measures for bronchiolitis may include:
  - o **Supplemental Oxygen:** Supplemental oxygen therapy is the mainstay of respiratory support in infants with bronchiolitis and hypoxemia. Oxygen may be administered via nasal cannula, face mask, or high-flow nasal cannula (HFNC) depending on the severity of hypoxemia and respiratory distress.
  - o **Non-Invasive Ventilation:** Non-invasive ventilation techniques such as continuous positive airway pressure (CPAP) or bilevel positive airway pressure (BiPAP) may be used to support respiratory efforts and improve oxygenation in infants with severe bronchiolitis and respiratory distress.
  - o Mechanical Ventilation: In cases of severe respiratory failure or respiratory arrest, invasive mechanical ventilation may be necessary to provide respiratory support and ensure adequate gas exchange in infants with bronchiolitis.

3.2.3.5. Prevention

- **Vaccination:** While there is currently no vaccine specifically for bronchiolitis, vaccination against RSV infection is an important preventive measure for infants at high risk of severe disease. Palivizumab, a monoclonal antibody against RSV, is recommended for certain high-risk infants during the RSV season to reduce the risk of severe RSV infection and hospitalization.
- **Hygiene Measures:** Simple hygiene measures can help reduce the risk of bronchiolitis and other viral respiratory infections in infants and

young children. These measures include:

- o **Hand Hygiene:** Regular handwashing with soap and water, especially before handling infants or preparing food, can help prevent the spread of viral pathogens that cause bronchiolitis.
- o **Respiratory Etiquette:** Covering the mouth and nose with a tissue or elbow when coughing or sneezing can help prevent the spread of respiratory droplets containing viral pathogens.
- o **Avoiding Exposure:** Limiting exposure to sick individuals, particularly during the peak RSV season, can help reduce the risk of bronchiolitis in infants and young children.

- **Environmental Measures:** Environmental factors such as tobacco smoke, air pollution, and overcrowding can increase the risk of bronchiolitis and other respiratory infections in infants and young children. Taking steps to reduce exposure to these environmental hazards can help prevent bronchiolitis and promote respiratory health:

- o **Avoiding Tobacco Smoke:** Avoiding exposure to tobacco smoke, both during pregnancy and after birth, can help reduce the risk of bronchiolitis and other respiratory infections in infants and young children.
- o **Improving Indoor Air Quality:** Ventilating indoor spaces, using air purifiers, and minimizing exposure to indoor pollutants such as dust, pet dander, and mold can help reduce the risk of bronchiolitis and other respiratory infections.
- o **Reducing Overcrowding:** Limiting exposure to crowded indoor spaces, particularly during the peak RSV season, can help reduce the risk of bronchiolitis and other viral respiratory infections in infants and young children.

3.2.3.6. Complications and Prognosis

- **Complications:** Most cases of bronchiolitis are mild and self-limiting, with infants recovering fully within one to two weeks. However, severe cases of bronchiolitis can lead to complications such as:

- o **Respiratory Distress:** Severe bronchiolitis can cause respiratory distress, characterized by rapid or labored breathing, retractions, nasal flaring, and cyanosis (bluish discoloration of the skin or lips due to hypoxemia).
- o **Dehydration:** Feeding difficulties due to nasal congestion or respiratory distress can lead to dehydration in infants with bronchiolitis, particularly if they are unable to tolerate oral fluids.
- o **Respiratory Failure:** In rare cases, severe bronchiolitis can progress to respiratory failure, characterized by severe hypoxemia, hypercapnia, and

respiratory arrest requiring mechanical ventilation.

- **Prognosis:** The prognosis of bronchiolitis is generally favorable, with most infants recovering fully within one to two weeks with supportive care. However, infants with underlying health conditions, prematurity, or severe bronchiolitis may have a higher risk of complications and may require hospitalization for close monitoring and respiratory support. Early recognition, prompt treatment, and appropriate supportive care are essential for optimizing outcomes and preventing complications in infants with bronchiolitis (Judson et al., 2022; Vohra & Nowak, 2023).

3.3. Lung Tissue Diseases

Some lung diseases affect the lung tissue, diminishing the amount of air entering the lungs. They include:

3.3.1. Pulmonary Fibrosis

Pulmonary fibrosis refers to a group of interstitial lung diseases characterized by progressive scarring of the lung tissue. The exact cause of pulmonary fibrosis is often unknown, and the term "idiopathic pulmonary fibrosis (IPF)" is used when the underlying cause cannot be identified. However, pulmonary fibrosis can also occur secondary to various factors, including environmental exposures, occupational hazards, autoimmune diseases, medication side effects, and genetic predisposition.

There are several types of pulmonary fibrosis, including:

- **Idiopathic Pulmonary Fibrosis (IPF):** The most common and severe form of pulmonary fibrosis, characterized by progressive scarring of the lung tissue with no identifiable cause.
- **Interstitial Pneumonia:** A group of lung diseases characterized by inflammation and scarring of the interstitium, including idiopathic interstitial pneumonia (IIP) and nonspecific interstitial pneumonia (NSIP).
- **Occupational Lung Diseases:** Pulmonary fibrosis can result from exposure to occupational hazards such as asbestos, silica, coal dust, and agricultural chemicals.
- **Connective Tissue Disease-Associated Interstitial Lung Disease (CTD-ILD):** Pulmonary fibrosis can occur in association with autoimmune diseases such as rheumatoid arthritis, systemic sclerosis (scleroderma), and polymyositis/dermatomyositis.
- **Drug-Induced Pulmonary Fibrosis:** Certain medications, particularly chemotherapy drugs, antibiotics, and anti-inflammatory agents, can cause pulmonary fibrosis as a side effect.

3.3.1.1. Pathophysiology

The pathophysiology of pulmonary fibrosis involves a complex interplay of genetic, environmental, and immunological factors leading to chronic inflammation, fibroblast activation, and excessive deposition of collagen and other extracellular matrix proteins in the lung tissue. The initial insult to the lungs, whether it be from environmental exposures, autoimmune reactions, or genetic abnormalities, triggers an inflammatory response that recruits immune cells and stimulates fibroblasts to produce collagen and other fibrotic proteins.

Over time, the accumulation of scar tissue in the lungs disrupts the normal architecture and function of the lung tissue, impairing gas exchange and leading to progressive respiratory insufficiency. The scarring may be patchy or diffuse, and it can affect both the airways (bronchiolar fibrosis) and the lung parenchyma (alveolar fibrosis). As the disease advances, the lungs become increasingly stiff and non-compliant, leading to restrictive lung function impairment and respiratory symptoms.

3.3.1.2. Causes and Risk Factors

- **Environmental Exposures:** Exposure to certain environmental pollutants and occupational hazards is a significant risk factor for pulmonary fibrosis. Common environmental exposures associated with pulmonary fibrosis include:
  - **Asbestos:** Inhalation of asbestos fibers can lead to the development of asbestosis, a type of pulmonary fibrosis characterized by the deposition of asbestos fibers in the lung tissue and progressive scarring.
  - **Silica:** Exposure to silica dust, commonly found in occupations such as mining, construction, and sandblasting, is a well-established cause of silicosis, a type of pulmonary fibrosis.
  - **Coal Dust:** Inhalation of coal dust in coal miners can lead to the development of coal workers' pneumoconiosis (CWP), also known as black lung disease, characterized by fibrotic changes in the lung tissue.
  - **Agricultural Chemicals:** Exposure to pesticides, herbicides, and other agricultural chemicals has been implicated in the development of pulmonary fibrosis in farmers and agricultural workers.
- **Occupational Hazards:** Occupational exposure to dust, fumes, and chemicals is a significant risk factor for pulmonary fibrosis. Workers in industries such as mining, construction, agriculture, manufacturing, and healthcare may be at increased risk of developing pulmonary fibrosis due to exposure to hazardous substances in the workplace.
- **Autoimmune Diseases:** Certain autoimmune diseases are associated with an increased risk of interstitial lung disease and pulmonary fibrosis. These include:
  - **Rheumatoid Arthritis (RA):** Rheumatoid arthritis is a systemic autoimmune disease characterized by chronic inflammation and joint destruction. Interstitial lung disease, including pulmonary fibrosis, is a common extra-articular manifestation of RA.
  - **Systemic Sclerosis (Scleroderma):** Systemic sclerosis is a connective tissue disease characterized by fibrosis of the skin and internal organs. Interstitial lung disease, particularly NSIP and usual interstitial pneumonia (UIP), is a common complication of systemic sclerosis.

- **Polymyositis/ Dermatomyositis:** Polymyositis and dermatomyositis are inflammatory myopathies characterized by muscle weakness and inflammation. Interstitial lung disease, including pulmonary fibrosis, can occur as a complication of these conditions.

- **Genetic Predisposition:** Genetic factors play a role in the development of pulmonary fibrosis, particularly in cases of familial or hereditary pulmonary fibrosis. Mutations in genes such as surfactant protein C (SFTPC), telomerase reverse transcriptase (TERT), telomerase RNA component (TERC), and mucin 5B (MUC5B) have been associated with an increased risk of pulmonary fibrosis.

3.3.1.3. Clinical Presentation

- **Symptoms:** The clinical presentation of pulmonary fibrosis can vary depending on the underlying cause, the extent of fibrosis, and the presence of comorbidities. Common symptoms of pulmonary fibrosis include:
  - **Progressive Dyspnea:** Gradually worsening shortness of breath, particularly during exertion, is the hallmark symptom of pulmonary fibrosis.
  - **Dry Cough:** A persistent, non-productive cough may develop as a result of irritation of the airways and lung tissue.
  - **Fatigue and Weakness:** Reduced exercise tolerance and generalized fatigue are common symptoms of pulmonary fibrosis, reflecting impaired gas exchange and oxygen delivery to the tissues.
  - **Chest Discomfort:** Some patients with pulmonary fibrosis may experience chest pain or discomfort, Particularly during breathing or coughing.
  - **Clubbing of the Fingers:** Clubbing, or enlargement and rounding of the fingertips, may occur in advanced cases of pulmonary fibrosis due to chronic hypoxemia and tissue hypoxia.
- **Clinical Course:** The clinical course of pulmonary fibrosis is variable and may be influenced by factors such as the underlying cause, disease severity, and response to treatment. In some cases, pulmonary fibrosis progresses slowly over several years, while in others, it may progress rapidly, leading to respiratory failure and death within a few months. The natural history of pulmonary fibrosis is often characterized by periods of relative stability interspersed with acute exacerbations or episodes of rapid decline in lung function.

3.3.1.4. Diagnosis

- **Clinical Evaluation:** Diagnosing pulmonary fibrosis begins with a thorough clinical evaluation, including a detailed medical history, physical examination, and assessment of respiratory symptoms.

The healthcare provider will inquire about the onset, duration, and progression of symptoms, as well as any underlying medical conditions, environmental exposures, or family history of lung disease.

- **Pulmonary Function Tests (PFTs):** Pulmonary function tests (PFTs) are essential for assessing lung function and diagnosing pulmonary fibrosis. Common PFT findings in pulmonary fibrosis include:
    - o **Restrictive Pattern:** Pulmonary fibrosis typically presents with a restrictive pattern on PFTs, characterized by reduced lung volumes (total lung capacity, vital capacity) and preserved or increased FEV1/FVC ratio.
    - o **Decreased Diffusing Capacity:** Diffusing capacity for carbon monoxide (DLCO) is often reduced in pulmonary fibrosis due to impaired gas exchange across the alveolar-capillary membrane.
- **Imaging Studies:** Imaging studies such as chest X-ray and high-resolution computed tomography (HRCT) are essential for evaluating the extent and severity of pulmonary fibrosis. Common imaging findings in pulmonary fibrosis include:
    - o **Interstitial Opacities:** HRCT typically shows reticular opacities, ground-glass opacities, and honeycombing in the lung parenchyma, indicating fibrotic changes and architectural distortion.
    - o **Peripheral and Basal Predominance:** Pulmonary fibrosis often has a peripheral and basal predominance on imaging, with fibrotic changes most prominent in the lower lobes and subpleural regions of the lungs.
- **Lung Biopsy:** In some cases, a lung biopsy may be necessary to confirm the diagnosis of pulmonary fibrosis and differentiate it from other interstitial lung diseases. Surgical lung biopsy or transbronchial lung biopsy may be performed to obtain lung tissue for histopathological examination, which can help identify characteristic features of pulmonary fibrosis such as fibroblastic foci, honeycombing, and chronic inflammation.

3.3.1.5. Classification and Severity

- **Classification of Pulmonary Fibrosis:** Pulmonary fibrosis can be classified based on various factors, including etiology, histopathological features, and radiological patterns. Common classifications of pulmonary fibrosis include:
    - o **Idiopathic Pulmonary Fibrosis (IPF):** IPF is characterized by progressive fibrosis of unknown cause and is the most common and severe form of pulmonary fibrosis.
    - o **Interstitial Pneumonia:** Interstitial pneumonia encompasses a group of lung diseases characterized by inflammation and scarring of the interstitium, including idiopathic

interstitial pneumonia (IIP) and nonspecific interstitial pneumonia (NSIP).

- **Usual Interstitial Pneumonia (UIP):** UIP is a specific histopathological pattern of pulmonary fibrosis characterized by alternating areas of fibrosis and normal lung tissue, often with honeycombing and fibroblastic foci.

- **Severity of Pulmonary Fibrosis:** The severity of pulmonary fibrosis can be assessed based on various factors, including symptoms, pulmonary function tests, imaging findings, and functional status. Common measures of disease severity in pulmonary fibrosis include:
    - **Forced Vital Capacity (FVC):** FVC is a measure of lung function that reflects the total volume of air exhaled forcefully after maximal inhalation. Reduced FVC is indicative of restrictive lung function impairment in pulmonary fibrosis.
    - **Diffusing Capacity for Carbon Monoxide (DLCO):** DLCO is a measure of gas exchange across the alveolar-capillary membrane. Reduced DLCO is indicative of impaired gas exchange and may correlate with disease severity in pulmonary fibrosis.
    - **Extent of Fibrosis on Imaging:** The extent and distribution of fibrotic changes on imaging studies such as HRCT can provide valuable information about disease severity and prognosis in pulmonary fibrosis.
    - **Exercise Tolerance:** Reduced exercise tolerance, as assessed by exercise testing or functional assessments such as the 6-minute walk test (6MWT), may indicate disease severity and functional impairment in pulmonary fibrosis.

3.3.1.6. Treatment

- **Pharmacological Therapy:** Pharmacological therapy for pulmonary fibrosis aims to slow disease progression, alleviate symptoms, and improve quality of life. The main classes of medications used to treat pulmonary fibrosis include:
    - **Antifibrotic Agents:** Antifibrotic agents such as pirfenidone and nintedanib have been shown to slow the progression of pulmonary fibrosis and reduce the decline in lung function in patients with IPF. These medications may also help alleviate symptoms and improve the quality of life in patients with pulmonary fibrosis.
    - **Corticosteroids:** Corticosteroids such as prednisone may be used to reduce inflammation and suppress the immune response in patients with inflammatory forms of pulmonary fibrosis, but their efficacy in IPF is limited, and long-term use is

associated with significant side effects.

- **Immunosuppressive Agents:** Immunosuppressive agents such as azathioprine and mycophenolate may be used in combination with corticosteroids for the treatment of autoimmune-related interstitial lung disease, but their efficacy in IPF is uncertain, and they may increase the risk of infection and other complications.

- **Oxygen Therapy:** Supplemental oxygen therapy is often necessary to maintain adequate oxygenation and relieve symptoms of hypoxemia in patients with advanced pulmonary fibrosis. Oxygen therapy may be delivered via nasal cannula, face mask, or portable oxygen concentrator, depending on the severity of hypoxemia and individual patient needs.
- **Pulmonary Rehabilitation:** Pulmonary rehabilitation programs are comprehensive interventions that combine exercise training, education, and support to improve symptoms, exercise capacity, and quality of life in patients with pulmonary fibrosis. Pulmonary rehabilitation may include:
    - **Exercise Training:** Aerobic exercise, strength training, and endurance exercises help improve cardiovascular fitness, muscle strength, and exercise tolerance in patients with pulmonary fibrosis.
    - **Education and Self-Management:** Patient education programs provide information on pulmonary fibrosis, medication management, breathing techniques, nutrition, and coping strategies for managing symptoms and exacerbations.
    - **Psychosocial Support:** Psychosocial support services such as counseling, support groups, and peer mentoring can help patients cope with the emotional and psychological impact of living with pulmonary fibrosis.
- **Lung Transplantation:** Lung transplantation may be considered in select cases of pulmonary fibrosis with advanced disease and significant respiratory compromise that is refractory to medical therapy and other interventions. Lung transplantation offers the potential for improved survival and quality of life in carefully selected patients with end-stage pulmonary fibrosis.

3.3.1.7. Management of Exacerbations

The management of acute exacerbations of pulmonary fibrosis involves prompt recognition, assessment, and treatment to minimize the impact on lung function and prognosis. Treatment of exacerbations may include:

- **Corticosteroids:** High-dose corticosteroids such as methylprednisolone may be used to reduce inflammation and stabilize lung function in patients with acute exacerbations of pulmonary fibrosis.
- **Oxygen Therapy:** Supplemental oxygen

therapy should be initiated promptly in patients with acute exacerbations and hypoxemia to maintain adequate oxygenation and prevent complications such as respiratory failure.

- o **Mechanical Ventilation:** In severe cases of acute exacerbations with respiratory failure, invasive mechanical ventilation may be necessary to support respiratory function and ensure adequate gas exchange (Judson et al., 2022; Vohra & Nowak, 2023).

3.3.2. Sarcoidosis

Sarcoidosis is a disease in which inflammation occurs in the lymph nodes, lungs, liver, eyes, skin, and/or other tissues.

3.3.2.1. Causes

- The exact cause of sarcoidosis is unknown. What is known is that when a person has the disease, tiny clumps of abnormal tissue (granulomas) form in certain organs of the body. Granulomas are clusters of immune cells.
- The disease can affect almost any organ. It most commonly affects the lungs.
- Health experts think that having certain genes makes it more likely for a person to develop sarcoidosis. Things that may trigger the disease include infections with bacteria or viruses. Contact with dust or chemicals may also be triggers.
- The disease is more common in African Americans and White people of Scandinavian heritage. More women than men have the disease.
- The disease often begins between ages 20 and 40. Sarcoidosis is rare in young children.
- A person with a close blood relative who has sarcoidosis is nearly 5 times as likely to develop the condition.

3.3.2.2. Symptoms

There may be no symptoms. When symptoms do occur, they can involve almost any body part or organ system.

Almost all people affected by sarcoidosis have lung or chest symptoms:

- Chest pain (most often behind the breastbone)
- Dry cough
- Shortness of breath
- Coughing up blood (rare, but serious)

Symptoms of general discomfort may include:

- Fatigue
- Fever
- Joint ache or pain (arthralgia)
- Weight loss

Skin symptoms may include:

- Hair loss
- Raised, red, firm skin sores (erythema nodosum), almost always on the front part of the lower legs
- Rash
- Scars that become raised or inflamed

Nervous system symptoms may include:

- Headache
- Seizures
- Weakness on one side of the face

Eye symptoms may include:

- Burning, itching, and discharge from the eye
- Dry eyes
- Pain
- Vision loss

Other symptoms of this disease may include:

- Dry mouth
- Fainting spells, if the heart is involved
- Nosebleed
- Swelling in the upper part of the abdomen
- Liver disease
- Swelling of the legs if heart and lungs are involved
- Abnormal heart rhythm if the heart is involved

3.3.2.3. Exams and Tests

The healthcare provider will perform a physical examination and ask about the symptoms.

Different imaging tests may help diagnose sarcoidosis:

- Chest X-ray to see if the lungs are involved or lymph nodes are enlarged
- CT scan of the chest
- Lung gallium scan (rarely done now)
- Imaging tests of the brain and liver
- PET scan of the whole body (or specific body parts)
- Echocardiogram or MRI of the heart

To diagnose this condition, a biopsy is needed. A biopsy of the lung using bronchoscopy is usually done. Biopsies of other body tissues may also be done.

The following lab tests may be done:

- Calcium levels (urine, ionized, blood)
- CBC
- Immunoelectrophoresis
- Liver function tests
- Quantitative immunoglobulins
- Phosphorus
- Angiotensin converting enzyme (ACE)

3.3.2.4. Treatment

Sarcoidosis symptoms will often get better without treatment, especially if there are only small lung abnormalities.

If the eyes, heart, nervous system, or lungs are affected, corticosteroids are usually prescribed. This medicine may need to be taken for 1 to 2 years.

Medicines that suppress the immune system are sometimes also needed.

In rare cases, people with very severe heart or lung damage (end-stage disease) may need an organ transplant.

With sarcoidosis that affects the heart, an implantable cardioverter-defibrillator (ICD) may be needed to treat heart rhythm problems.

3.3.2.5. Outlook (Prognosis)

Many people with sarcoidosis are not seriously ill and get better without treatment. Up to half of all people with the disease get better in 3 years without treatment. People whose lungs are affected may develop lung damage.

Overall the death rate from sarcoidosis is less than 5%. Causes of death include:

- Bleeding from the lung tissue
- Heart damage, leading to heart failure and abnormal heart rhythms
- Lung scarring (pulmonary fibrosis)

3.3.2.6. Possible Complications

Sarcoidosis may lead to these health problems:

- Fungal lung infections (aspergillosis)
- Glaucoma and blindness from uveitis (rare)
- Kidney stones from high calcium levels in blood or urine
- Osteoporosis and other complications of taking corticosteroids for long periods of time
- High blood pressure in the arteries of the lungs (pulmonary hypertension) (Judson et al., 2022; Vohra & Nowak, 2023)

3.4. Lung Circulation Diseases

The lungs are full of blood vessels that absorb the oxygen from the air. If the vessels are damaged, it means the body may not get sufficient oxygen, and may have difficulty in getting rid of harmful carbon dioxide. These diseases include:

3.4.1. Pulmonary Hypertension

A pulmonary artery blood pressure increase that is not normal is called pulmonary hypertension. This essential blood vessel comes from the right side of the heart and delivers oxygen-rich blood to the lungs. If a person's circulation has high blood pressure, or hypertension, close to the lungs, this condition is likely to worsen and result in major health issues.

Hypertension is not synonymous with pulmonary hypertension. High blood pressure can impact several body systems, but it primarily affects the circulatory system. This condition is known as hypertension. It is recommended that an individual's resting pulmonary blood pressure should be between 8 and 20 millimeters of mercury (mm Hg) (Figure 3.5).

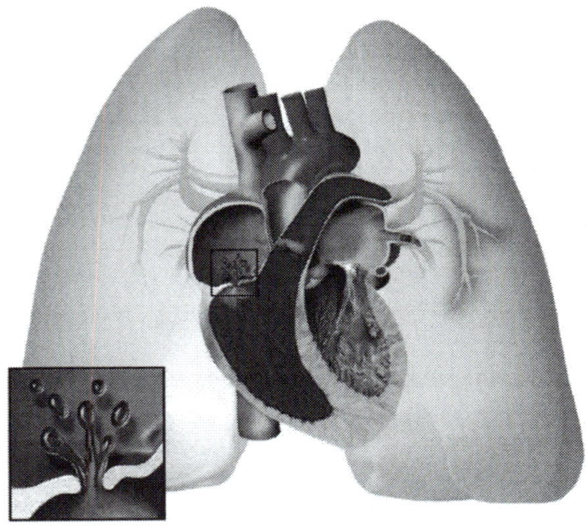

Figure 3.5. *Pulmonary hypertension causes your pulmonary arteries to become narrow. This makes it harder for oxygen-poor blood to reach your lungs.*

Source: *By BruceBlaus – Own work, CC BY-SA 4.0, https://commons.wikimedia.org/w/index.php?curid=61278364.*

3.4.1.1. Types

There are two types of pulmonary hypertension:

i. **Primary Pulmonary Hypertension:** This is a relatively rare condition that does not occur due to an underlying condition.

ii. **Secondary Pulmonary Hypertension:** This stems from an underlying condition, such as a congenital heart anomaly or chronic obstructive pulmonary disease (COPD).

3.4.1.2. Symptoms

The main symptom of pulmonary hypertension is shortness of breath or dyspnea. Breathlessness can affect a person's ability to walk, talk, and physically exert themselves.

Some other primary symptoms include fatigue, fainting, and dizziness.

It is important to note that pulmonary hypertension might produce no symptoms at all until the condition reaches a more severe stage.

3.4.1.3. Complications

- Right sided heart failure, also known as cor pulmonale, is the main complication of pulmonary hypertension.
- The back pressure on the heart and the increased effort needed to maintain blood flow can lead to a heart disease called right ventricular hypertrophy.
- This causes a collapse in the right ventricle of the heart due to thickened arterial walls. This causes the heart to overwork, the ventricle to get bigger, and blood pressure to increase.
- This is a life-threatening complication, as it can lead to heart failure. Heart failure is the main cause of death for people with pulmonary hypertension.
- Other complications include blood entering the lungs and coughing up blood, or hemoptysis. Both of these complications can be fatal.
- Blood clots and an irregular heartbeat, or arrhythmia, are other possible complications of pulmonary hypertension.
- If a person suspects that they have pulmonary hypertension, they should seek medical attention as soon as possible.
- Receiving prompt medical help can reduce the risk and severity of complications.

3.4.1.4. Causes

The thickening of the blood vessel walls in the lung causes pulmonary hypertension.

This narrows the space within the vessel through which blood can travel, increasing the pressure.

A complex set of factors leads to the thickening of blood vessels in the lungs, including:

- problems with connective tissue, such as sclerosis
- congenital heart anomalies, or structural issues that have been present since birth
- inherited genetic causes, such as a *BMPR2* gene mutation
- the use of drugs or other toxins
- liver disease, such as cirrhosis, which occurs due to scarring of the liver
- long term kidney failure
- HIV
- pulmonary embolism, wherein blood clots form in or move to the lungs
- sarcoidosis, in which the immune system causes lumps to form in organs throughout the body
- sickle cell anemia

- lung tumors
- metabolic disorders, including thyroid disorders
- left heart diseases, such as heart valve disease and aortic stenosis
- parasitic infection, including tapeworms such as *Echinococcus*
- lung diseases such as COPD
- regular exposure to high altitudes

3.4.1.5. Diagnosis

A range of factors can cause pulmonary hypertension, and the condition may occur alongside different types of heart or lung disease. As a result, the cause of the pulmonary hypertension can often be difficult to diagnose.

A doctor will ask about family and medical history and carry out a physical exam.

If they suspect that a person has pulmonary hypertension, they will usually suggest a series of tests, including:

- **A Chest X-Ray:** A doctor usually combines this with CT or MRI scans to help find the underlying cause of pulmonary hypertension.
- **Electrocardiogram:** This measures the electrical activity of the heart.
- **Right Sided Heart Catheterization:** This measures pulmonary blood pressure.

A doctor diagnoses pulmonary hypertension when the pressure in the pulmonary artery is higher than 25 mm Hg at rest or 30 mm Hg during exertion.

The 6-minute walk test (6MWT) allows a doctor to assess the progression of pulmonary hypertension and assign a stage to the condition. Staging demonstrates the severity of the condition on a scale of 1 to 4.

Stage 1 refers to a symptomless presentation of the condition, in which physical activity does not cause discomfort. Stage 4 means that a person experiences the symptoms of pulmonary hypertension even while at rest.

The 6MWT measures how far a person with suspected pulmonary hypertension can walk in 6 minutes, as well as how their body responds to the activity.

After staging the condition, the doctor will devise an appropriate treatment plan. They can also use the 6MWT to gauge the outlook of the condition.

3.4.1.6. Treatment

Treatment for pulmonary hypertension depends on the underlying cause, any co-occurring health problems, and the severity of the condition.

Therapies that may help a person manage their condition include low-intensity exercise such as walking. This can help them improve their capacity for physical exertion.

Continuous oxygen therapy may be necessary to help maintain oxygen saturation in the blood, especially among those who also have lung disease.

During a high-altitude flight, people may need oxygen therapy to compensate for reduced oxygen levels.

In oxygen therapy, a doctor administers additional oxygen from outside the body. They will deliver the oxygen from a tank through an oxygen mask or tubes in the nose and windpipe.

3.3.1.6.1. Drugs for Pulmonary Hypertension

Several drugs, either in isolation or in combination with each other, can support the management of pulmonary hypertension. For example:

- **Diuretics:** These help a person reduce fluid retention and swelling. They are also known as water pills.
- **Digoxin:** A person can use these to manage heart failure. Digoxin helps control heart rate and rhythm and increases the amount of blood that the heart can pump with each heartbeat.
- **Blood Thinning Drugs Such as Warfarin:** These can help reduce the risk of blood clots, which are more likely in people with pulmonary hypertension.
- **Calcium Channel Blockers Such as Diltiazem:** These help the blood vessels widen to improve blood flow.
- **Phosphodiesterase-5 (PDE5) Inhibitors:** These also increase blood flow by making blood vessels wider. Sildenafil is one example of a PDE5 inhibitor.
- **Endothelin Receptor Antagonists Such as Bosentan and Ambrisentan:** These limit the constriction of arteries that can develop when a person has too much natural peptide.

Inhaled options, such as iloprost (Ventavis) or treprostinil (Tyvaso), can help relieve breathlessness.

3.3.1.6.2. Surgical Solutions

More invasive treatments may be necessary when medication is not having the desired effect.

Surgical options include:

- **Atrial Septostomy:** In this procedure, a surgeon will introduce a shunt to the area between the heart chambers. This improves the output of the heart while a person awaits transplant surgery.
- **Lung Transplant:** This is a procedure to replace one lung or both lungs.
- **A Combined Heart and Lung Transplant:** This procedure is an intensive double transplant.

Chronic thromboembolic pulmonary hypertension is one presentation of high blood pressure in the lungs that also involves a number of blood clots in the arteries.

Some people with chronic thromboembolic pulmonary hypertension may undergo a procedure called a pulmonary thromboendarterectomy. This is specialized heart surgery to remove blood clots from coronary arteries.

Although many treatments are available to ease the symptoms, improve the outlook, and slow its progression, there is currently no cure for pulmonary hypertension (Judson et al., 2022; Vohra & Nowak, 2023).-

A Closer Look

Lung Cancer

Lung cancer is a complex and devastating disease characterized by the uncontrolled growth of abnormal cells within the lungs. It is the leading cause of cancer-related mortality worldwide, responsible for a significant number of deaths each year. While smoking remains the most prominent risk factor for lung cancer, exposure to environmental pollutants, genetic predisposition, and other factors also contribute to its development.

The disease is broadly classified into two main types: non-small cell lung cancer (NSCLC) and small cell lung cancer (SCLC), each with distinct characteristics and treatment approaches. NSCLC comprises the majority of lung cancer cases and includes subtypes such as adenocarcinoma, squamous cell carcinoma, and large cell carcinoma. SCLC, although less common, tends to be more aggressive and is often diagnosed at an advanced stage.

Symptoms of lung cancer can vary but commonly include persistent cough, chest pain, shortness of breath, coughing up blood, fatigue, and unintended weight loss. Unfortunately, these symptoms often do not manifest until the disease has progressed to an advanced stage, making early detection challenging.

Diagnosis of lung cancer typically involves a combination of imaging studies (such as chest X-rays, CT scans, and PET scans), tissue biopsy, and molecular testing to determine the histological subtype of the tumor and assess its genetic profile. Staging of the disease, which evaluates the extent of tumor spread and involvement of nearby structures or distant organs, is crucial for determining treatment options and prognosis.

Treatment strategies for lung cancer depend on several factors, including the type and stage of the disease, the patient's overall health, and their treatment preferences. Common treatment modalities include surgery, chemotherapy, radiation therapy, targeted therapy, and immunotherapy, often used alone or in combination to achieve the best possible outcomes.

Advances in precision medicine and immunotherapy have revolutionized the treatment landscape for lung cancer, offering new hope for patients with advanced or metastatic disease. Targeted therapies, which specifically target genetic mutations or alterations driving tumor growth, have shown remarkable efficacy in select patient populations. Immunotherapy, which harnesses the body's immune system to recognize and destroy cancer cells, has also demonstrated promising results in improving survival and quality of life.

Despite these advancements, lung cancer remains a formidable challenge, with many patients facing a poor prognosis, particularly those diagnosed at later stages. Early detection through screening programs, smoking cessation initiatives, and continued research into novel treatment approaches are critical in combating this deadly disease and improving outcomes for affected individuals. Efforts to raise awareness, reduce risk factors, and promote early detection and treatment are essential in the ongoing fight against lung cancer (Judson et al., 2022; Vohra & Nowak, 2023).

Summary

- Lung disease refers to several types of diseases or disorders that prevent the lungs from functioning properly. Lung disease can affect respiratory function, or the ability to breathe, and pulmonary function, which is how well the lungs work. There are many different lung diseases, some of which are caused by bacterial, viral, or fungal infections. Other lung diseases are associated with environmental factors, including asthma, mesothelioma, and lung cancer.
- Asthma is a chronic disease that causes the airways of the lungs to swell and narrow. It leads to breathing difficulties, such as wheezing, shortness of breath, chest tightness, and coughing.
- Chronic obstructive pulmonary disease (COPD) is a chronic inflammatory lung disease that causes obstructed airflow from the lungs. Symptoms include breathing difficulty, cough, mucus (sputum) production and wheezing. It is typically caused by long-term exposure to irritating gases or particulate matter, most often from cigarette smoke. People with COPD are at increased risk of developing heart disease, lung cancer, and a variety of other conditions.
- Bronchiolitis is swelling and mucus buildup in the smallest air passages in the lungs (bronchioles). It is usually due to a viral infection. Bronchiolitis usually affects children under the age of 2, with a peak age of 3 to 6 months. It is a common, and sometimes severe illness. Respiratory syncytial virus (RSV) is the most common cause. More than half of all infants are exposed to this virus by their first birthday.
- Bronchiectasis is a long-term condition where the airways of the lungs become widened, leading to a build-up of excess mucus that can make the lungs more vulnerable to infection. The most common symptoms of bronchiectasis include: a persistent cough that usually brings up phlegm (sputum) and shortness of breath.
- Pulmonary fibrosis is a lung disease that occurs when lung tissue becomes damaged and scarred. This thickened, stiff tissue makes it harder for the lungs to work properly. Pulmonary fibrosis worsens over time. Some people can stay stable for a long time, but the condition gets worse faster in others.
- Sarcoidosis in the lungs is called pulmonary sarcoidosis. It causes small lumps of inflammatory cells, called granulomas, in the lungs. They can affect how the lungs work. Experts don't know what causes this condition.
- Pulmonary hypertension is high blood pressure in your pulmonary arteries, which carry oxygen-poor blood from your heart to your lungs. The earliest symptom is shortness of breath during your usual routine. The most common causes are heart disease, lung disease and hypoxia. Early diagnosis and treatment can help you enjoy a better quality of life.

References

1. Boulet, L. P., & Godbout, K. (2020). Diagnosis of asthma in adults. In A. W. Burks, S. T. Holgate, R. E. O'Hehir, et al. (Eds.), *Middleton's Allergy: Principles and Practice* (9th ed., chap. 51). Philadelphia, PA: Elsevier.

2. Clifton, I. J., & Ellames, D. A. B. (2022). Respiratory medicine. In I. D. Penman, S. H. Ralston, M. W. J. Strachan, R. P. Hobson, et al. (Eds.), *Davidson's Principles and Practice of Medicine* (24th ed., chap. 17). Philadelphia, PA: Elsevier.

3. Cloutier, M. M., Dixon, A. E., Krishnan, J. A., Lemanske Jr., R. F. Pace, W., & Schatz, M. (2020). Managing asthma in adolescents and adults: 2020 asthma guideline update from the National Asthma Education and Prevention Program. *JAMA, 324*(22), 2301–2317. https://doi.org/10.1001/jama.2020.21974.

4. Iannuzzi, M. C. (2020). Sarcoidosis. In L. Goldman & A. I. Schafer (Eds.), *Goldman-Cecil Medicine* (26th ed., chap. 89). Philadelphia, PA: Elsevier.

5. Judson, M. A., Koth, L. L., & Baughman, R. P. (2022). Sarcoidosis. In V. C. Broaddus, J. D. Ernst, T. E. King, et al. (Eds.), *Murray and Nadel's Textbook of Respiratory Medicine* (7th ed., chap. 93). Philadelphia, PA: Elsevier.

6. Kraft, M. (2020). Approach to the patient with respiratory disease. In L. Goldman & A. I. Schafer (Eds.), *Goldman-Cecil Medicine* (26th ed., chap. 77). Philadelphia, PA: Elsevier.

7. Liu, A. H., Spahn, J. D., & Sicherer, S. H. (2020). Childhood asthma. In R. M. Kliegman, J. W. St. Geme, N. J. Blum, S. S. Shah, R. C. Tasker, K. M. Wilson, et al. (Eds.), *Nelson Textbook of Pediatrics* (21st ed., chap. 169). Philadelphia, PA: Elsevier.

8. Marcdante, K. J., Kliegman, R. M., & Schuh, A. M. (2023). Asthma. In K. J. Marcdante, R. M. Kliegman, & A. M. Schuh (Eds.), *Nelson Essentials of Pediatrics* (9th ed., chap. 78). Philadelphia, PA: Elsevier.

9. Raghu, G., & Martinez, F. J. (2020). Interstitial lung disease. In L. Goldman & A. I. Schafer (Eds.), *Goldman-Cecil Medicine* (26th ed., chap. 86). Philadelphia, PA: Elsevier.

10. Ryu, J. H., Selman, M., Lee, J. S., Colby, T. V., & King, T. E. (2022). Idiopathic pulmonary fibrosis. In V. C. Broaddus, J. D. Ernst, T. E. King, et al. (Eds.), *Murray and Nadel's Textbook of Respiratory Medicine* (7th ed., chap. 89). Philadelphia, PA: Elsevier.

11. Silhan, L. L., & Danoff, S. K. (2018). Nonpharmacologic therapy for idiopathic pulmonary fibrosis. In H. R. Collard & L. Richeldi (Eds.), *Interstitial Lung Disease* (chap. 5). Philadelphia, PA: Elsevier.

12. Vohra, T. T., & Nowak, R. M. (2023). Asthma. In R. M. Walls (Ed.), *Rosen's Emergency Medicine: Concepts and Clinical Practice* (10th ed., chap. 59). Philadelphia, PA: Elsevier.

Chapter

SYMPTOMS OF MENTAL ILLNESS OR EMOTIONAL PROBLEMS

4

Contents

Introduction

Effective identification, diagnosis, and treatment of mental illness or emotional problems depend on an understanding of their symptoms. A wide range of conditions that impact people's thoughts, feelings, behaviors, and general well-being are collectively referred to as mental illnesses. Persistent mood swings that severely affect everyday functioning and quality of life, such as protracted feelings of melancholy, hopelessness, or irritability, are among the classic signs of mental illness. These mood disorders can show up as a variety of symptoms, such as energy swings, irregular sleep or eating patterns, and a loss of interest in or enjoyment from previously enjoyed activities. Furthermore, cognitive symptoms are prevalent and can include anything from racing thoughts or persistent worries that interfere with daily tasks to problems with memory, concentration, or decision-making. Moreover, there could be behavioral shifts, like social disengagement, heightened agitation or impulsivity, or engaging in self-destructive activities like substance abuse or self-harm. The physical manifestations of stress or emotional distress can include headaches, stomachaches, and exhaustion. Interpersonal problems are frequently seen, such as relationship problems, communication or trust issues, and feelings of isolation or loneliness. It is critical to understand that symptoms of mental illness can differ greatly from person to person and that it can affect people of all ages, socioeconomic backgrounds, and lifestyles. Through early detection and comprehension of these indications, individuals, families, and medical professionals can promptly take action and offer suitable assistance and therapy to facilitate recuperation and enhance general health.

Orientation and Directional Terms

Term	Definition	Illustration
Autism	Autism is clinically regarded as a spectrum disorder, meaning that it can manifest very differently in each person.	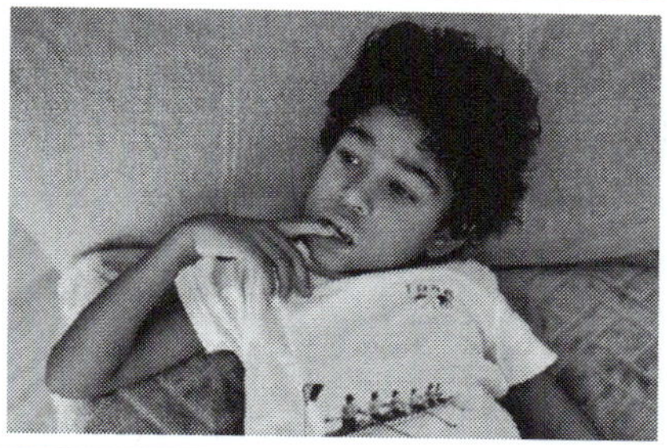
Schizophrenia	Schizophrenia is a serious mental illness that can affect a person's thoughts, feelings, and behaviors.	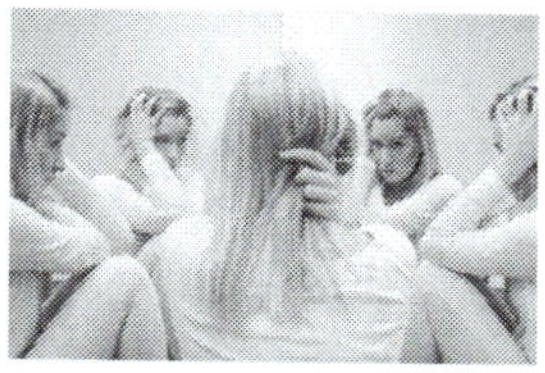
Depression	Depression (major depressive disorder) is a common and serious medical illness that negatively affects how you feel, the way you think and how you act.	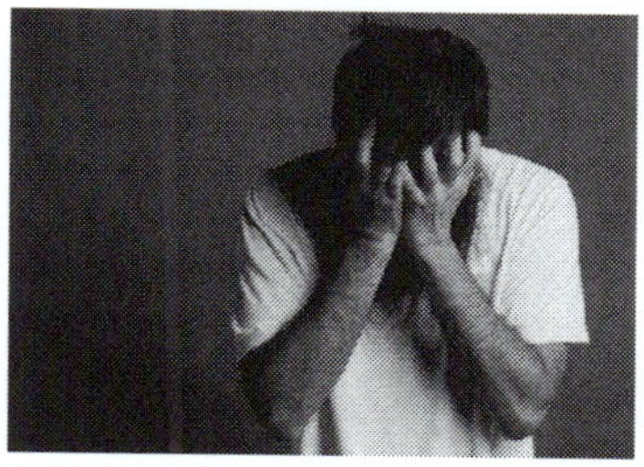
Obsessive-compulsive disorder	Obsessive-compulsive disorder (OCD) is a mental and behavioral disorder that causes people to have recurring, unwanted thoughts, ideas, or sensations (obsessions).	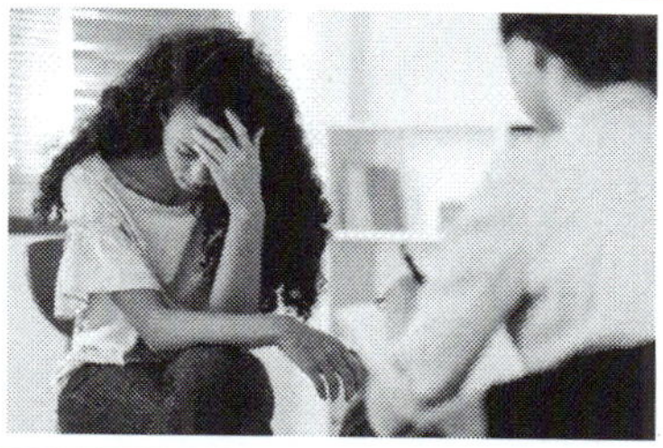
Anger	Anger is a normal emotion that can be useful when expressed appropriately. However, uncontrolled anger can have negative effects on your health and relationships.	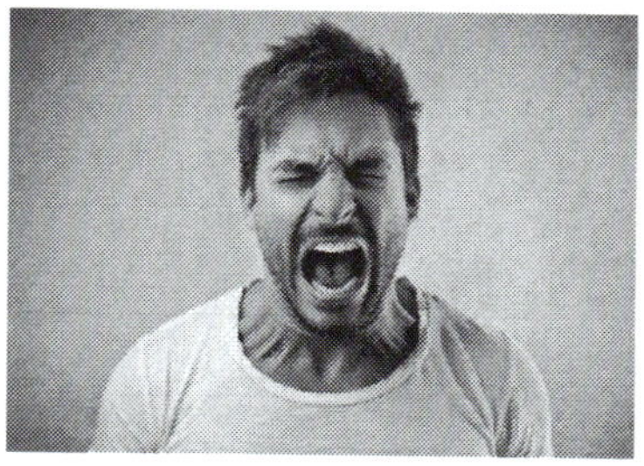

4.1. Mental Illness

Mental illness is defined by the American Psychiatric Association as a medical condition characterized by "changes in emotion, thinking, or behavior—or a combination of these." It is critical to understand the distinctions between mental health and mental illness. Your capacity to carry out daily tasks, maintain positive relationships, and deal with challenges head-on are all considered indicators of your mental well-being.

On the other hand, diagnosable mental health conditions that cause noticeable changes in one's thoughts, feelings, and behavior are referred to as mental illnesses. These alterations significantly distress people and make it difficult to function.

- There is no stigma associated with mental illness, and treatment and support are accessible, much like with other medical conditions like diabetes or heart disease.
- Mental illnesses are disorders or diseases that impact an individual's thoughts, emotions, behavior, and relationships with others and their environment. They occur frequently. Many individuals either have one or know someone who does.
- Mild to severe symptoms are possible. They may also differ among individuals. It often makes day-to-day living difficult. But you can frequently turn your life around when a specialist makes a diagnosis and assists with receiving treatment.
- A mental illness is characterized as a medical condition that alters a person's thinking, feelings, or behavior—or all three—and results in distress and functional difficulties for the individual. Like many other illnesses, mental illness can range in severity from mild to severe. Even in cases where their condition is mild, people with mental illnesses don't always appear sick. Some people might exhibit more overt signs like agitation, disorientation, or withdrawal. There are numerous mental health conditions, such as schizophrenia, depression, autism, attention deficit hyperactivity disorder (ADHD), and obsessive-compulsive disorder. Every illness affects a person differently in terms of their thoughts, feelings, and/or behaviors. We will talk about specific mental illnesses in this module at times, as well as general mental illnesses. Compared to other mental illnesses, depression, schizophrenia, and ADHD will be covered in more detail.
- Not every brain disease falls under the mental illness category. Though they are classified as neurological diseases rather than mental illnesses, conditions like epilepsy, Parkinson's disease, and multiple sclerosis are still classified as brain disorders. It is interesting to note that there is some blurring of the distinctions between these other neurological or brain disorders and mental illnesses. As researchers continue to look into the brains of those who suffer from mental illnesses, they are discovering that these disorders do, in fact, have a biological basis and are linked to changes in the chemistry, structure, and function of the brain.

4.1.1. Mental Illness in the Population

Many people believe that mental illness is uncommon, that it only affects people in drastically different situations than their own, and that it will never touch them. Studies on the epidemiology of mental illness show how inaccurate this belief is. Indeed, according to the surgeon general, mental illnesses are so prevalent that few U.S. Families remain unaffected by them.

4.1.1.1. Mental Illness in Adults (Figure 4.1)

Figure 4.1. *Scientists estimate that one in every four people is affected by mental illness either directly or indirectly.*

Source. *By Edward Boatman – Noun Project – https://thenounproject.com/icon/3746, CC0, https://commons.wikimedia.org/w/index.php?curid=64906637.*

It is highly likely that you have known someone who has dealt with mental illness, even if you or a family member have not personally experienced it. It is estimated that one in four individuals experience mental illness, either directly or indirectly. Consider the following statistics to get an idea of just how widespread the effects of mental illness are in society:

- According to recent estimates, approximately 20% of Americans, or about one in five people over the age of 18, suffer from a diagnosable mental disorder in a given year.
- Four of the 10 leading causes of disability—major depression, bipolar disorder, schizophrenia, and obsessive-compulsive disorder—are mental illnesses.
- About 3% of the population have more than one mental illness at a time.
- About 5% of adults are affected so seriously by mental illness that it interferes with their ability to function in society. These severe and persistent mental illnesses include schizophrenia, bipolar disorder, other severe forms of depression, panic disorder, and obsessive-compulsive disorder.
- Approximately 20% of doctor's appointments are related to anxiety disorders such as panic attacks.
- 8 million people have depression each year.
- 2 million Americans have schizophrenia disorders, and 300,000 new cases are diagnosed each year.

4.1.1.2. Mental Illness in Children and Adolescents

Adolescents and children are not immune to mental illness. There are 12 million kids under 18 who suffer from mental illnesses. The National Mental Health Association has compiled some statistics about mental illness in children and adolescents:

- Mental health problems affect one in every five young people at any given time.
- An estimated two-thirds of all young people with mental health problems are not receiving the help they need.
- Less than one-third of the children under age 18 who have a serious mental health problem receive any mental health services.
- As many as 1 in every 33 children may be depressed. Depression in adolescents may be as high as 1 in 8.
- Suicide is the third leading cause of death for 15- to 24-year-olds and the sixth leading cause of death for 5- to 15-year-olds.
- Schizophrenia is rare in children under age 12, but it occurs in about 3 of every 1,000 adolescents.
- Between 118,700 and 186,600 youths in the juvenile justice system have at least one mental illness.
- Of the 100,000 teenagers in juvenile detention, an estimated 60% have behavioral, cognitive, or emotional problems.

4.1.2. Warning Signs for Mental Illness

Each mental illness has its own characteristic symptoms. However, some general warning signs might alert you that someone needs professional help. Some of these signs include

- marked personality change
- inability to cope with problems and daily activities
- strange or grandiose ideas
- excessive anxieties
- prolonged depression and apathy
- marked changes in eating or sleeping patterns
- thinking or talking about suicide or harming oneself
- extreme mood swings—high or low
- abuse of alcohol or drugs
- excessive anger, hostility, or violent behavior

4.2. Diagnosing Mental Illness

4.2.1. Mental Health Professionals

A person needs to be assessed by a licensed practitioner with experience in mental health to receive a diagnosis of mental illness. Psychiatric nurses, mental health counselors, psychiatrists, psychologists, and social workers are examples of mental health professionals. Pediatricians, internists, and family physicians are typically qualified to diagnose common mental illnesses like ADHD, anxiety disorders, and depression. A mental health professional who is not a psychiatrist will frequently refer a patient to one, depending on the patient and his or her symptoms. A physician (M.D.) is a psychiatrist-who has taken additional courses in the study of mental diseases and mental health. Psychiatrists assess a patient's mental health alongside their physical health and can recommend medication. Only M.Ds and psychiatrists are able to prescribe drugs to treat mental health conditions.

4.2.2. Mental Illnesses Are Diagnosed by Symptoms

In contrast to other medical diagnoses, mental illness cannot be diagnosed by a blood test or by culture of certain microorganisms. In the interim, mental health practitioners will have to diagnose mental illnesses based on a patient's symptoms. Perhaps in the future, scientists will create distinct physiological tests for mental illnesses. It is common practice to base a diagnosis on a patient's symptoms rather than a quantitative medical test, such as a urinalysis, X-rays, throat swab, or blood chemistry test. Based solely on symptoms, doctors can diagnose a wide range of illnesses, such as Parkinson's disease, Alzheimer's disease, and migraines. Doctors use symptom analysis to gain a good idea of the nature of other diseases, like mononucleosis or asthma, and then perform a physiological test to confirm the diagnosis or provide more information.

When working with someone who may be experiencing mental health issues, a mental health professional will collaborate with the person to ascertain the symptoms, duration of the symptoms, and impact on the person's life. To get information, mental health providers frequently interview patients to learn about their symptoms, including how long they have been present and how severe they are. To get a more complete picture, the medical professional will frequently also speak with the patient's family members. The patient's medical history and a physical examination will probably be performed by a doctor to rule out additional health issues.

Experts in mental health assess symptoms to diagnose mental disease. To diagnose a particular mental illness, they use the criteria listed in the Diagnostic and Statistical Manual of Mental Disorders (DSM-IV; currently, the fourth edition), published by the American Psychiatric Association. The DSM-IV provides a general description and a list of typical symptoms for each mental illness. The DSM-IV is consulted by mental health practitioners to verify whether a patient's symptoms correspond to a particular mental disorder. Mental health professionals understand that while the DSM-IV offers useful information to aid in the diagnosis of mental illness, it is crucial to observe patients over an extended period of time to fully comprehend the patient's mental illness and its impact on their life (Corrigan & Lundin, 2001)

4.3. Mental Illness and the Brain

The phrase "mental illness" makes it abundantly evident that there is a mental health issue. As scientists continue to look into mental illnesses and their causes, they are learning more and more about how the biological processes that make the brain function are altered when a person has a mental illness. But is it just the mind in an abstract sense, or is there a physical basis for mental illness?

4.3.1. The Basics of Brain Function

It is helpful to consider how the brain normally works before considering the issues that arise in the brain when someone has a mental illness. The brain is an extraordinarily intricate organ. Although it only accounts for 2% of our body weight, it uses up 20% of the oxygen we breathe and 20% of the energy we absorb. It regulates almost every aspect of human experience, including movement, perception of our surroundings, involuntary bodily functions like breathing, and emotional regulation. The brain undergoes hundreds of thousands of chemical reactions every second, which are the basis for the ideas, deeds, and behaviors we use to react to the stimuli around us. To put it briefly, the brain controls the bodily functions and tendencies that enable us to live (Figure 4.2).

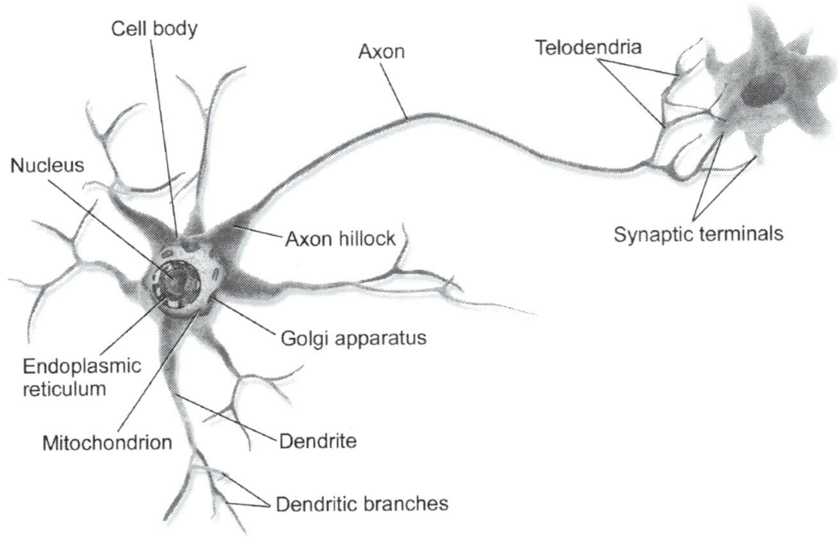

Figure 4.2. *The neuron, or nerve cell, is the functional unit of the nervous system. The neuron has processes called dendrites that receive signals and an axon that transmits signals to another neuron.*

Source: *By BruceBlaus - Own work, CC BY 3.0, https://commons.wikimedia.org/w/index.php?curid=28761830.*

The neuron is the basic functional unit of the brain; how does it process all this information and come up with a response? A neuron is a type of specialized cell with precise connections to muscle cells, other neurons, and sensory receptors that enable it to perform a variety of actions. Four anatomically and functionally distinct regions make up a typical neuron: the cell body, dendrites, axons, and axon terminals.

The neuron's metabolic core is located in the cell body. The majority of the cell's protein synthesis takes place in the nucleus, which is housed in the cell body.

A neuron's cell body normally contains a number of fibers called dendrites that extend from it. These functions, which resemble tree branches when they branch out, are the primary means of receiving information from other nerve cells.

The axon is also derived from the cell body. Axons can reach lengths of up to one meter; in most circumstances, they are significantly longer than dendrites. The portion of the neuron that is dedicated to transmitting signals to other cells and away from the cell body is called the axon. A fatty insulating substance known as myelin envelops some large axons, allowing electrical signals to move through them more quickly.

The axon splits into numerous fine branches near its end, each of which has a specialized swelling known as an axon terminal or presynaptic terminal. The dendrites of another neuron are close to where the axon terminals end. The message from the axon terminals of one neuron is received by the dendrites of that neuron (Figure 4.3).

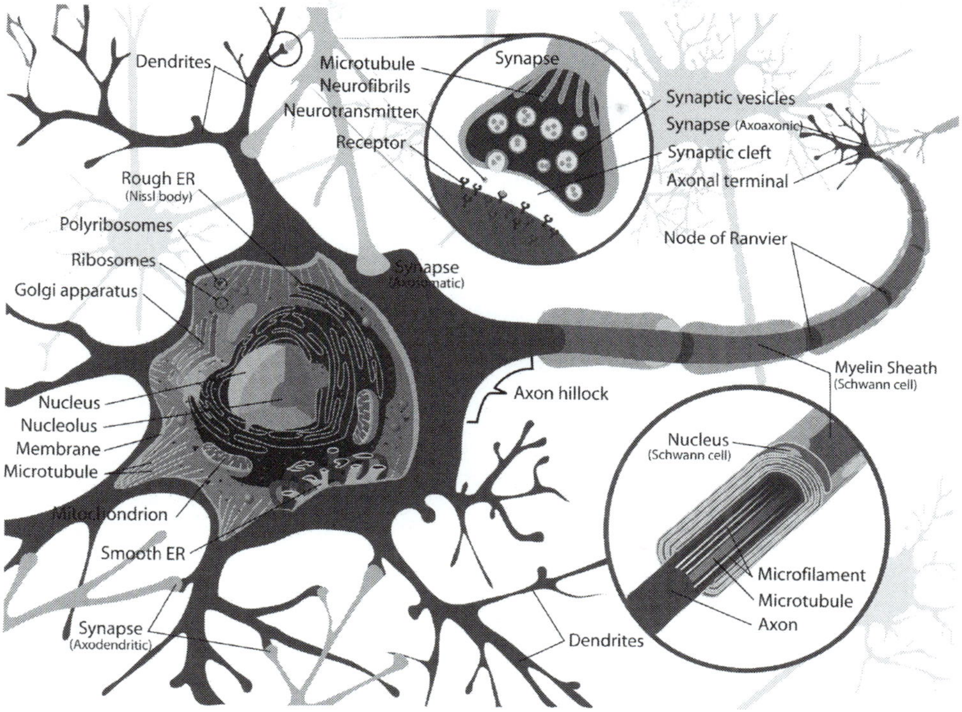

Figure 4.3. *Diagram of a synapse.*

Source: By LadyofHats – Own work. Image renamed from Image: Complete neuron cell diagram.svg, Public Domain, https://commons.wikimedia.org/w/index.php?curid=3970826

The synapse is the location where an axon terminal ends up next to a receiving dendrite. The presynaptic neuron is the cell that transmits information, and the postsynaptic neuron is the cell that receives it. It is crucial to understand that there is no cytoplasmic connection between the two neurons at the synapse, nor is there a physical connection. The synaptic space, also known as the synaptic cleft, is the intercellular region that separates the presynaptic and postsynaptic neurons. An average neuron connects to other neurons through about 1,000 synapses. According to estimates, the human brain contains more synapses than stars in our galaxy. Moreover, synaptic connections change over time. In reaction to events in life, neurons create new synapses or fortify existing ones. Learning is based on this dynamic shift in neural connections (Figure 4.4).

Both chemical and electrical signals are used by neurons to communicate. A presynaptic neuron's axon carries information in the form of an electrical impulse away from the cell body of the neuron and toward the axon terminals. The electrical signal is unable to pass through the synaptic cleft or synaptic space once it reaches the presynaptic axon terminal. Rather, the postsynaptic cell is affected by chemical changes that are triggered by the electrical signal and can travel across the synapse. Vesicles, which are membrane sacs, travel toward the axon terminal membrane when an electrical impulse reaches the presynaptic axon terminal. The vesicles merge with the membrane upon reaching it, releasing their contents into the synaptic space. Neurotransmitters are chemical compounds that are present in the vesicles. Numerous neurotransmitter molecules are present in each vesicle. The released neurotransmitter molecules attach to unique proteins on the postsynaptic neuron known as receptors after drifting across the synaptic cleft. A molecule of a neurotransmitter will only attach to a particular type of receptor.

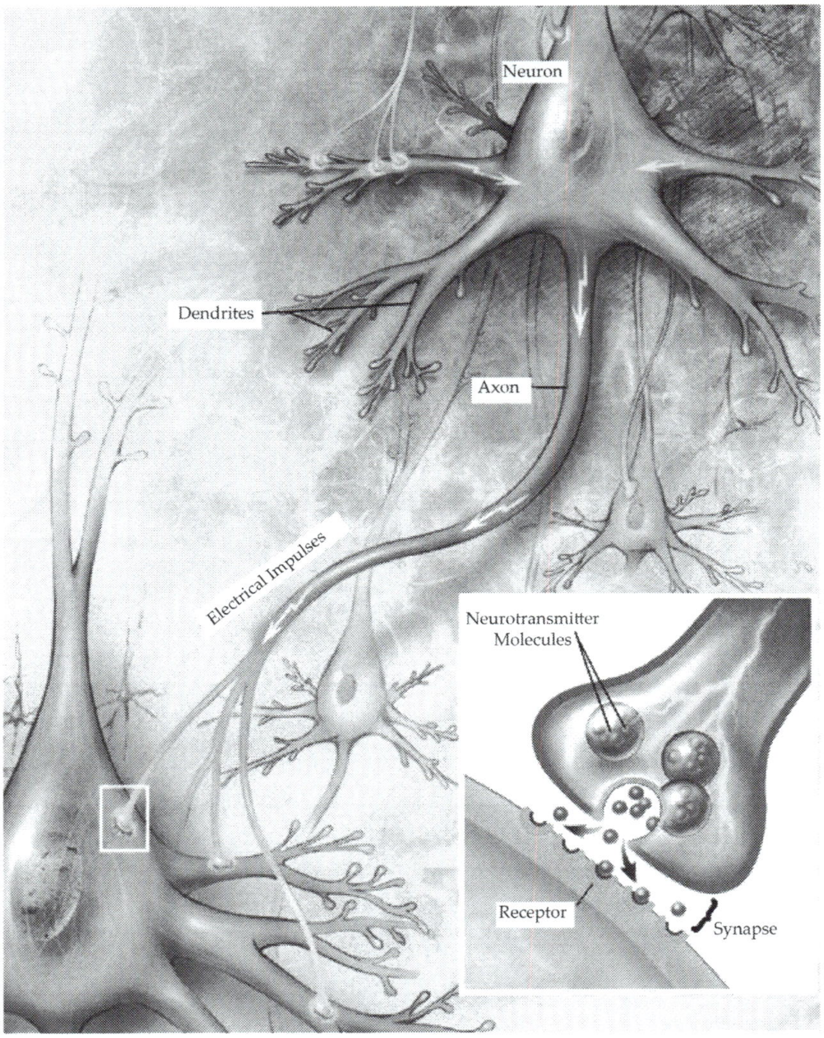

Figure 4.4. *Neurons relay their information using both electrical signals and chemical messages in a process called neurotransmission.*

Source. *By user: Looie496 created file; Illustrator: Christy Krames, MA, CMI, for US National Institutes of Health, National Institute on Aging – https://web.archive.org/web/20070713113018/http://www.nia.nih.gov/Alzheimers/Publications/UnravelingTheMystery/Part1/NeuronsAndTheirJobs.htm, Public Domain, https://commons.wikimedia.org/w/index.php?curid=8882110.*

A neuron produces an electrical impulse when neurotransmitters bind to their receptors. The electrical impulse then travels toward the cell body from the dendritic ending. The neurotransmitter releases from the receptor and returns to the synaptic space after stimulating an electrical impulse in the postsynaptic neuron. The neurotransmitter is transported back into the presynaptic neuron by certain proteins known as transporters or reuptake pumps. Repackaged into vesicles, the neurotransmitter molecules are ready for release the next time an electrical impulse reaches the presynaptic axon terminal. Neurotransmitter molecules that are not taken up again into the presynaptic neuron are broken down by synaptic space enzymes.

Although the nervous system makes use of a wide range of neurotransmitter molecules, each neuron is only capable of synthesizing and secreting one particular kind of neurotransmitter. The brain contains a variety of neurotransmitters, some of which are glutamate, GABA, serotonin, dopamine, and norepinephrine. A few of these names will come up concerning specific mental illnesses, but the specifics of each neurotransmitter's distribution and function in the brain are outside the purview of this module.

4.3.2. Investigating Brain Function

The symptoms that an individual displays serve as the basis for the diagnosis and treatment of mental illness by mental health professionals. When these specialists treat a patient, their aim is to get rid of any symptoms that are making it difficult for the patient to live their life normally. Conversely, research scientists aim to achieve something different. They are interested in finding out what structural or chemical alterations take place in the brains of those suffering from mental illnesses. Scientists can create more effective treatments or discover a cure if they can figure out what exactly goes on in the brain (Figure 4.5).

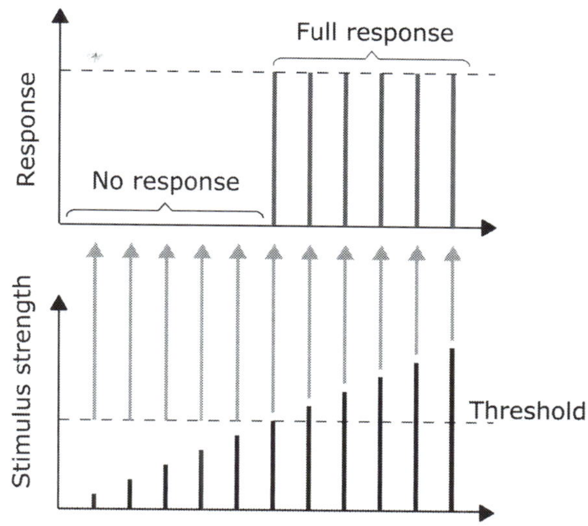

Figure 4.5. *Scientists use a variety of imaging techniques to investigate brain structure and function.*

Source. *By Blacktc – Translated from, CC BY 4.0, https://commons.wikimedia.org/w/index.php?curid=78013076.*

Depending on the questions they want to answer, scientists employ different methods to study the brain. For some inquiries, researchers look into particular genes or proteins in the neurons using molecular or biochemical techniques. To better understand how the activity or structure of the brain changes, scientists are interested in visualizing changes in the brain. In the past, scientists could only study brains after a person had passed away, but new imaging techniques now allow them to study the brain in living animals, including humans. It is critical to understand that mental illness cannot be diagnosed using these brain imaging methods. A person's presenting symptoms are used to diagnose mental illnesses. The following paragraphs' descriptions of imaging techniques won't help the mental health practitioner diagnose or treat the patient more successfully. Additionally, some of the methods involve slight radiation exposure for the patients and are invasive. Typically, children and adolescents are not involved in research studies that employ these tests.

Positron emission tomography (PET) is a widely used method to investigate brain activity and how mental illness alters the brain. PET scans track the movement and spatial distribution of a radioactive substance injected into living subjects' tissues. The method can be used to look into the connection between alterations in brain activity and behavioral and physiological effects while the patient is conscious. PET scans have a spatial resolution of roughly 4 millimeters and are capable of detecting very small (nanomolar) concentrations of tracer molecules. Furthermore, two or three-dimensional reconstruction of images from a PET scan can be done by computers.

Compounds labeled with positron-emitting isotopes must be used for PET. An electron has a negative charge, whereas a positron has a positive charge. An electron and a positron have the same mass and spin. To create these isotopes, protons are accelerated into the nuclei of nitrogen, carbon, oxygen, or fluorine using a cyclotron. The isotope is unstable due to the extra proton. The proton needs to decay into a neutron and a positron to return to its stable state. The unstable positron dissipates energy as it moves away from the site of generation. When the positron and electron eventually collide, two gamma rays that are 180 degrees apart are released. When the gamma rays hit two detectors, the event is recorded. Because the detectors only react to simultaneous emissions, the source of the gamma rays can be precisely mapped by scientists. The radioactive substances utilized in PET have a very brief half-life. Depending on the particular compound, the half-life (or the amount of time it takes for half of the radioactive label to break down) of the widely used radioisotopes can vary from less than two hours to about two minutes. Humans can safely use this technique because a PET scan only needs a small amount of short-lived radioisotopes—a few micrograms—to perform.

Where the neurons are most active in the brain is one of the many questions about brain function that PET scans can address. Different radiolabeled compounds are used by scientists to look into various biological questions. Radiolabeled glucose, for instance, can be used to pinpoint the areas of the brain that light up in response to a particular stimulus. Compared to inactive neurons, active neurons consume more glucose. More positrons are released by active neurons, which appear on PET scans as red or yellow instead of blue or purple in regions where the neurons are not very active. (While various computer enhancement methods may employ a different color scheme, it is common to use a spectrum with blue denoting low activity and red denoting high activity. Researchers can use PET to track alterations in a patient's brain activity in particular regions when they suffer from a mental illness. Researchers can also look into how treatment affects the brains of those with mental illnesses.

Researchers employ a variety of methods to study how mental illness alters the brain, including PET imaging. Scientists receive different information from different techniques. Magnetic resonance imaging is an additional crucial method (MRI). It is used to look at structural changes in the brain, as opposed to PET, which shows changes in activity levels. For instance, ventricles, or spaces within the brain, are larger in people with schizophrenia than they are in healthy people, according to MRI studies. Electroencephalography (EEG), functional magnetic resonance imaging (fMRI), and single photon emission computed tomography (SPECT) are additional methods that scientists use to study brain function in a living organism. Every method has benefits of its own and offers unique insights into the composition and operations of the brain (National Institute of Mental Health, 1999; American Psychiatric Association. Diagnostic and Statistical Manual of Mental Disorders, 2000; National Institute of Mental Health, 2001).

4.4. The Causes of Mental Illnesses

Right now, scientists are still unsure of the exact causes of mental illnesses. It is hardly surprising that determining the causes of mental illnesses is a difficult task when you consider the structural and organizational complexity of the brain as well as the complexity of effects that mental illnesses have on thoughts, feelings, and behaviors. The relationships between people's behaviors, thoughts, and feelings and how their actions can occasionally spiral out of control are explored in different ways by the disciplines of neuroscience, psychiatry, and psychology. Scientists are attempting to determine the causes of mental illnesses with the help of this multidisciplinary research. Scientists can create new therapies or attempt to find a cure once they have identified the underlying causes of mental illnesses.

4.4.1. The Biology of Mental Illnesses

The majority of scientists think that issues with neurotransmission—the flow of information between brain neurons—are the cause of mental illnesses. For instance, people with depression have reduced levels of the neurotransmitter serotonin. This discovery prompted the creation of specific drugs to treat the condition. The mechanism of action of selective serotonin reuptake inhibitors (SSRIs) is to decrease the quantity of serotonin reabsorbed by presynaptic neurons. As a result, there is more serotonin in the synaptic space available to bind to the postsynaptic neuron's receptor. Depression may also be accompanied by changes in other neurotransmitters, in addition to serotonin, which complicates the underlying cause of the illness (Figure 4.6).

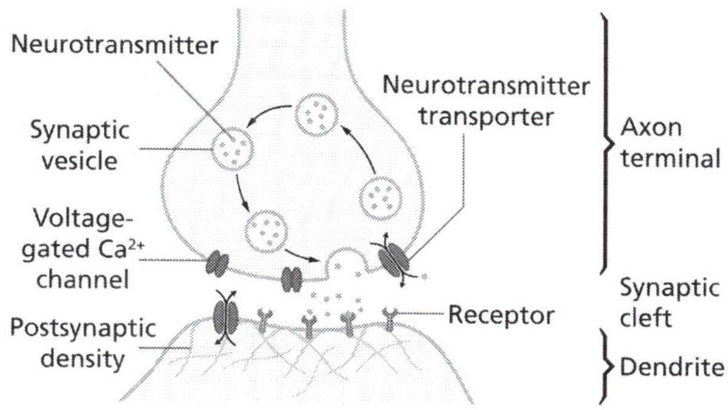

Figure 4.6. *Scientists understand that mental illnesses are associated with changes in neurochemicals. For example, in people who have depression, less of the neurotransmitter serotonin (small circles) is released into the synaptic space than in people who do not have depression. Certain medications called selective serotonin reuptake inhibitors (SSRIs) relieve symptoms of depression by causing an increase in the amount of serotonin in the synaptic space.*

Source: *By Thomas Splettstoesser (www.scistyle.com) – Own work, CC BY-SA 4.0, https://commons.wikimedia.org/w/index.php?curid=41349083.*

Dopamine, glutamate, and norepinephrine neurotransmitter abnormalities are thought to be present in schizophrenia patients. The fact that cocaine addicts occasionally exhibit schizophrenia-like symptoms is one clue that dopamine may play a significant role in the neurotransmitter disease. Cocaine stimulates dopamine-containing brain neurons to raise the concentration of dopamine in the synapses.

4.4.2. Risk Factors for Mental Illnesses

While the exact causes of mental illnesses are still unknown, scientists have discovered risk factors for people. These factors can be classified as social, genetic, or environmental. Indeed, the likelihood of someone developing mental illness is probably influenced by a combination of all these factors. The risk of developing mental illness is influenced by a combination of social, environmental, and genetic factors.

The chance of developing a mental illness can be raised by environmental factors such as head injuries, poor nutrition, and exposure to toxins like lead and tobacco smoke.

The likelihood that someone will experience mental illness is also influenced by their genes. The conditions that are most likely to have a genetic basis are ADHD, bipolar disorder, autism, and schizophrenia. One indication that genetics may play a part in determining an individual's susceptibility to ADHD is the finding that children with the disorder are significantly more likely to have a parent or sibling who also has the disorder. According to twin studies, identical twins are much more likely than fraternal twins to have ADHD. The same is true for depression and schizophrenia. Scientists believe that interactions between multiple genes may cause mental illnesses rather than changes in a single gene. Furthermore, the severity of a mental illness may depend on a confluence of social, environmental, and genetic factors.

Social factors also present risks and can harm an individual's, especially a child's, mental health. Social factors include;

- severe parental discord
- death of a family member or close friend
- parent's mental illness
- parent's criminality
- overcrowding
- economic hardship
- abuse
- neglect
- exposure to violence (National Institute of Mental Health, 1999; American Psychiatric Association. Diagnostic and Statistical Manual of Mental Disorders, 2000; National Institute of Mental Health, 2001)

4.5. Treating Mental Illnesses

While the majority of mental illnesses are currently incurable, they can typically be managed well enough to reduce symptoms and restore the patient's ability to function in social, occupational, and educational settings. An individual must see a licensed mental health professional in order to start treatment. Speaking with the patient to learn more about the symptoms, their duration, and how they are affecting their life is the first step a doctor or other mental health specialist will take. A physical examination will also be performed by the doctor to rule out any further health issues. For instance, certain symptoms (like mood swings) may be brought on by hormonal or neurological issues linked to long-term conditions like heart disease, or they may be a side effect of specific drugs. The doctor will create a treatment plan after assessing the patient's general health and diagnosing the ailment. Depending on the illness and how severe it is, treatment options may include both medication and psychotherapy.

4.5.1. Medications

Mental illnesses are frequently treated with medications. We are learning more about those medications through magazine and television advertisements. Medication for mental illness must be taken for a few days or weeks for it to fully work. When a patient starts taking medication, it is critical for a physician to keep an eye on their health. The doctor may adjust the dosage or prescribe an alternative medication with fewer side effects if the medication is causing unwanted side effects. A different medication may be prescribed by the doctor if the current one does not relieve the symptoms (Figure 4.7).

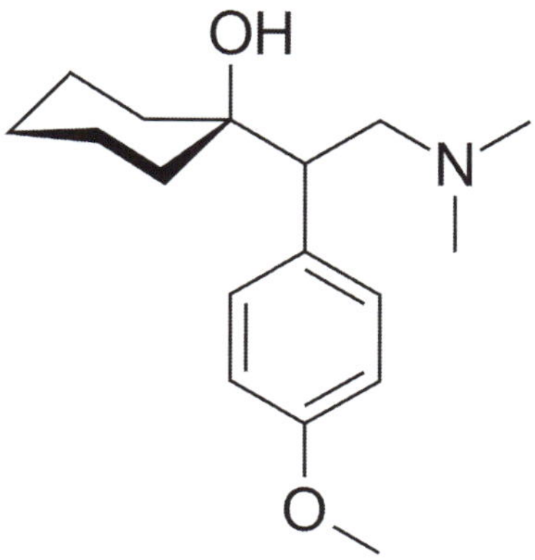

Figure 4.7. *Medicines are one part of an effective treatment plan for mental illnesses.*

Source. *By Vaccinationist – Own work, Public Domain, https://commons.wikimedia.org/w/index.php?curid=23472542.*

Because of the side effects, people with mental illnesses occasionally refuse to take their medications. It is critical to keep in mind that every medication has both advantages and disadvantages. Antibiotics, for instance, have completely changed how certain bacterial illnesses are treated. Antibiotics, however, frequently disrupt the good bacteria in the human body, resulting in adverse reactions like nausea and diarrhea. Like other medications, psychiatric drugs can lessen the symptoms of mental illness, but they can also have unintended side effects. When taking medication for a medical condition, be it mental health or another illness, patients should consult with their doctors to fully understand the prescription, its purpose, how to take it, and potential side effects.

From time to time, stories in the media link psychiatric medication side effects to potentially dangerous outcomes, like suicide. In these situations, it is typically very difficult to assess the relative contributions of the mental illness and the medication to the suicidal behavior. Like other medications, those used to treat mental illness may have side effects. To reduce side effects, the psychiatrist or doctor can typically change the medication or dose.

4.5.2. Psychotherapy

Psychotherapy is a type of treatment where the patient and a mental health professional—a psychologist, psychiatrist, or other mental health professional—discuss issues and feelings. Patients can identify solutions and comprehend the causes of their issues through this conversation. There are various forms of psychotherapy. The therapy can help patients

- change thought or behavior patterns,
- understand how past experiences influence current behaviors,
- solve other problems in specific ways, or
- learn illness self-management skills.

Psychotherapy can take place between a therapist and a patient, between a therapist and a patient's family, or between a therapist and a group. Psychotherapy and medication are often the most effective combination for treating mental illness. Medication eases the symptoms of severe mental illnesses, while psychotherapy assists patients in managing their condition.

Similar to how there are no drugs that can treat mental illnesses instantly, psychotherapy is a continuous process. Depending on the nature of the illness or issue, a person may attend psychotherapy for a few visits or several years. Psychotherapy should generally last longer the more serious the issue.

4.5.3. The Stigma of Mental Illness

"People with mental illnesses are crazy, insane, and wacky. "Those with mental illnesses are morally repugnant. "Those with mental illnesses ought to be permanently committed to an asylum because they are dangerous. "Those who suffer from mental illness require care from someone." "We may even be guilty of saying things like these ourselves. How often have we heard remarks like these or seen these kinds of portrayals in films, TV series, or books? Are these depictions accurate, or are they just a result of our ignorance and fear? (Figure 4.8).

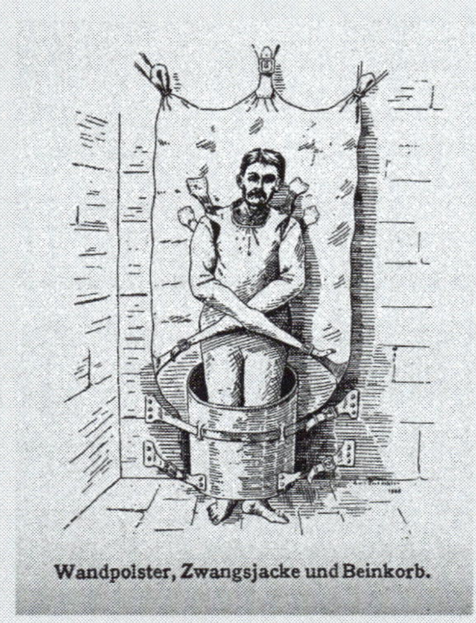

Figure 4.8. *Words can hurt. Many derogatory words and phrases are used in relation to mental illness. However, these words maintain the stereotyped image and not the reality of mental illness. Try not to use such words, and encourage students not to use them. It is more appropriate to refer to "a person who has a mental illness" when speaking about someone.*

Source: *By https://wellcomeimages.org/indexplus/obf_images/50/3f/676196b0c9e055181c7b13798313.jpgGallery: https://wellcomeimages.org/indexplus/image/V0016643ER.htmlWellcome Collection gallery (2018-03-22): https://wellcomecollection.org/works/wu29r4y5 CC-BY-4.0, CC BY 4.0, https://commons.wikimedia.org/w/index.php?curid=36505597.*

Stigmas are negative stereotypes about groups of people. Common stigmas about people who are mentally ill are:

- Individuals who have a mental illness are dangerous.
- Individuals who have a mental illness are irresponsible and can't make life decisions for themselves.
- People who have a mental illness are childlike and must be taken care of by parents or guardians.
- People who have a mental illness should just get over it.

All those stereotypes about those with mental illnesses are based on misinformation. There are very few dangerous mental illness sufferers in our society. Most are able to live freely, work, and go to school. No more so than a person with a different chronic illness like diabetes, asthma, or heart disease can someone with a mental illness just decide to get over it. Similar to other diseases, mental illness arises from a physical issue within the body.

Discrimination against individuals with mental illness results in unfair treatment in housing, employment, and education. Overcoming these stigmas is a tough challenge for those with mental illness, as the negative attitudes they face can be more disabling than the illness itself. The shame and guilt brought on by these stigmas lead to low self-esteem, dependence on others, and feelings of isolation and hopelessness. The fear of stigma also prevents many from seeking treatment that could greatly improve their symptoms.

One effective method for reducing stigmas surrounding mental illness is by providing accurate information. Advocacy groups actively fight against the stereotypes placed on individuals with mental illnesses, urging the media to portray them more accurately and encouraging the public to stop believing negative misconceptions. A powerful way to combat these stereotypes is through personal interactions with individuals managing serious mental illnesses successfully, such as holding down jobs, supporting themselves, and actively participating in their communities. Interacting with those with mental illnesses can challenge and change a person's preconceived notions and attitudes towards mental illness.

Though there is still a long way to go before people acknowledge that mental illness is a disease with a biological basis, attitudes regarding mental illness are gradually shifting. According to a National Mental Health Association survey, 55% of those who have never had a depression diagnosis acknowledge that it is an illness and not something that people should "snap out of." Compared to the 38% of survey participants in 1991 who identified depression as a disease, this represents a significant increase.

4.5.4. The Consequences of Not Treating Mental Illness

Many individuals seek medical treatment without hesitation for physical illnesses like bronchitis, asthma, diabetes, or heart disease. Unfortunately, the same cannot be said for those suffering from mental illnesses. Studies show that a large number of young people with mental health issues do not receive the necessary treatment, with estimates stating that two-thirds of them do not receive help. Similarly, less than one-third of children under 18 with serious mental health problems receive any form of mental health services. The problem of untreated mental illnesses extends to adults as well.

In September 2000, a conference on children's mental health was organized by the U.S. Surgeon General. Dr. David Satcher, the former surgeon general, highlighted the significance of mental health in children, emphasizing that missed prevention opportunities, fragmented services, and limited resources were causing suffering for children and families. Dr. Satcher also addressed the stigma surrounding mental illness as a major concern.

Mental illness in children and teenagers can have serious repercussions. A lot of mental health practitioners talk about the deficits that build up when children's mental illness goes untreated. Firstly, learning can be negatively impacted by mental illness in students. Teens with mental illnesses who do not receive prompt, aggressive treatment often find themselves falling further and further behind in their academics. When they grow up, they have a lower likelihood of becoming fully integrated members of society and a higher likelihood of dropping out of school. Furthermore, we now understand that young people with depressive disorders have an increased risk of illness as well as ongoing interpersonal and psychosocial challenges following their depressive episodes. In addition, a large number of adults with mental illnesses have childhood-onset issues. Childhood depression may be a sign of more serious illness later in life. Once believed to only affect children and adolescents, attention deficit hyperactivity disorder may continue into adulthood and be linked to issues in the social, legal, and professional spheres.

The impact of mental illness on society is significant due to its high incidence. Employers lose more than $23 billion annually as a result of employee absenteeism and decreased productivity during depressions alone. Disability-adjusted life years, or DALYs, are units of measurement used by the World Health Organization to quantify the burden of all diseases. These years are lost due to premature death or disability. Mental illness was the cause of more than 15% of all DALYs. Over $69 billion was spent on the direct treatment of mental illnesses in the US in 1996. The United States lost $79 billion as a result of the indirect costs of mental illness resulting from lost productivity at work, in schools, or in homes. S. the 1990s economy.

For patients, their families, and society as a whole, treatment—including psychotherapy and medication management—is reasonably priced. Benefits include decreased need for psychiatric hospitalization, fewer sick days and disability claims, fewer trips to other doctor's offices, diagnostic centers, and hospitals for physical ailments based on psychological distress, and more stable employment. On the other hand, failing to treat mental health issues can result in broken relationships, poor performance at work or loss of employment, mental anguish, substance misuse, needless medical procedures, psychiatric hospitalization, and suicide (National Institute of Mental Health, 1999; American Psychiatric Association. Diagnostic and Statistical Manual of Mental Disorders, 2000; National Institute of Mental Health, 2001).

4.6. Common Mental Health Disorders

Diagnosing mental illness is a complex process that does not have a simple solution. Tests to determine if a person has a mental illness are not always accurate. Each mental illness comes with its own set of signs and symptoms that are connected to biological dysfunction. The sections below outline the symptoms and effects of three highlighted mental illnesses in this curriculum supplement: depression, attention deficit hyperactivity disorder, and schizophrenia.

4.6.1. Depression

Depression, also known as depressive disorders, is one of the main causes of disability both domestically and internationally. In any given year, it is estimated to impact 90.5% of adult Americans. Depression affects almost twice as many women as men. According to epidemiological studies, up to 2% of children and 8% of adolescents in the US experience depression.

4.6.1.1. The Symptoms of Depression

Depression is more than just feeling depressed or unhappy. These emotions are common to everyone, but they do not always indicate depression. In actuality, there are three primary categories of depressive disorders, not just depression. They are:

- major depressive disorder,
- dysthymia, and
- bipolar disorder (manic-depression).

While some depressive symptoms are typical during a transient "blue mood," major depressive disorder is identified when a person experiences five or more symptoms almost daily for two weeks. Symptoms of depression include:

- a sad mood
- a loss of interest in activities that one used to enjoy
- a change in appetite or weight
- oversleeping or difficulty sleeping
- physical slowing or agitation
- energy loss
- feelings of worthlessness or inappropriate guilt
- difficulty concentrating
- recurrent thoughts of death or suicide

Depression can have a severe impact on people's lives, causing difficulties in functioning at work or school and a lack of interest in typical family and social activities. If left untreated, a major depressive episode in adults can last an average of nine months. Additionally, at least half of those who experience a major depressive episode are likely to have another episode in the future.

In children, depression lasts an average of seven to nine months with symptoms similar to those in adults. Symptoms in children may include

- sadness
- loss of interest in activities they used to enjoy
- self-criticism
- feelings that they are unloved
- hopelessness about the future
- thoughts of suicide
- irritability
- indecisiveness
- trouble concentrating
- lack of energy

Headaches, stomachaches, and general aches and pains are more common in children and adolescents with depression than in adults. Major depressive disorder affects most children and adolescents, but most also suffer from anxiety disorders, substance abuse disorders, or disruptive or antisocial behavior. Adolescents and children with depression have a higher suicide risk than other young people. Depression episodes are likely to recur, just like in adults.

While more chronic, dysthymia is less severe than major depressive disorder. Dysthymia is characterized by a depressed mood that lasts for at least two years in adults, or one year in children or adolescents, along with at least two other symptoms of depression. While these symptoms might not be as incapacitating, they do prevent affected individuals from feeling well or functioning normally. Dysthymia frequently starts in early adulthood, adolescence, or childhood. In children and adolescents, dysthymia typically lasts four years without treatment.

Bipolar disorder, also known as manic-depression, is a third type of depressive disorder where individuals experience alternating episodes of major depression and mania, characterized by abnormally elevated mood or irritability. During manic periods, the person will also have three or more of the following symptoms:

- overly inflated self-esteem,
- decreased need for sleep,
- increased talkativeness,
- racing thoughts,
- distractibility,
- increased goal-directed activity or physical agitation, and
- excessive involvement in pleasurable activities that have a high potential for painful consequences.

Adolescents who are manic may do dangerous or careless things like speeding and having inappropriate sex.

Bipolar disorder typically emerges during the teenage years or early adulthood. In adults, episodes of mania and depression are distinct and occur every few years. However, children and teens with bipolar disorder may experience rapid mood swings between depression and mania multiple times a day. Diagnosing bipolar disorder in young individuals can be challenging as the symptoms can be similar to those of other mental disorders like ADHD, conduct disorder, or oppositional defiant disorder.

4.6.1.2. The Causes of Depression (Depressive Disorders)

Although the precise causes of depression are unknown, it is likely a result of a combination of biological, environmental, and social factors, much like other mental illnesses. For a long time, researchers believed that depression was caused by low brain concentrations of specific neurotransmitters, such as norepinephrine, serotonin, or dopamine. Scientists now think that depression is caused by a much more complex interplay of factors. Family studies have indicated that there may be genetic reasons for depression in children and adolescents, as evidenced by the fact that 20 to 50% of these individuals have a history of depression in their family and that children of depressed parents are more than three times more likely to suffer from a depressive disorder than children of nondepressed parents. Depression may be brought on by abnormal endocrine function, particularly of the hypothalamus or pituitary. Other risk factors for depressive disorders in youths include:

- stress,
- cigarette smoking,
- loss of a parent,
- the breakup of a romantic relationship,
- attention disorders,
- learning disorders,
- abuse,
- neglect, and
- other trauma including experiencing a natural disaster.

Although the precise causes of depression are unknown, it is likely a result of a combination of biological, environmental, and social factors, much like other mental illnesses.

Researchers have examined alterations in the brain linked to depression. PET imaging studies have revealed that while brain activity in some regions of the brain is significantly reduced in depressed individuals, activity in other regions of the brain increases when compared to the same individual following successful treatment. Additionally, depression has been linked to decreased neurotransmitter (i.e., serotonin and dopamine) receptor binding potential in specific brain regions, according to PET imaging studies. Researchers examining the alterations in bipolar patients' brains discovered reductions in the size of the cerebellum (the area of the brain responsible for balance and coordinated movements), modifications in the metabolism of certain substances, and a drop in activity in particular brain regions (prefrontal cortex) during the depressive episode.

4.6.1.3. Treating depression

- Depression is treated with a range of antidepressant drugs and psychotherapies. For the majority of patients, a combination of medicine and psychotherapy is the most successful course of treatment.
- Medication is an effective treatment for depression in up to 70% of cases. The neurotransmission pathway is often the target of medications used to treat depression disorders. For instance, certain drugs have an impact on the activity of neurotransmitters like norepinephrine and serotonin. Different pharmacological treatments are needed for different depressive disorders. For instance, people with bipolar disorder are frequently treated with a combination of mood-stabilizing and antidepressant medications during their depressive phase and a mood-stabilizing drug, such as lithium, during their manic phase.
- Typically, medications can alleviate symptoms of depression within 6 to 8 weeks. If one medication is

ineffective, doctors can prescribe a different antidepressant. Like other mental health medications, patients are closely monitored by their doctors for symptoms and side effects. Patients who continue medication for at least six months after recovering from major depression have a 70% lower risk of relapse.

- Patients who receive psychotherapy can learn more efficient coping mechanisms for the issues in their lives. Typically, these therapies require 6 to 20 weekly meetings. If within three or four months there is no improvement in the symptoms, these treatment plans should be adjusted.
- Although doctors can use other techniques, the combination of medication and psychotherapy is the standard of care and is effective in most cases. When psychotherapy and antidepressants are ineffective, electroconvulsive therapy (ECT), also known as electroshock therapy, is a very successful treatment. ECT is not frequently administered to minors and young adults. The patient is put to sleep before receiving an electrical shock to particular brain regions during an ECT procedure. The shock is not felt by the patient consciously. Although ECT can produce dramatic and quick relief, its effects typically wear off rather quickly. People typically take antidepressants after electroconvulsive therapy (ECT).
- The combination of medications and psychotherapy is effective in the majority of cases.
- The herbal remedy St. John's wort is an over-the-counter treatment for mild to moderate depression. Nevertheless, a lot of the assertions lacked solid scientific support. The efficacy and security of St. John's wort are still unclear, and using it is generally discouraged.

4.6.1.4. Coping with Depression

Anxiety, worthlessness, powerlessness, and hopelessness are common feelings in people with depression (or other depressive disorders). Some individuals feel like giving up because of these depressing thoughts and emotions that come with the illness. As the treatment starts to work, these thoughts start to fade. Some strategies that can help while the patient waits for treatment to take full effect, these include:

- setting realistic goals in light of the depression and assuming a reasonable amount of responsibility
- breaking large tasks into small ones, setting some priorities, and doing what one can as one can
- trying to be with other people and to confide in someone—it is usually better than being alone and secretive
- participating in activities that may make one feel better
- getting some mild exercise, going to a movie or a ball game, or participating in religious, social, or other activities
- expecting one's mood to improve gradually, not immediately (feeling better takes time)
- postponing important decisions until the depression has lifted and discussing big decisions with

family or friends who have a more objective view of the situation

- remembering that positive thinking will replace the negative thinking that is part of the depression as one's depression responds to treatment
- letting one's family and friends help (National Institute of Mental Health, 1999; American Psychiatric Association. Diagnostic and Statistical Manual of Mental Disorders, 2000; National Institute of Mental Health, 2001).

4.6.2. Suicide

Suicide is a tragically possible side effect of untreated depression. Suicide accounted for over 30,000 deaths in the US in 1997, and it was the third most common cause of death for those aged 10 to 24. More than 90% of these individuals suffered from a mental illness, most commonly from a substance abuse disorder or a depressive disorder. According to data from the National Institute of Mental Health, up to 7% of teenagers with major depressive disorder go on to commit suicide.

Danger signs that a teen may be considering suicide include:

- undergoing dramatic personality change
- giving away prized possessions
- writing notes or poems about death
- talking about suicide, even jokingly
- making comments such as, "I can't take it anymore" or "I won't be a problem for you much longer"
- previously attempting suicide
- running away from home
- having other symptoms or risk factors for depression, such as difficulty getting along with parents and friends, difficulty in school, or acting bored or withdrawn.

Suicidal children and teenagers describe feelings of worthlessness, hopelessness, rage, depression, and anxiety. They feel powerless to alter annoying situations or discover a fix for their issues. Family disputes and the suicide death of a friend, relative, or acquaintance are risk factors for child and adolescent suicide in addition to depression. Children and teenagers may require intervention in the event of another person's suicide to avoid social isolation, trauma, or guilt feelings. Programs designed to address these issues and which school professionals offer can be very beneficial in identifying grieving youth who may require assistance.

Establishing phone crisis hotlines, limiting access to suicide tools (such as guns), counseling the media to stop "copycat" suicides, testing teenagers for suicide risk factors, and educating medical professionals on better diagnosing and treating mood disorders are all examples of public health strategies to prevent suicide. The screening and training strategies are more beneficial than the other methods in preventing youth suicides, according to research on the efficacy of these approaches.

4.6.3. Attention Deficit Hyperactivity Disorder (ADHD)

The most often identified behavioral disorder in children is attention deficit hyperactivity disorder (ADHD). Approximately 41.1% of youths aged 9 to 17 are estimated to be affected by ADHD in any given six-month period. ADHD is two to three times more common in boys than in girls. Despite being most commonly linked to children, ADHD can still exist in adults. According to one researcher, up to two-thirds of the children he evaluated for ADHD still had the disorder in their twenties, and many of the individuals who no longer met the criteria for ADHD still experienced severe difficulties at work or in other social situations.

4.6.3.1. The Symptoms of ADHD

The three main signs of ADHD are an inability to control one's level of activity (hyperactivity), pay attention to tasks (inattention), and restrain one's behavior (impulsivity). ADHD sufferers may exhibit impulsive/hyperactive behavior most of the time, hyperactive/impulsive behavior most of the time, or a combination of the two. Children and adolescents with ADHD

- are often unpopular among their peers
- have trouble in school
- have higher injury rates than their peers
- have difficulty paying attention to details
- are easily distracted
- find it difficult and unpleasant to finish their schoolwork
- put off things that require continued mental effort
- make careless mistakes
- are disorganized
- appear not to listen when spoken to
- fail to follow through on tasks

Before diagnosing ADHD, the DSM-IV lists many conditions in addition to the symptoms mentioned above. For a diagnosis of ADHD, the behaviors must

- appear before age seven
- continue for at least six months
- be more frequent or severe than in other children of the same age
- cause dysfunction in at least two areas of life, such as school, home, work, or social settings

Diagnostic interview techniques that have been tried and tested are a reliable way to diagnose ADHD. There isn't currently a reliable, independent test for ADHD, though.

ADHD commonly coexists with other behavioral, emotional, or learning issues in children, including depression, anxiety disorders, oppositional defiant disorder, and learning disabilities.

4.6.3.2. The Causes of ADHD

Although the precise causes of ADHD are unknown, research has shown that the disorder is not caused by factors that many people associate with its development. For instance, small head injuries, birth trauma, food allergies, excessive sugar intake, excessive television viewing, subpar education, or inadequate parenting do not contribute to ADHD. It is unknown what causes ADHD in one person. Instead, several important risk factors that have an impact on behavior expression and neurodevelopment have been linked. ADHD risk can be raised by factors like maternal alcohol and tobacco use that impact fetal brain development. Iron deficiency and other environmental pollutants have also been linked to brain damage.

Researchers have looked into how the neurotransmitter dopamine contributes to the development of ADHD because it is essential for controlling movement, boosting motivation and alertness, and causing sleeplessness. The finding that ADHD typically runs in families is compelling evidence in favor of a genetic component to the illness. At least one close relative suffers from ADHD, which is common among children with the disorder. According to one set of studies, a child's likelihood of developing ADHD is 11–18 times higher in identical twins than in nontwin siblings.

Studies on specific genes linked to ADHD have concentrated on two genes: the dopamine transporter gene (DAT1) on chromosome 5 and the dopamine receptor gene (DRD) on chromosome 11. Studies on the relationship between these genes and others and ADHD are still ongoing. The likelihood that someone has ADHD is most likely influenced by some genes as well as environmental variables.

According to imaging studies, boys with ADHD and boys without the disorder have different brain morphologies. Researchers discovered that boys with ADHD typically have smaller brains in specific regions. Research has indicated that the overall brain volume of girls with ADHD is smaller than that of control subjects; these findings are consistent with findings regarding the brains of boys with ADHD. The incapacity to suppress thoughts, a symptom of attention deficit hyperactivity disorder (ADHD), may be related to alterations in specific brain regions, according to scientific conjecture.

4.6.3.3. Treating ADHD

To treat ADHD, a range of drugs and behavioral therapies are employed. The most commonly used drugs are amphetamines, d-amphetamine, and methylphenidate (Ritalin). These medications act as stimulants, altering the amount of the neurotransmitter dopamine present at the synapses. When using one of these medications, nine out of ten kids get better.

These medications are thought to be fairly safe when taken as directed by licensed medical professionals. Diminished appetite and sleeplessness are side effects linked to moderate dosages. Usually starting early in the course of treatment, these side effects frequently go away over time. According to certain research, stimulants used to treat ADHD slow down growth rate without affecting final height.

Various interventions are utilized to treat ADHD, including cognitive-behavioral therapy, social skills training, support groups, and training for parents and educators. Combining medication with psychotherapy has been found to be more effective than either treatment alone in enhancing social skills, improving parent-child relationships, boosting reading achievement, and mitigating aggressive symptoms.

To improve social skills, parent-child relationships, reading achievement, and aggressive symptoms, treating ADHD with a combination of medication and psychotherapy is more effective than treating the disorder with either treatment alone.

Some parents and therapists have attempted a range of nutritional interventions in addition to the well-proven therapies mentioned above to treat ADHD. Some children respond well to these kinds of treatments, according to a few studies. However, no proven nutritional intervention has been demonstrated to be consistently effective in treating ADHD.

4.6.3.4. Coping with ADHD

ADHD interferes with a person's daily life, as the symptoms suggest. In addition to the treatment options available to help individuals and alleviate symptoms, the following basic strategies can also be helpful.

- Asking the teacher or boss to repeat instructions (rather than guessing what they were).
- Breaking large assignments or job tasks into small, simple tasks. Set a deadline for each task and give a reward as each one is completed.
- Making a list of what needs to be done each day. Plan the best order for doing each task. Then make a schedule for doing them. Use a

calendar or daily planner to keep on track.

- Working in a quiet area. Do one thing at a time. Take short breaks.
- Writing things that need to be remembered in a notebook with dividers. Carry the book at all times.
- Posting notes as reminders of things to do.
- Storing similar things together.
- Creating a routine. Get ready for school or work at the same time, in the same way, every day.
- Exercising, eating a balanced diet, and getting enough sleep (National Institute of Mental Health, 1999; American Psychiatric Association. Diagnostic and Statistical Manual of Mental Disorders, 2000; National Institute of Mental Health, 2001).

4.6.4. Schizophrenia

About 0.2 million Americans, or 1% of the population, suffer from schizophrenia. Both men and women are impacted equally. Most cases of the illness occur in young adults who are in their teens or twenties. Schizophrenia is rare until adolescence, even though it can strike children over five. In children, the illness typically progresses gradually and is frequently accompanied by delays in the development of speech or motor skills. Compared to adult-onset schizophrenia, childhood-onset schizophrenia typically has a worse prognosis and is more difficult to treat.

4.6.4.1. The Symptoms of Schizophrenia

There are a lot of false beliefs and myths regarding schizophrenia. People with schizophrenia are not multiple or split personalities, nor are they psychotic or incoherently insane all the time. While people with schizophrenia are frequently portrayed in the media as violent, in actuality, very few of these individuals pose a threat to others. Actually, rather than being violent themselves, people with schizophrenia are more likely to be victims of violence.

Schizophrenia has severe symptoms. A diagnosis of schizophrenia requires that at least two of the symptoms below be present during a significant portion of a one-month period:

- delusions (false beliefs such as conspiracies, mind control, or persecution);
- hallucinations (usually voices criticizing or commenting on the person's behavior);
- disorganized speech (incomprehensible or difficult to understand);
- grossly disorganized or catatonic behavior; and
- negative symptoms such as flat emotions, lack of facial expressions, and inattention to basic self-care needs such as bathing and eating.

However, if the delusions are particularly strange or if the hallucinations include one or more voices continuously commenting on the subject's actions or thoughts, the presence of any one of the first two symptoms is sufficient to diagnose schizophrenia.

The DSM-IV specifies additional criteria for a diagnosis of schizophrenia:

- social or occupational dysfunction,
- persistence of the disturbance for at least six months,
- exclusion of a mood disorder,
- exclusion of a substance abuse or medical condition that causes similar symptoms, and

- consideration of a possible pervasive developmental disorder.

The majority of individuals with schizophrenia typically go through one or more relapses following their initial psychotic episode. Relapses are times when an illness's symptoms—such as hallucinations and delusions—are more severe. Negative symptoms of emotion or self-care are typically still present during remissions. 10% or so of patients never fully recover from their severe illnesses and never return to their pre-illness states. Up to one-third to one-half of those with schizophrenia experience significant improvement or even full recovery from their condition, according to several long-term studies.

4.6.4.2. The Causes of Schizophrenia

Similar to the other mental illnesses covered here, the cause of schizophrenia is still a mystery to scientists. The disease is most likely caused by a combination of genetic and environmental factors, just like other mental illnesses. Many studies point to the involvement of imbalances in the brain's chemical neurotransmitter systems, such as those involving glutamate, norepinephrine, GABA, and dopamine, in the development of schizophrenia.

Studies on adoption, twins, and families lend credence to the notion that genetics plays a significant part in the illness. For instance, compared to the general population, children of individuals with schizophrenia are 13 times more likely to develop the disorder, and identical twins are 48 times more likely. Researchers are still searching for genes that could contribute to schizophrenia. Researchers studying schizophrenia are interested in a gene that produces an enzyme that degrades dopamine at the synapses. The function of this and other genes is still being investigated.

Imaging studies have shown that the brain structure and function of people with schizophrenia differ from those of control subjects. According to research on brain imaging, the brains of young people with schizophrenia differ structurally from those of people without the disorder. Reduced amounts of gray matter, which makes up the majority of the brain and is primarily composed of neuron cell bodies and dendrites, enlarged brain ventricles—the cavities or spaces in the brain that are filled with cerebrospinal fluid—and other abnormalities are some of the changes that have occurred. The cerebrum, the upper portion of the brain that is divided into halves, has also shrunk in volume. The frontal lobes, or the front portion of the cerebral lobes, exhibit less brain activity in the identical twin with schizophrenia than in the twin without the disorder, according to PET scans of the twins. Over the course of five years, one team of researchers used MRI to periodically scan the brains of teenagers with childhood-onset schizophrenia and an age-matched control group. They found that teens with schizophrenia lose four times the amount of neurons in a specific region of the brain that teens in the control group lose.

4.6.4.3. Treating Schizophrenia

Schizophrenia cannot be cured, but there are effective treatments that help most affected individuals manage their condition. Antipsychotic medication in addition to various psychotherapeutic interventions is the ideal course of treatment.

Antipsychotic medications, such as chlorpromazine and haloperidol, have been prescribed by physicians since the 1950s to treat schizophrenia-related hallucinations and delusions. More recently, it has been shown that newer antipsychotic medications—also referred to as atypical—like risperidone and clozapine are more efficacious. Prompt and consistent therapy, incorporating antipsychotic medication, is crucial for enhancing the disease's trajectory in the long run. Patients who stop taking their medication run the risk of getting sick again.

The most successful schizophrenia patients combine psychosocial rehabilitation (training in life skills) with medication. Schizophrenic patients benefit from therapies that combine behavioral and cognitive skills, education, and support from their families and communities to address particular issues. These approaches enhance the quality of life and functioning of the patients (National Institute of Mental Health, 1999; American Psychiatric Association. Diagnostic and Statistical Manual of Mental Disorders, 2000; National Institute of Mental Health, 2001).

4.7. Emotional Problems

For all of us, health is an essential and natural concern. It is a dynamic process that varies continuously. Being well is a blessing and a necessity. A healthy person can accomplish more work in less time and doesn't put off doing their tasks. He can complete tasks on time and with reasonable efficiency. His work gains vitality and strength from his good health. He also takes pleasure in his food and lives life to the fullest. We can manage job success, physical activity, emotional issues, and stress management if we take responsibility for our own wellbeing. Wellness is an improvement in quality of life with personal growth or positive behaviors and attitudes.

Taking care of your health is a valuable asset. You can do this by engaging in regular physical exercise, going for early morning walks, playing, eating a balanced diet, getting enough rest, and managing your stress levels. Neglecting your health can lead to disorders, such as mental illness, which can impact your ability to learn and grow intellectually. Mental disorders affect a person's behavior, emotions, and mood. While it is normal to experience a range of emotions, if these feelings start to disrupt your life, you may be experiencing a mental or emotional disorder.

Disorders can start in childhood or adolescence and may remain undiagnosed or untreated for many years. Emotional turmoil can lead to a mental disorder, often caused by abnormalities in brain development or function. If your emotions and feelings are not functioning properly, it may be a psychological issue. Excessive emotional thinking and dramatic behavior can be clear signs of an emotional disorder.

Emotional disorders are not highly specialized; rather, there is a relationship between the disorders and specific circumstances such as physical abuse, poverty, neglect, parental stress, excessive expectations, rule changes, confusion, and so forth. Eight emotional issues that arise in daily life are defined here along with their corresponding solutions.

4.7.1. Anorexia and Bulimia

Eating disorders cause unhealthy weight loss. Anorexics and bulimics may have a skewed perception of their bodies, leading them to purge or restrict calories in an attempt to achieve unattainable weight targets. Meal skipping, reduced portion sizes, and a growing number of restricted food options are common effects of calorie restriction. Remorse over what you eat can cause you to purge through food, exercise, or prescription drugs like laxatives. Malnutrition can occur and may cause damage to normal development and growth.

Anorexia can affect anyone, even though it more commonly affects women. Any gender, race, ethnicity, age, social class, and economic status can develop anorexia.

Many times, people who develop anorexia begin with the very understandable desire to lead a healthier lifestyle. But eventually, compulsive ideas about working out, dieting, and losing weight take over. These result in excessive weight loss and unhealthy behaviors. One may become secretive about their eating habits and restrictions as a result of the eating disorder. Eating disorders can develop subtly, and parents and physicians frequently fail to identify them. Anorexics regulate their body weight. They may:

- Eat only a small number of "safe" foods, usually low in calories and fat
- Avoid eating food on their plate by moving it around or cutting it up into tiny pieces
- Not eat food they cook for others
- Do things to keep their mind off their hunger, such as chewing gum or drinking large amounts of water
- Exercise in excess

Anorexics may also:

- Wear baggy clothes to hide their body
- Spend more time alone and away from friends and family
- Tire more quickly
- Seem depressed or anxious
- Be more emotional, or quick to cry or get angry

Malnutrition can cause anorexia over time, which can impact the entire body. It most obviously affects the heart, brain, bones, reproductive, and digestive systems. A lack of food can cause both physical and mental changes in the body.

Physical changes with anorexia:

- Always feeling cold because the body has lost the fat it needs to keep warm.
- Dizziness, fainting, or near fainting.
- More noticeable bones because of a loss of normal fat layers and muscle.
- Hair loss.
- Brittle hair and fingernails.
- Dry and rough skin.
- Affected menstrual periods. If anorexia develops before a girl's first period, periods may not start. For girls developing anorexia later, periods may stop.
- Stomach pain, constipation and bloating.
- Stunted growth that could be permanent.
- Anemia (low count of red blood cells) causing tiredness, weakness and dizziness.

Mental changes with anorexia:

- Feeling depressed, anxious or irritable
- Decreased concentration
- Increased difficulty completing tasks, such as schoolwork

When it comes to mental illnesses, anorexia has the highest death rate. Suicide or malnutrition (the body not getting enough nutrients) are two possible causes of death.

Bulimia is an eating disorder characterized by binge eating excessive amounts of food followed by an attempt to somehow neutralize the effects of the binge. Usually, the individual gets rid of (purges) the food they've consumed.

Bulimics frequently consume large quantities of food in a short period of time during a binge. A person's binge usually comes to an end when they run out of food, experience stomach pains after eating, or are distracted. Because the person experiencing the binge frequently feels helpless and out of control, binges are typically emotionally upsetting.

Bulimia sufferers often experience guilt and fear of gaining weight after bingeing. Through vomiting or other means, they rid their bodies of the food in an attempt to alleviate their guilt and fear. They might also resort to rigorous dieting or intense exercise. This "control" period continues until the subsequent binge. After then, the cycle resumes.

In contrast to bulimics, binge-eaters experience extreme guilt after consuming large amounts of food quickly, but they do not purge after a binge.

While bulimia is most commonly seen in teenage girls and young adult women, it can affect individuals regardless of gender, race, age, ethnicity, or social and economic background.

Individuals with bulimia experience dissatisfaction with their body, leading them to engage in bingeing behaviors as a response to anxiety and other emotions. Those with bulimia may exhibit underweight, overweight, or average weight.

People with bulimia have difficulty controlling their eating behavior. They may

- Become very secretive about binge eating.
- Spend a lot of time thinking about and planning the next binge. For example, they may
- Set aside certain times to binge and purge
    - o Avoid social activities to binge and purge
    - o Steal food or hide it in different places, such as under their bed or in closets
    - o Exercise or use laxatives to "purge" their body of food consumed

People with bulimia often face other problems as well, such as

- Depression and thoughts of suicide
- Substance use

Bulimia harms a person's physical and mental health. For example,

- Teeth start to decay from contact with stomach acids during vomiting.
- Weight goes up and down.
- Menstrual periods may become irregular or stop.
- The face and throat may look puffy and swollen.
- Dizziness and fainting may occur.
- Dehydration caused by loss of body fluids occurs.
- Upset stomach, constipation, and sore throat.
- Damage to vital organs such as the liver and kidneys; heart problems.
- Death.

Eating disorders have no known cause. Still, there are a few things that could be involved. These include certain personality traits, environmental factors, and a family history of eating disorders or mood disorders.

Recovery from an eating disorder is more likely the earlier it is identified. Therapy is based on numerous factors. These include the eating disorder's stage, the person's readiness to change, and the support of family members.

Treatment for eating disorders requires a team approach to be successful. Numerous medical professionals collaborate as a team. Every single one addresses a particular facet of the illness.

A pediatrician should be consulted before starting treatment so they can evaluate the physical effects of the eating disorder. In the event that the effects are severe, hospitalization may be required. Successful treatment of the eating disorder requires first restoring good nutrition and physical health.

The team assists a patient in returning to a healthy weight as part of their anorexia treatment. Regaining weight is essential to a full recovery. A person may require hospital admission for nourishment if they refuse to eat. When treating bulimia, the medical team may decide to admit the patient to the hospital to address comorbid conditions like electrolyte imbalance or dehydration or to break the binge-purge cycle (National Institute of Mental Health, 1999; American Psychiatric Association. Diagnostic and Statistical Manual of Mental Disorders, 2000; National Institute of Mental Health, 2001).

4.7.2. Antisocial Personality Disorder

Although the official diagnosis of true antisocial personality disorder cannot be made until the adolescent is eighteen, most teens with this disorder have shown this pattern of behavior before the age of fifteen. Before the age 18, this pattern of behavior is diagnosed as conduct disorder (see under 4.7.5. Disruptive Behavior Disorders). Without expert assistance and a loving family, they might develop into immature, careless adults with a startling lack of morality as adults.

- **Signs of Antisocial Personality Disorder**
    - Irritability and aggressiveness
    - Frequent fighting
    - Lying, cheating and other deceitful behavior
    - Impulsivity
    - Reckless disregard for personal safety or the safety of others
    - Lack of remorse for hurtful acts
    - Failure to apply oneself in school
    - History of truancy, delinquency, vandalism, theft, unlawful acts

4.7.3. Bipolar Disorder

Recently, there has been much discussion about mental health, and almost all parents and caregivers are worried about it. Many of us believe that our children will manage somehow if they are loved and understood. In addition, we are aware that 1 in 6 youth suffer from a mental illness that is incurable without medical attention.

Approximately 1% to 2% of all U. S. children under the age of eighteen suffer from bipolar disorder, a condition marked by sporadic changes in behavior and mood. Here are some things to consider about bipolar disorder and how to recognize symptoms in your child. Children and teenagers with bipolar disorder can eventually get better with treatment.

Bipolar disorder, formerly known as manic depression, is a brain illness that results in abrupt mood swings. Individuals diagnosed with bipolar disorder (bipolar I, bipolar II, or cyclothymia) experience manic episodes characterized by heightened mood, irritability, and high energy levels. Sometimes, they might also experience depressive episodes where they feel down, discouraged, and hopeless. Even during acute manic or depressive episodes, children and adolescents are more prone to experience mood swings.

Children who have bipolar disorder may also exhibit symptoms that are eerily similar to those of other common childhood disorders, including major depressive disorder, anxiety disorders, conduct disorders, and substance use disorders, as well as attention deficit hyperactivity disorder (ADHD) and disruptive mood dysregulation disorder (DMDD). Additionally, childhood trauma is very important for mental health. These are just a few of the explanations for why, even in cases where children exhibit multiple symptoms suggestive of bipolar disorder, medical professionals frequently struggle to reach a definitive diagnosis.

Children who suffer from bipolar disorder experience abrupt and severe swings in their sleep, mood, and energy levels, which can interfere with their ability to think clearly and interact socially.

When a child is experiencing mania, they might:

- Act incredibly happy, silly or even giddy
- Feel more irritable or impatient than usual
- Talk rapidly, hopping from subject to subject
- Need much less sleep than usual without feeling tired
- Struggle to stay focused on one task or topic
- Show strong interest in dangerous/risky activities
- Make snap decisions that seem out of character
- Lose or break things they value (mobile phones, bikes, jewelry, etc.)
- Experience more conflicts or misunderstandings with others

When they're in a depressed mood, kids with bipolar disorder might:

- Feel sad, discouraged or hopeless
- Show more anger and irritability than usual
- Complain of pain, such as stomach troubles or headaches
- Sleep much more than usual—or have trouble getting to sleep
- Experience "brain fog" that makes it hard for them to concentrate
- Have much less energy than normal for them
- Turn away from friends, family and activities they usually love
- Eat too much or too little
- Talk or think about death or suicide

4.7.4. Emotional Eating

Beyond sating hunger and meeting nutritional needs, food is used by both adults and children for other purposes. Actually, a lot of the time, kids who are obese eat because it fulfills them.

Think about if your own parents in your home relied on food for comfort. This is a typical occurrence that starts at birth. Breast milk or infant formula is usually given to a crying or agitated baby, and feeding him becomes a means of soothing and quieting him. Children are frequently given cookies or other desserts at birthdays and holidays when they are surrounded by family and feel loved; these treats then come to represent this love and caring.

These days, your own child may turn to food as a comfort when he is feeling anxious, possibly because of an impending math test or because he is being teased at school. On the other hand, children may eat for a variety of other reasons besides comfort.

Youngsters sometimes reach for food when they experience any of the following

- Boredom
- Insecurity
- Anger

- Depression
- Loneliness
- Happiness
- Stress
- Fatigue
- Frustration
- Resentment

Your child may come to enjoy food, but the results might not be exactly what he was hoping for. Ironically, he might feel worse after a food binge knowing that it can exacerbate his weight problem if he overeats to ease feelings of insecurity or depression, for example, or maybe because he is stressed about giving an oral report at school. He may feel guilty or ashamed even before the food has had a chance to break down.

Determining whether your child is eating for the correct reasons is actually one of your biggest parenting challenges. Consider the following: Does he eat outside of regular mealtimes and snacks? Does he constantly munch? What possible causes of his overeating exist that require your intervention?

When parents reward their kids with food—does getting an A on an exam sometimes mean going to the ice cream shop?—they unintentionally contribute to their kids' obesity. Praise and rewards can be given in healthier ways. Consider rewarding a young child with a few stickers or planning a shopping trip to purchase a new pair of shoes or a toy.

Don't undervalue the significance of verbal affirmation. Inform your child when he is acting appropriately. Observe how encouraging remarks can help him feel better about himself and be inspired to keep choosing the best course of action for his weight and health. Look for alternative methods to express gratitude, even if he's struggling to stick to his diet ("You walked more than half a mile today, that's so great!"). Don't bother him or give him the impression that he failed when he regresses. Encourage him to press on, regardless of his occasional complaints ("I want a soft drink, not ice water"), and to persevere through the situation. Give him all of the assistance he requires and merits.

4.7.5. Disruptive Behavior Disorders

Of all the coexisting conditions, disruptive behavior disorders are among the easiest to recognize because they involve actions that are easy to observe, like throwing tantrums, physically attacking other children, arguing excessively, stealing, and other acts of defiance or resistance to authority. These disorders, which include CD and ODD, usually become noticeable when they affect peer and family relationships or academic performance, and they often get worse over time.

Disruptive behavior disorders (DBD), ODD, and CD are all regarded as distinct conditions that can occur separately. However, behaviors characteristic of DBD can closely resemble ADHD—particularly when impulsivity and hyperactivity are involved. Coexisting ODD and CD are present in up to one-third of children with ADHD and up to 25% of children with CD, respectively. Because their defiant behavior causes so many conflicts with adults and other people they interact with, children with both conditions typically lead more difficult lives than those with ADHD alone. On the other hand, your child's chances of learning to control these behaviors may increase with early detection and treatment.

4.7.5.1. Oppositional Defiant Disorder

Many kids with ADHD occasionally act in an oppositional manner. The Diagnostic and Statistical Manual of Mental Disorders, Fourth Edition (DSM-IV) published by the American Psychiatric Association defines oppositional defiant disorder as characterized by recurrent episodes of "negativistic, defiant, disobedient, and hostile behaviors toward authority figures." In addition to arguing with adults frequently, losing his temper easily, disobeying rules, blaming others for his own mistakes, purposefully upsetting others, and acting in other ways that are angry, resentful, and vindictive, a child with ODD may also exhibit these behaviors. He will probably run into disciplinary issues and social conflicts at school on a regular basis. Many times these symptoms get worse over time, sometimes to the point where a conduct disorder diagnosis is made, especially in the absence of early diagnosis and treatment.

4.7.5.2. Conduct Disorder

Conduct disorder is a more severe condition than ODD. It is characterized by a repetitive and persistent pattern of behavior that involves violating the basic rights of others or major age-appropriate social rules. Symptoms of CD may include serious aggression towards people, harm to animals, destruction of property, stealing, running away from home, skipping school, or breaking social rules without consequences. Many children with CD may have previously been diagnosed with ODD, especially if they were physically aggressive at a younger age. Children with CD often continue to exhibit symptoms of ODD, such as argumentativeness and resistance. These behaviors, combined with impulsivity and hyperactivity of ADHD, may lead to these children being perceived as delinquent. They are more likely to be suspended from school and have more police contact compared to children with ADHD alone or ADHD with ODD.

Compared to adults with ADHD alone or ADHD plus ODD, children with ADHD whose CD symptoms began early also typically have worse outcomes as adults, especially when it comes to delinquency, criminal activity, and drug abuse.

Behavioral strategies tailored to the needs of children with ADHD and disruptive behavior disorders can be used both at home and in the classroom. These strategies usually involve teaching your child to recognize his own anger cues and to use them as cues to start different coping mechanisms, such as "Take five deep breaths and consider the three best options for how to respond before lashing out at a teacher"), and give himself praise (saying to himself, "Well done, you saw the cue and applied your tactics!"), for exercising self control. In the meantime, you and your child's teachers can learn how to better handle ODD or CD-type behavior by bargaining, making concessions, working through problems with your child, anticipating and averting potentially explosive situations, and setting priorities so that less critical issues are put off until more critical ones have been resolved. Professional behavior therapists or other mental health specialists recommended by your child's pediatrician, school psychologist, or other family-related professionals can teach these extremely specific techniques.

It might be decided to put your child in a special classroom at school that is designed for more rigorous behavior management if he has a diagnosis of coexisting ODD or CD and well-planned classroom behavioral techniques in his mainstream classroom have not worked. Still, schools are required to educate your child in a mainstream classroom whenever feasible and to revisit your child's education plan regularly to determine whether or not it is still the best fit for him.

An increasing body of research suggests that the stimulant drugs used to treat core ADHD symptoms may also benefit coexisting CD and ODD. It has been demonstrated that stimulants can lessen stealing, vandalism, hostile peer interactions, and physical and verbal aggression. Stimulant drugs may lessen the aggression that prevents kids from forming relationships with people their own age, even though they don't teach them new skills like recognizing and responding to others' social cues. Because of this, when it comes to medication treatment for children who have both ADHD and a co-occurring disruptive behavior disorder, stimulants are typically the first option.

Introducing stimulants to address coexisting ODD or CD at an early stage is highly beneficial. If a child with disruptive behavior disorder does not receive treatment for their aggressive behavior, they may gravitate towards others who also exhibit discipline issues. As they enter adolescence, they may reject treatment that could assist in changing their behavior, potentially causing them to be excluded by their peers. By this point, they may have become accustomed to their defiant nature and feel out of place when stimulants curb their reckless behavior. Treating these behaviors during elementary school or earlier can greatly reduce the chances of your child developing a negative self-image.

Your child's pediatrician may decide to reassess the situation and substitute other medications for the stimulant if your child has received treatment with two or more types of stimulants and his aggressive symptoms remain the same or worse. His pediatrician may continue to prescribe stimulants in combination with one of these other agents if the stimulant medication alone produced some but not enough improvement (National Institute of Mental Health, 1999; American Psychiatric Association. Diagnostic and Statistical Manual of Mental Disorders, 2000; National Institute of Mental Health, 2001).

4.7.6. Fears and Phobias

Fears are common as children develop and learn about the world around them, often encountering new situations and obstacles.

One common childhood fear is the fear of being alone in the dark. A fear of animals, like big barking dogs, is also included. Certain kids have a fear of thunderstorms, high places, and fires. Others worry about terrorism or war because they are aware of the images in the media. They might start worrying about the well-being of people around them if there has been a recent serious illness or death in the family.

The fears in your child may come and go. Most phobias in childhood are small. However, even when they worsen, they usually go away on their own with time, comfort, and support. However, there are instances when fears can turn into phobias because they are so intense, enduring, and narrowly focused.

Strong, illogical fears are known as phobias, and they can seriously disrupt a child's regular daily activities. For instance, a 6-year-old who has a dog phobia may become so anxious about potential dog encounters that they won't venture outside at all. A 10-year-old child may insist on spending the night with his parents due to fear stemming from news reports about a serial killer.

4.7.6.1. Social Phobias

Some kids get phobias related to the people they come into contact with on a daily basis. Their extreme shyness may prevent them from relating to most adults, especially strangers, and from forming friends at school. They might purposefully stay away from social events like club meetings, birthday celebrations, and sporting events. They might find it awkward to converse with anyone outside of their close family.

In children, separation anxiety is also prevalent. This anxiety can occasionally get worse when the family transfers to a new neighborhood or daycare. These kids might develop anxiety related to attending school or summer camp. They may experience physical symptoms from their phobias, such as headaches or stomachaches.

4.7.6.2. Treatment for Childhood Fears & Phobias

Thankfully, the majority of phobias are easily treated. If your child's anxiety keeps getting in the way of their enjoyment of life, they may benefit from seeing a child psychologist or psychiatrist who treats phobias.

4.7.6.3. Behavioral Therapy

- Many therapists recommend exposing your child to the source of their anxiety in small, non-threatening doses as part of a phobia treatment plan.
- A child who is afraid of dogs may start by talking about this fear and by watching pictures or videos of dogs, under the supervision of a therapist. After that, they might observe a neighborhood dog from the protection of a window. Then, they might spend a few minutes in the same room as a kind, amiable puppy with a parent or therapist by their side. They will eventually be able to stroke the dog. They will gradually become more comfortable around bigger, stranger dogs.
- This process, known as desensitization, involves your child becoming less sensitive to their fear each time they face it. Eventually, they will no longer feel the need to avoid the situation that triggers their phobia.
- Psychotherapy can occasionally aid in children's development of greater confidence and decreased fear. Children can benefit from breathing techniques and relaxation exercises when they are under stress.
- Phobias are treated initially with behavior therapy. Your child's doctor may suggest medication as part of the treatment plan in rare instances where behavioral therapy isn't providing enough assistance. This would serve as an additional therapeutic tool rather than behavioral therapy as the only one. Among these medications are antidepressants, which work to lessen the anxiety and panic that frequently accompany these issues (National Institute of Mental Health, 1999; American Psychiatric Association. Diagnostic and Statistical Manual of Mental Disorders, 2000; National Institute of Mental Health, 2001)

4.7.7. Fecal Soiling

Boys are more likely than girls to experience fecal soiling, which is referred to medically as encopresis in children over the age of four. It affects approximately 10.5% of young schoolchildren. Although less common than inadvertent urination or small leaks, it can cause greater distress for both parents and children. Not only is the smell more overpowering and unsettling, but in our culture, even two-year-olds are expected to "know better" than to sully their pants.

Fecal soiling, however, is typically not a choice; rather, it happens when a child resists having bowel movements due to emotional stress, resistance to toilet training, or physical pain. Constipation results from this resistance, or stool retention, and when the pressure builds up, it causes involuntary leakage or soiling. If this keeps happening, the child may find it more difficult to feel the urge to urinate because the muscles involved in ejecting stool may start to stretch and local nerve sensations may decrease. The intestines might become less able to contract, which would make bowel movements even more difficult and increase the likelihood of fecal soiling.

Most of the time, treating the underlying issue that is making your child resist a bowel movement is the best course of action when it comes to dealing with the problem of fecal soiling caused by constipation. If you support him while he defecates or lessens the pressure to use the potty, for example, he might stop holding onto his stool. Additionally, if his bowel movements become more regular, his fecal soiling may go away.

But make sure to schedule a visit with your child's pediatrician if the issue persists after one or two mishaps. He will look over your child's medical history to see if the soiling is due to a physical condition instead of stool retention. Accidental soiling can occasionally result from allergies, ulcerative colitis, congenital megacolon or Hirschsprung's disease (a congenital condition that prevents a child from feeling the sensation of having a full bowel), or even from a diet that contains an excessive amount of dairy products or high-fat foods.

Emotional or psychological causes should be taken into consideration if the physical causes have also been ruled out. Fecal soiling can happen when a child experiences anxiety or emotional distress related to an uncontrollable aspect of their life, like family disputes, academic setbacks, or social interaction issues. If soiling persists, it might also be necessary to take into account sexual and physical abuse.

Of course, it is not out of the question for any young child to experience an incident like this once or twice. Whatever the reason, your child needs to understand that he is not to blame for what happened and that you are aware of it as well.

Similar to bedwetting, the best course of action is to tidy up right away, try to minimize feelings of shame and embarrassment and give him the knowledge he needs to better regulate his bowel movements and maintain clean clothes. After ensuring that your child's feelings are safeguarded, you can move forward with determining the root cause, keeping in mind that a solution might not be available right away (National Institute of Mental Health, 1999; American Psychiatric Association. Diagnostic and Statistical Manual of Mental Disorders, 2000; National Institute of Mental Health, 2001).

A Closer Look

Agitation

Agitation is a common and distressing symptom characterized by a state of heightened arousal, restlessness, and emotional tension. It can manifest in various ways, ranging from pacing, fidgeting, and hand-wringing to verbal outbursts, aggression, and hostility. Agitation often accompanies underlying medical or psychiatric conditions and can significantly impair an individual's ability to function and interact with others.

Agitation can arise from a wide range of factors, including medical conditions, psychiatric disorders, substance use, environmental stressors, and medication side effects. Common medical causes include pain, infection, dehydration, metabolic imbalances, and neurological conditions such as dementia, traumatic brain injury, or stroke. Psychiatric disorders such as anxiety, depression, bipolar disorder, and psychosis may also present with agitation as a prominent symptom.

The symptoms of agitation can vary widely but often include physical restlessness, pacing, hand-wringing, or tapping. Individuals may exhibit verbal agitation through yelling, cursing, or screaming, or they may display aggressive behaviors such as hitting, pushing, or throwing objects. Emotional symptoms may include heightened irritability, anxiety, or fear, as well as emotional lability or mood swings. In severe cases, agitation can lead to self-injurious behaviors or harm to others.

Managing agitation requires a comprehensive approach tailored to the underlying cause and individual needs. Non-pharmacological interventions such as providing a calm and structured environment, reducing sensory stimuli, using distraction techniques, or engaging in therapeutic activities (e.g., music, and relaxation exercises) can help de-escalate agitation. Pharmacological interventions, including antipsychotic medications, benzodiazepines, or sedatives, may be necessary in cases of severe agitation or when non-pharmacological measures are ineffective or contraindicated. However, the use of medications should be carefully considered, weighing potential risks and benefits, and monitored closely to minimize adverse effects (National Institute of Mental Health, 1999; American Psychiatric Association. Diagnostic and Statistical Manual of Mental Disorders, 2000; National Institute of Mental Health, 2001).

Summary

- Mental illnesses are diseases or conditions that affect how you think, feel, act, or relate to other people or to your surroundings.
- Many people feel that mental illness is rare, something that only happens to people with life situations very different from their own, and that it will never affect them.
- Suicide is the third leading cause of death for 15- to 24-year-olds and the sixth leading cause of death for 5- to 15-year-olds.
- Schizophrenia is rare in children under age 12, but it occurs in about 3 of every 1,000 adolescents.
- Some of the predominant neurotransmitters in the brain include glutamate, GABA, serotonin, dopamine, and norepinephrine.
- PET measures the spatial distribution and movement of a radioactive chemical injected into the tissues of living subjects.
- Genetic, environmental, and social factors interact to influence whether someone becomes mentally ill.
- Medications are often used to treat mental illnesses. Through television commercials and magazine advertisements, we are becoming more aware of those medications.
- Depression is more than just being in a bad mood or feeling sad. Everyone experiences these feelings on occasion, but that does not constitute depression.
- Children and adolescents who are suicidal report feelings of depression, anger, anxiety, hopelessness, and worthlessness.
- Attention deficit hyperactivity disorder (ADHD) is the most commonly diagnosed behavioral disorder of childhood. In any six-month period, ADHD affects an estimated 4.1% of youths ages 9 to 17.
- Schizophrenia is not a multiple or split personality, nor are individuals who have this illness constantly incoherent or psychotic.

References

1. Agency for Healthcare Policy and Research. (1999). Treatment of depression—Newer pharmacotherapies. Summary, Evidence Report/Technology Assessment, Number 7. Retrieved from: http://www.ahcpr.gov/clinic/deprsumm.htm (accessed on 16 July 2024).
2. American Psychiatric Association. (2000). *Diagnostic and Statistical Manual of Mental Disorders, 4th Edition, Text Revision (DSM-IV-TR)*. Washington, DC: American Psychiatric Press.
3. Castellanos, F. X., Giedd, J. N., Berquin, P. C., Walter, J. M., Sharp, W., Tran, T., & Rapoport, J. L. (2001). Quantitative brain magnetic resonance imaging in girls with attention-deficit/hyperactivity disorder. *Archives of General Psychiatry, 58*, 289–295.
4. Castellanos, F. X., Giedd, J. N., Marsh, W. L., Hamburger, S. D., Vaituzis, A. C., Dickstein, D. P., & Rapoport, J. L. (1996). Quantitative brain magnetic resonance imaging in attention-deficit hyperactivity disorder. *Archives of General Psychiatry, 53*, 607–616.

5. Commission on Behavioral and Social Sciences Education, National Research Council. (2000). *How People Learn: Brain, Mind, Experience, and School*. Washington, DC: National Academies Press.
6. Corrigan, P., & Lundin, R. (2001). *Don't Call Me Nuts*. Tinley Park, IL: Recovery Press.
7. Egan, M. F., Goldberg, T. E., Koachana, B. S., Callicott, J. H., Mazzanti, C. M., Straub, R. E., & Weinberger, D. R. (2001). Effect of COMT Val 108/158 Met genotype on frontal lobe function and risk for schizophrenia. *Proceedings of the National Academy of Sciences USA, 98*, 6917–6922.
8. George, M. (1993). Depression PET scan. Retrieved from: http://www.nimh.nih.gov/hotsci/scandep.html (accessed on 16 July 2024).
9. Joint Committee on National Health Education Standards. (1995). *National Health Education Standards: Achieving Health Literacy*. Atlanta, GA: American Cancer Society.
10. Loucks-Horsley, S., Love, N., Hewson, P. W., & Stiles, K. E. (1998). *Designing Professional Development for Teachers of Science and Mathematics*. Thousand Oaks, CA: Corwin Press.
11. National Institute of Mental Health. (1996). Attention deficit hyperactivity disorder. Retrieved from: http://www.nimh.nih.gov/publicat/adhd.cfm (accessed on 16 July 2024).
12. National Institute of Mental Health. (1999a). Schizophrenia. Retrieved from: http://www.nimh.nih.gov/publicat/schizoph.cfm (accessed on 16 July 2024).
13. National Institute of Mental Health. (1999b). Archival record—Early recognition and treatment of schizophrenia and bipolar disorder in children and adolescents.
14. National Institute of Mental Health. (2000a). Depression in children and adolescents: A fact sheet for physicians.
15. National Institute of Mental Health. (2000b). Depression. Retrieved from: http://www.nimh.nih.gov/publicat/depression.cfm (accessed on 16 July 2024).
16. National Institute of Mental Health. (2000c). NIMH research on treatment for attention deficit hyperactivity disorder (ADHD): The multimodal treatment study—Questions and answers.
17. National Institute of Mental Health. (2001a). The numbers count: Mental disorders in America.
18. National Institute of Mental Health. (2001b). The impact of mental illness on society.
19. National Institute of Mental Health. (2001c). Depression research at the national institute of mental health.
20. National Institute of Mental Health. (2001d). The invisible disease: Depression.
21. National Institute of Mental Health. (2001e). Bipolar disorder. Retrieved from: http://www.nimh.nih.gov/publicat/bipolar.cfm (accessed on 16 July 2024).
22. National Institute of Mental Health. (2001f). Attention deficit hyperactivity disorder.
23. National Institutes of Health. (1998). Diagnosis and treatment of attention deficit hyperactivity disorder. NIH consensus statement.
24. National Mental Health Association. (2001). Depression survey reveals dramatic changes in public opinion: Disease or state of mind?
25. National Research Council. (1996). *National Science Education Standards*. Washington, DC: National Academies Press.

26. Pearlson, G. D. (2000). Neurobiology of schizophrenia. *Annals of Neurology, 48*, 556–566.

27. Pfizer Inc. (2000). Mental illness stigma and bias assailed at historic White House conference. *Pfizer Views*, Making News. Retrieved from: http://www.viewsmakingnews.com/policy/mental_health.shtml (accessed on 16 July 2024).

28. Rapoport, J. L., Castellanos, F. X., Gogate, N., Janson, K., Kohler, S., & Nelson, P. (2001). Imaging normal and abnormal brain development: New perspectives for child psychiatry. *Australian and New Zealand Journal of Psychiatry, 35*, 272–281.

29. Rapoport, J. L., Giedd, J., Kumra, S., Jacobsen, L., Smith, A., Lee, P., Nelson, J., & Hamburger, S. (1997). Childhood-onset schizophrenia. Progressive ventricular change during adolescence. *Archives of General Psychiatry, 54*, 897–903.

30. Ratey, J. (1998). An update on medications used in the treatment of attention deficit disorder. *FOCUS Archives, National Attention Deficit Disorder Association*.

31. Sowell, E. R., Toga, A. W., & Asarnow, R. (2000). Brain abnormalities observed in childhood-onset schizophrenia: A review of the structural magnetic resonance imaging literature. *Mental Retardation and Developmental Disabilities Research Reviews, 6*, 180–185.

32. Stoll, A. L., Renshaw, P. F., Yurgelun-Todd, D. A., & Cohen, B. M. (2000). Neuroimaging in bipolar disorder: What have we learned? *Biological Psychiatry, 15*, 505–517.

33. Thompson, P. M., Vidal, C., Giedd, J. N., Gochman, P., Blumenthal, J., Nicolson, R., Toga, A. W., & Rapoport, J. L. (2001). Mapping adolescent brain change reveals dynamic wave of accelerated gray matter loss in very early-onset schizophrenia. *Proceedings of the National Academy of Sciences USA, 98*, 11650–11655.

34. U.S. Department of Health and Human Services. (2000). Mental health: A report of the surgeon general.

35. U.S. Public Health Service. (2000). Report of the surgeon general's conference on children's mental health: A national action agenda. Retrieved from: http://www.surgeongeneral.gov/cmh/childreport.htm (accessed on 16 July 2024).

36. Veggeberg, S. K. (1997). The big story in depression: What isn't happening. *Brainwork—The Neuroscience Newsletter*.

37. Yatham, L. N., Liddle, P. F., Shiah, I. S., Scarrow, G., Lam, R. W., Adam, M. J., Zis, A. P., & Ruth, T. J. (2000). Brain serotonin2 receptors in major depression: A positron emission tomography study. *Archives of General Psychiatry, 57*, 850–858.

Chapter

5

SYMPTOMS OF FEMALE REPRODUCTIVE HEALTH PROBLEMS

Contents

Introduction

The state of the male and female reproductive systems at every stage of life is referred to as reproductive health. Organs and hormone-producing glands, such as the pituitary gland in the brain, comprise these systems. The reproductive organs, or gonads, of males and females, respectively, are the testicles and ovaries, which keep their respective systems healthy. Because they make and release hormones, they also serve as glands.

Many illnesses, including cancer, uterine fibroids, endometriosis, ovarian cysts, infertility, sexually transmitted diseases (STDs), and more, can have an impact on a woman's reproductive system.

Symptoms of female reproductive and hormonal health problems include:

1. Bleeding or spotting between periods
2. Itching, burning, or irritation (including bumps, blisters, or sores) of the vagina or genital area
3. Pain or discomfort during sex
4. Excessively heavy bleeding or severe pain with periods
5. Severe pelvic/abdominal pain
6. A change in vaginal discharge (amount, color or odor)
7. Feeling of fullness in the lower abdomen
8. Frequent urination or feeling of urgency to urinate
9. Lower back pain
10. Pelvic Pain
11. Known reproductive problems such as infertility, past miscarriages or early labor
12. Excessive hair growth on the face, chest, stomach, thumbs, or toes
13. Baldness or thinning hair
14. Acne, oily skin, or dandruff
15. Patches of thickened dark brown or black skin

Orientation and Directional Terms

Term	Definition	Illustration
Adenomyosis	Adenomyosis is a gynecological condition that occurs when the lining of the uterus grows into the muscular wall of the uterus. This can cause the uterus to thicken and enlarge, which can lead to heavy menstrual bleeding.	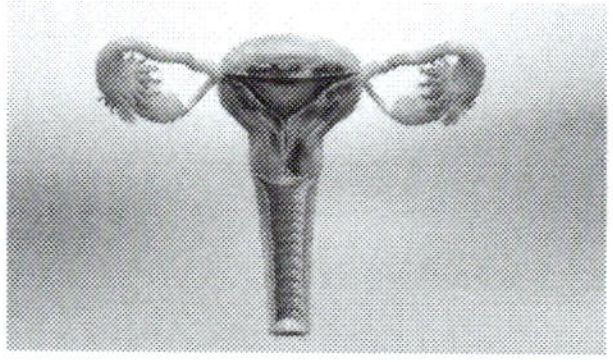
Dysmenorrhea	Dysmenorrhea is moderate to severe pain that occurs during menstruation. It usually starts when menstruation begins and lasts for less than three days.	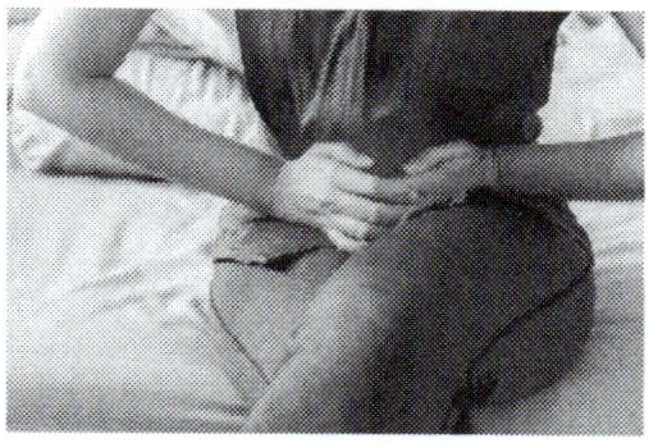
Dyspareunia	Dyspareunia is the medical term for painful sexual intercourse that can be caused by medical or psychological factors. It can be felt before, during, or after sex, and can be internal or external.	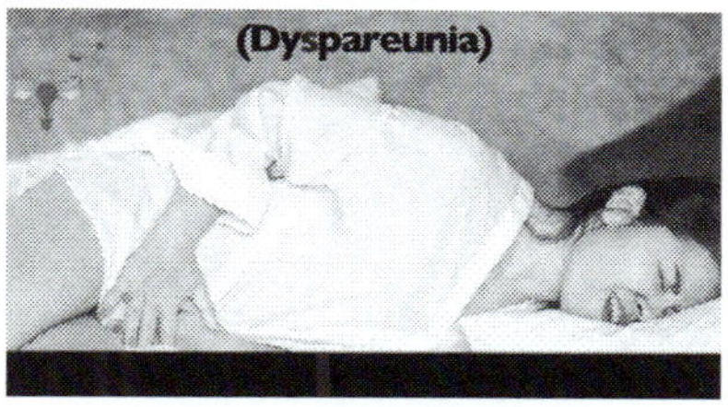
Infertility	Infertility is defined as the inability to get pregnant after one year or more of unprotected sex. The most common cause of infertility in women is problems with ovulation, which occurs in 40% of women with infertility issues.	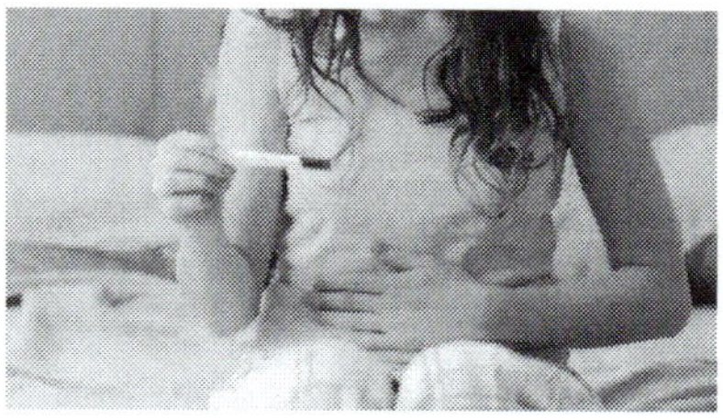
Pelvic pain	Pelvic Pain Is Often Due To Conditions That Affect The Reproductive System, Such As Endometriosis, Fibroids, Or An Ectopic Pregnancy.	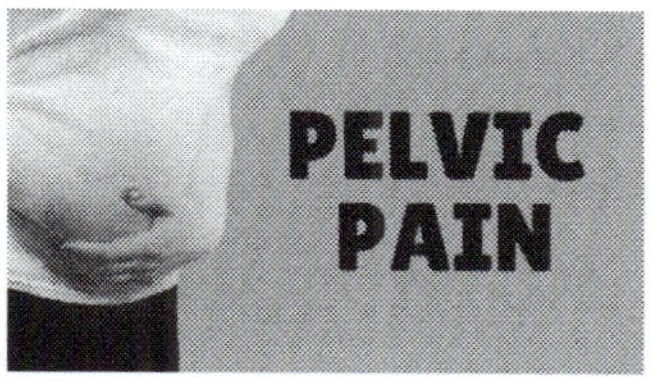
Uterine fibroids	Uterine fibroids are non-cancerous muscle tumors that grow in or around the uterus. They can range in size from microscopic to melon-sized and can affect up to half of all women by age 50.	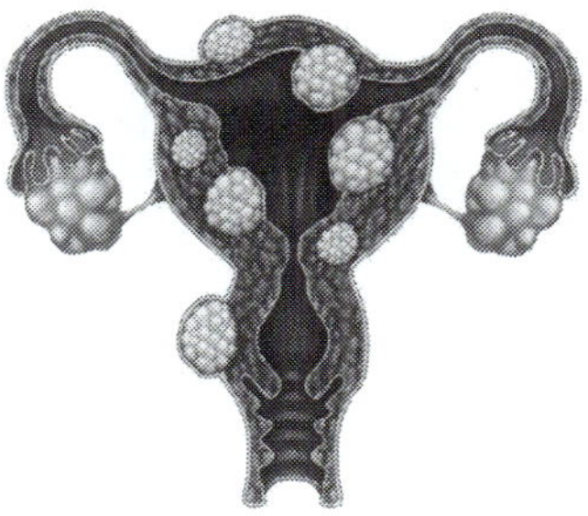

5.1. Endometriosis

A long-term, benign condition called endometriosis is defined by the growth and presence of endometrial tissue outside of the uterus. Although endometrial tissue can also be found outside of the pelvis, the pelvic cavity is the primary site of endometriosis, with the ovary being the most frequently affected organ. The illness typically affects women during their reproductive years and has an impact on both fertility and quality of life.

5.1.1. Epidemiology and Risk Factors

Because the clinical presentation of endometriosis varies and surgery is usually required for a definitive diagnosis, it is challenging to determine the prevalence of the condition. It is thought to impact roughly 6–10% of women, but the prevalence is higher (35–50%) among those who are in pain, infertile, or both. The underdiagnosis of endometriosis is linked to a 4–11-year delay from the onset of symptoms to diagnosis. Prolonged exposure to endogenous estrogen is the primary risk factor. Conditions with high proliferative stimulus on the endometrium include nulliparity, early age at menarche, late menopause, shorter menstrual cycles, and heavy menstrual bleeding. Conversely, prolonged lactation, late menarche, and multiple pregnancies are protective.

Affected women's first-degree relatives have a three- to nine-fold increased risk of getting the illness. Studies on twins and families point to a genetic component. About half of the variation in endometriosis risk is due to genetic factors, with a 51% hereditability estimate.

Women with endometriosis have been found to have polymorphisms in genes related to immunomodulatory proteins, cytokines, estrogen receptors, attachment and invasion factors, and detoxification processes.

Since a higher prevalence has been reported in Asian and Caucasian women compared to Black and Hispanic women, race may also play a role. The remaining primary risk factors include blockage of menstrual flow (e.g., Mullerian anomalies), pigmentary characteristics, sun exposure patterns, alcohol consumption, and environmental variables (e.g., exposure to dioxin and polychlorinated biphenyls). Numerous pathogenic mechanisms linked to endometriosis, including inflammation, estrogen activity, menstrual cyclicity, and prostaglandin metabolism, can be influenced by diet; however, there is conflicting information on the potential protective value of fruits and vegetables as well as the negative effects of dairy, red meat, and unsaturated fats. Exercise appears to lower the risk of endometriosis, most likely because it has anti-inflammatory properties.

The risk of endometrioid and clear cell subtypes of ovarian cancer is 2 to 3 times higher in women who have endometriosis. Further research is required to confirm the association between endometriosis and other cancers, including thyroid, kidney, brain, endocrine, and cutaneous melanoma.

5.1.2. Pathophysiology

There is currently no known cause of endometriosis, and no one theory can account for every case of the condition. The most widely accepted theories state that retrograde menstruation, blood and lymphatic dissemination, and the metaplasia of celomic epithelium and stem cells are the sources of endometriotic cell establishment.

The idea of retrograde menstruation, which was put forth by Sampson in the 1920s, affirms that endometrial fragments move through fallopian tubes during the menstrual cycle. Roughly 90% of healthy women experience this phenomenon; however, only a small percentage of them have endometriosis, indicating the possibility of other contributing factors like immunologic abnormalities, uterine hyperperistalsis, and genetic defects. Studies showing a higher prevalence of endometriosis in women with uterine abnormalities that impede the menstrual flow, such as uterine septum and cervical stenosis, provide additional evidence for this etiology. Moreover, endometrial cells can spread from the endometrium via blood or lymphatic circulation, just like tumor cells do. The most compelling evidence for this theory comes from reports of endometriotic lesions in the brain, lung, and bone that have been histologically proven to occur in locations other than the uterus. Since both peritoneal and endometrial cells originate from the celomatic wall's epithelium, Meyer (1919) postulated that endometriosis might arise from the metaplastic transformation of peritoneal cells.

A more recent theory proposes that endometrial cells can be transformed from hematopoietic, bone marrow, or mesenchymal stem cells. It has also been suggested that endometrial stem cells may play a part. During menstruation, endometrial-derived stem/progenitor cells that are found in the basalis layer and are in charge of the tissue's ability to regenerate can shed through the fallopian tube into the peritoneal cavity and form endometriotic implants (Figure 5.1).

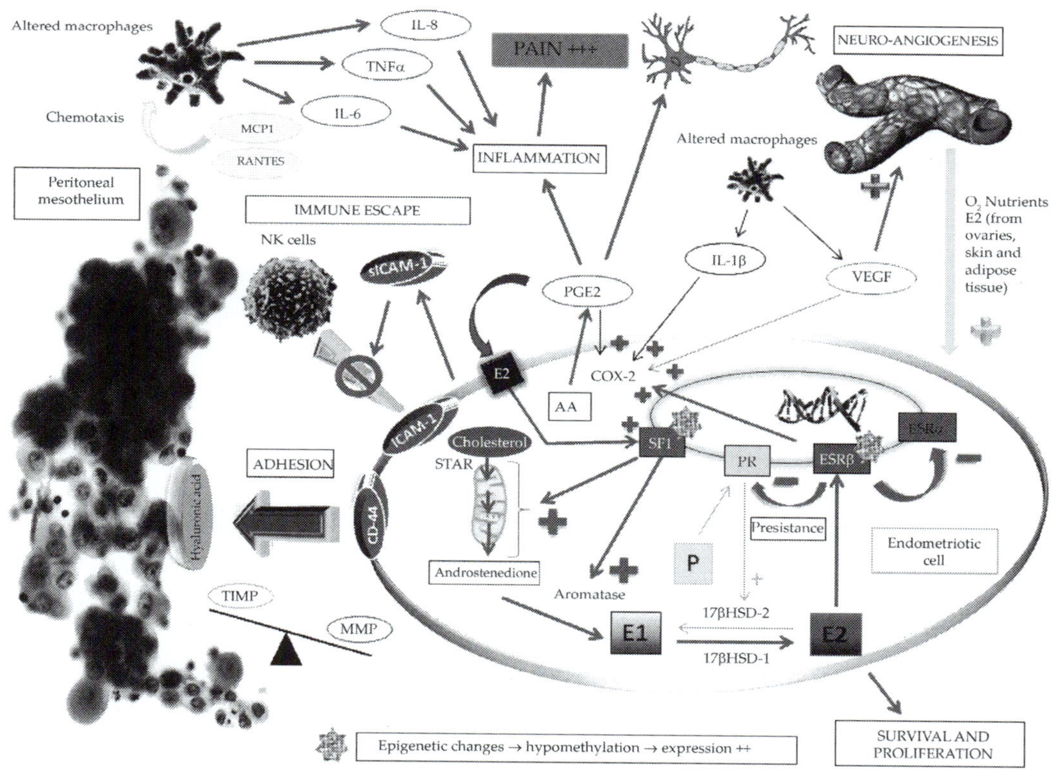

Figure 5.1. *Main pathogenetic theories of endometriosis.*

Source: Monnin N, Fattet AJ, & Koscinski I. (2023). Endometriosis: Update of pathophysiology, (Epi) genetic and environmental involvement. Biomedicines, 11(3), 978. https://doi.org/10.3390/biomedicines11030978.

5.2.1.1. Immune Dysfunction and Inflammation

The formation of a local immune response in the peritoneal cavity against endometrial cells is greatly aided by the immune system. Normally, immune cells like lymphocytes, natural killer (NK) cells, and macrophages remove refluxed endometrial cells from the peritoneum. Reduced clearance of refluxed endometrial cells is caused by impaired cellular and humoral immunity, which has been documented in endometriotic tissue. The higher incidence of autoimmune disorders in endometriosis patients lends credence to the theory that an altered immune response contributes to the pathogenesis of the disease. Natural killer cells, macrophages, neutrophils, humoral immunity, cytokines, and growth factors are the primary immune changes. Growth factors and cytokines appear to facilitate ectopic endometrial invasion, implantation, and growth (proliferating and angiogenesis). Tumor necrosis factor-α (TNF-α), RANTES (regulated on activation, normal T-cell expressed and secreted), IL-1, IL-6, IL-8, monocyte chemotactic protein-1 (MCP-1), and vascular endothelial growth factor are the primary factors involved (VEGF).

Overproduction of prostaglandins, cytokines, chemokines, and growth factors is linked to inflammation. High concentrations of these inflammatory mediators likely facilitate the attachment of fragments of endometrial tissue to the peritoneal surface; proteolytic membrane metalloproteinases (MMP-2, MMP-3, MMP-7, and MMP-9), which are elevated in endometriosis, may then facilitate the fragments' implantation.

The onset and progression are significantly influenced by oxidative stress: reactive oxygen species (ROS) trigger the synthesis of some disintegrin and metalloproteases (ADAM) family metallopeptidases, including ADAM 17. This results in the proteolytic release of the active form of Notch proteins and their transport to the nucleus, where they activate the transcription of genes linked to fibrosis. Endometriosis is typified by an increase in fibrosis as a result of ADAM17/Notch signaling.

In endometriosis, apoptosis is also modified to promote the survival and regrowth of ectopic tissue. Additionally, because the peritoneal environment is less vascularized than the endometrial eutopic tissue, neoangiogenesis is required for the formation and maintenance of endometriotic lesions. The presence of VEGF, which has been found in high concentrations in the peritoneal fluid of endometriosis-affected women, appears to be crucial to this process. Neoangiogenesis and neuroangiogenesis are closely associated: it has been shown that factors that promote innervation, such as nerve growth factor (NGF), are overexpressed in neoangiogenesis.

Along with inflammation, neoangiogenesis and neuroangiogenesis play a role in the pathophysiology of pain related to this disorder.

5.2.1.2. Hormonal Influences

Progesterone resistance and increased estrogen sensitivity are two of the primary pathogenetic events of endometriosis. The aromatase and 17β17β-hydroxysteroid dehydrogenases are expressed in endometriotic implants. Androstenedione is converted into estrone and estrone into estradiol by 17β-HSD type 1. Rather than expressing 17β-HSD type 2, which inactivates estrogens, endometriosis cells do not. This combination enables a high local concentration of bioavailable estrogens to be exposed to the implants. A positive feedback mechanism between the production of estrogen and inflammation is established when there is an excess of local estradiol, which leads to the proliferation of lesions and stimulates the production of prostaglandin E_2.

Progesterone resistance is another feature of endometriosis, in addition to estrogen dependence. When compared to eutopic endometrium, endometriotic implants show a reduction in progesterone receptors overall and an absence of progesterone receptor-B (Figure 5.2).

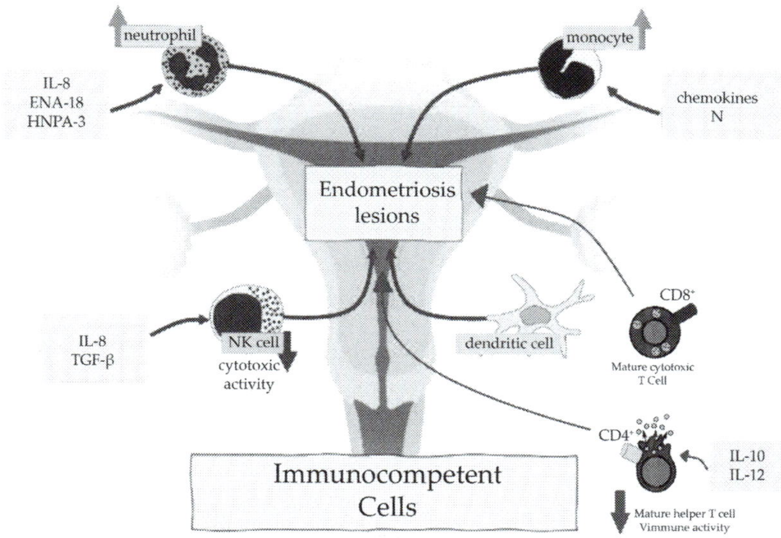

Figure 5.2. Pathogenetic mediators of endometriosis.

Source: Lamceva J, Uljanovs R, & Strumfa I. (2023). The main theories on the pathogenesis of endometriosis. International Journal of Molecular Sciences, 24(5), 4254. https://doi.org/10.3390/ijms24054254.

5.2.1.3. Anatomic Sites

Anywhere, including the pelvic and extrapelvic regions, can develop endometriosis. In over half of the cases, the ovaries are bilaterally involved and the most affected organ is the left one.

The hallmark of ovarian endometriosis is the presence of cysts, or endometriomas, or OMAs, ranging in size from 5 mm to 15 cm and surrounded by duplicated ovarian parenchyma. The inside of the cyst is lined with endometrium and contains a dark substance that is filled with hemosiderin-containing blood and histiocytes. It is believed that endometrioma originates from an ovarian cortex invagination at the location of the ovary's initial adhesion to the peritoneum.

The formation of menstrual debris from the superficial ovarian implants of endometriosis, which line the inside of the cyst as a result of the invagination, or the metaplastic transformation of the invaginated mesothelium of the ovarian cortex, which transforms into mature endometrial cells, could be the cause of the accumulation of chocolate fluid inside the cyst.

Deep infiltrating endometriosis (DIE) often involves the uterosacral ligaments, fossa ovarica, anterior and posterior cul-de-sac, and posterior broad ligament. The cervix, bladder, rectovaginal septum, and vagina are among the other, less common sites. Although cases of endometriosis of the gastrointestinal tract, urinary tract, upper, and lower respiratory systems, diaphragm, pleura, pericardium, brain, and abdominal scars are uncommon, extrapelvic endometriosis is not.

The most common extrapelvic location is the thoracic involvement, which can result in catamenial pneumothorax because of pleural endometrial tissue bleeding during the menstrual cycle. Extrapelvic endometriosis is difficult to diagnose and should be suspected in women who have period-related symptoms due to its wide range of clinical expression and symptoms that resemble those of other pathological conditions (de Ziegler et al., 2010; Ahn et al., 2015; Clemenza et al., 2018; Agarwal et al., 2019).

5.1.3. Classification of Endometriosis

Endometriosis classification remains controversial, with no single system being able to adequately classify the disease—often because research has focused on only one aspect of it—such as anatomy, histology, surgery, and fertility. The following is a list of the most popular classifications:

- The current most used classification in clinical practice divides endometriosis into three categories: superficial or peritoneal (SUP), characterized by the presence of implants located on the surface of the peritoneum, ovarian (OMA) and deep endometriosis (DIE) (lesions infiltrating deeper than 5 mm under the peritoneum).
- American Fertility Society (AFS) classification: created in 1979, revised in 1985 as rAFS and modified in 1996 as revised American Society for Reproductive Medicine (rASRM) score, it is the classification most widely established throughout the world. It was a point-scoring system, based on laparoscopic findings. Depending on the number, location, and size of the endometriotic lesions, the disease was classified in four stages: mild, moderate, severe, and extensive (Revised American Fertility Society Classification of Endometriosis 1985). Although widely used, this system has not been demonstrated to be related to symptoms frequency and severity or reproductive prognosis.
- Adamyan classification concerns retrocervical location of endometriosis: stage I indicates retrocervical endometriosis with no vaginal involvement, stage II involves vagina, stage III involves vagina and rectum with cul-de-sac distortion, and stage IV includes cul-de-sac obliteration.
- Chapron classification (2003) describes deep infiltrating endometriosis (DIE), subdividing it into anterior and posterior compartments for better surgical management.
- Enzian classification can be used for deep endometriosis. Retroperitoneal structures are divided into compartment A (rectovaginal septum and vagina), compartment B (sacrouterine ligament to the pelvic wall), and compartment C (rectum and sigmoid colon) and F (retroperitoneal distant locations). The severity of the disease is defined for all the compartments by the invasion: grade 1 invasion<1 cm, grade 2 invasion 1–3 cm, and grade 3 invasion >3 cm.
- Koninckx et al. created a classification based on type (subtle, typical, cystic, deep) and size of lesions.

5.1.4. Symptoms and Clinical Manifestations of Endometriosis

Endometriosis is a disease characterized by the growth of tissue outside the uterus that resembles the lining of the uterus and causes pain, bloating, infertility, and other symptoms. Endometriosis patients may experience crippling symptoms that interfere with daily living, or they may not experience any symptoms at all.

Endometriosis symptoms often include:

- Pain, during menstrual periods but also all month long
- Abnormal, heavy, or irregular bleeding
- Abdominal, pelvic, leg, and back pain
- Pelvic heaviness
- Pain during sex (dyspareunia)
- Infertility
- Bloating (referred to as "endo belly")
- Fatigue
- Constipation or diarrhea
- Pain during bowel movements (dyschezia)
- Pain during urination (dysuria)
- Chest pain and shortness of breath

5.1.4.1. Pain

The most typical endometriosis symptom is pain. But not every endometriosis sufferer feels pain in the same way.

Pain associated with endometriosis can be felt in many different places, such as the back, hips, legs, pelvis, and more. In addition, a variety of triggers, including sex, urination, bowel movements, menstruation, and more, can cause pain.

Everybody experiences endometriosis pain differently. While some people may experience pain on a regular basis, others may not.

Pain from endometriosis varies in intensity as well. While some people only feel slight discomfort, others suffer from incapacitating pain.

Endometriosis symptoms can range from mild to extremely incapacitating. As a result, a large number of patients have no symptoms at all, and endometriotic lesions are unintentionally discovered during surgery for unrelated purposes. The most typical symptoms include dysmenorrhea, dyspareunia, back pain, and persistent pelvic pain, but painful defecation and urinary disorders can also arise.

Different clinical manifestations may indicate different lesions in different locations. For instance, dyspareunia with peritoneal or deeply infiltrating endometriosis, painful defecation with posterior cul-de-sac and rectovaginal septum implants, and urinary symptoms with bladder endometriosis are frequently associated with severe dysmenorrhea. Bowel endometriosis can cause cramping in the intestines, diarrhea, constipation, and dyschezia.

Although the exact cause of pain is still unknown, it most likely has multiple origins. The main mechanisms that appear to be involved are inflammation, neurogenesis, and adhesions.

Hyperalgesia, or an unusually high perception of pain concerning the stimulus experienced, is a common symptom of endometriosis. This phenomenon may be attributed to the direct infiltration of endometriotic stromal cells into the peripheral nerves as well as the local activation of nerve fibers by neurogenic factors. Women with endometriosis have increased levels of neuroendocrine (NE) cells in their eutopic endometrium; the strong synaptophysin (SYN) expression may stimulate nociceptors and nerve fibers, causing pain signals.

Pain symptoms may also be exacerbated by adhesions that are the result of the disease or prior surgery.

Even though the aforementioned mechanisms contribute to endometriosis's clinical manifestation, more research is required to completely comprehend the cause of pain in these patients.

5.1.4.2. Painful Sex, Irregular Bleeding, Infertility

To understand the effects of endometriosis on people's lives, one study conducted interviews with 35 individuals who had the disease and looked at their answers. Persistent pain was not the most common symptom of endometriosis; infertility, painful sex, and irregular bleeding were.

Infertility affects about one-third of endometriosis-affected women. The question of whether these patients have a lower ovarian reserve is debatable because some researchers have discovered low levels of anti-mullerian hormone (AMH) in the blood. Multifactorial genesis also contributes to infertility.

5.1.4.3. Endo Belly

Painful abdominal bloating and distention (stretching), also known as "endo belly," is another typical endometriosis symptom.

This symptom was once dismissed as having nothing to do with endometriosis. Nonetheless, studies show that it is among the most prevalent endometriosis symptoms. The symptom profile gets more accurate as more endometriosis patients speak out for themselves and as scientists gain more understanding of the condition.

5.1.4.4. Inflammation and Immune Factor

The function of peritoneal fluid (PF) in fertility is significant and intricate. Increased levels of cytokines, interleukins, and reactive oxygen species (ROS) are present in the PF of endometriosis patients, which can lower fertility through a variety of mechanisms. Specifically, sperm cell motility is affected by IL-1 and IL-6, and their motility is reduced by macrophage migration inhibitory factor; sperm cellular DNA may be harmed by TNF-α; sperm binding to the zona pellucida is reduced by TNF-α, RANTES, and macrophage migration inhibitory factor; and sperm migration inhibitory factor and IL-6 may prevent capacitation. The endometrium produces the neuropeptides urocortin and CRH, which are involved in the inflammatory and reproductive processes of endometrial decidualization. Specifically, CRH through CRH receptor type 1 (CRH-R1, antalarmin) increases IL-1 and IL-6 production and interacts with prostaglandins during the decidualization process, potentially starting local inflammation events, vascular permeability, extracellular matrix remodeling, inflammatory factor secretion, and implantation site facilitation. A disturbed local CRH/Ucn/CRH-R1 pathway may also account for the decreased fertility that endometriosis patients exhibit. Women with endometriosis exhibit abnormal expression of CRH and Ucn during the menstrual cycle, a decreased response to CRH and Ucn, and impaired expression of CRH-R1 mRNA in their endometrium.

5.1.4.5. Mechanical Factor

In cases where the fallopian tubes are involved, fibrosis and adhesions resulting from prior surgical interventions as well as the pathology itself may play a mechanical role in accomplishing the goal of pregnancy.

5.1.4.6. Iatrogenic Factor

It is important to recognize the potential for iatrogenic damage to occur at the ovarian level after surgical procedures, particularly when repeated and bilateral procedures are performed.

5.1.5. Diagnosis of Endometriosis

When endometriosis is discovered four to eleven years after symptoms first appear, it is frequently misdiagnosed. Delays in diagnosis can lead to adhesion formation and disease progression, which can worsen chronic pelvic pain and potentially impair fertility.

Although a laparoscopy and histological confirmation are necessary for a conclusive diagnosis, the diagnosis of endometriosis is based on the patient's medical history, symptoms, signs, physical examination, and imaging techniques.

5.1.5.1. Clinical History

Every woman who has endometriosis suspicions should have a thorough clinical history taken. Investigating the following factors in particular is crucial: age, parity, endometriosis in the family history, bleeding patterns, infertility, pain (dysmenorrhea, dyspareunia, dysuria, dyschezia, and chronic pelvic pain), hematuria and/or hematochezia, and past endometriosis treatments.

5.1.5.2. Pelvic Examination

High-accuracy physical examinations are used to diagnose endometriosis. Bimanual exploration makes it possible to identify palpable nodules, stiffened and/or thickened pelvic anatomy, particularly in the uterosacral ligaments, vagina, rectovaginal space, pouch of Douglas, adnexa, rectosigmoid, or posterior wall of the bladder, as well as ovarian masses suggestive of endometriomas. A speculum examination should be part of the pelvic exam to look for any evidence of powderburn lesions on the cervix or the posterior fornix of the vagina.

5.1.5.3. Ultrasound Examination

The initial imaging method used to diagnose and monitor endometriosis is transvaginal ultrasonography. A round or ovoid unilocular cystic formation with thick, regular walls and homogenous hypoechoic content—also referred to as "ground glass"—without papillary projection, poor peripheral vascularization, and no central vascularization is the typical appearance of an endometrioma.

Other endometriotic lesions, such as adhesions and infiltrating endometrial nodules affecting the anterior, lateral, and posterior pelvic compartments, can also be identified and described using transvaginal ultrasound.

By applying pressure to the posterior fornix with the vaginal probe and causing the uterus to slide anteriorly with respect to the intestinal wall, the sliding signing maneuver can detect adherent syndrome and the obliteration of the Douglas pouch.

Transrectal ultrasonography can be used on virgin women in place of transvaginal ultrasound.

Table 5.1. Revised ASRM Classification of Endometriosis

Table for calculating American Society for Reproductive Medicine revised classification of endometriosis

Patient's name ____________________ Date ____________

Stage 1 (minimal) ________ 1 to 5 Laparoscopy ________

Stage II (mild) ________ 6 to 15 Laparotomy ________

Stage III (moderate) ________ 16 to 40 Photography ________

Stage IV (severe) ________ >40 Recommended treatment ________

Total ________ Prognosis ________

Peritoneum	Endometriosis	<1 cm	1 to 3 cm	>3 cm
	Superficial	1	2	4
	Deep	2	4	6
Ovary	R superficial	1	2	4
	Deep	4	16	20
	L superficial	1	2	4
	Deep	4	16	20
	Posterior cul-de-sac obliteration	Partial		Complete
		4		40
Ovary	Adhesions	<1/3 enclosure	1/3 to 2/3 enclosure	>2/3 enclosure
	R filmy	1	2	4
	Dense	4	8	16
	L filmy	1	2	4
	Dense	4	8	16
Tube	R filmy	1	2	4
	Dense	4*	8*	16
	L filmy	1	2	4
	Dense	4*	8*	16

Source: Sharma, S., & Tripathi, A. (2022). Endometriosis: The Enigma That It Continues to Be. IntechOpen. doi: 10.5772/intechopen.108774.

5.1.5.4. Magnetic Resonance Imaging

When endometriosis is suspected, magnetic resonance imaging is a noninvasive investigative technique. Because of its high cost, low sensitivity, and limited availability, magnetic resonance imaging (MRI) ought to be used as a backup method for diagnosing pelvic endometriosis, following ultrasonography, and prior to surgery for the best possible preoperative staging.

Depending on the age of the bleeding, endometriosis foci show varying signal intensities on T2- and T1-weighted images. While fibrotic endometrial lesions show relatively low signal intensity on both T1- and T2-weighted images, subacute bleeding may result in very high signal intensity on T1-weighted images and relatively low signal intensity on T2-weighted images.

5.1.6. Differential Diagnosis of Endometriosis (Figure 5.3)

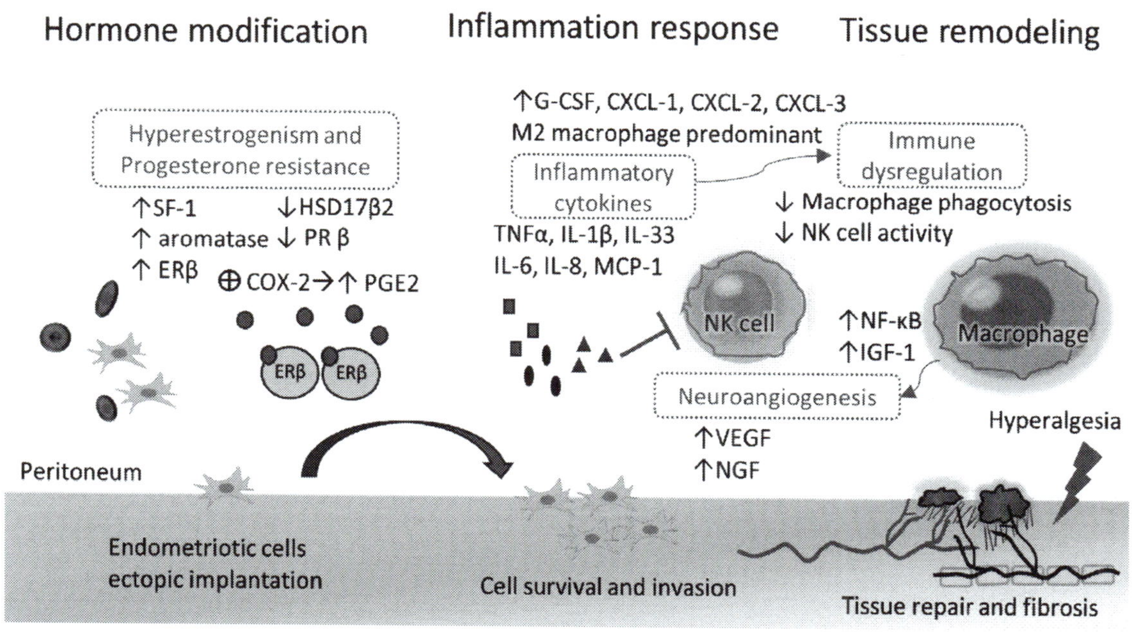

Figure 5.3. *Mechanisms of endometriosis.*

Source: Chen L-H, Lo W-C, Huang H-Y, & Wu H-M. (2023). A lifelong impact on endometriosis: Pathophysiology and pharmacological treatment. International Journal of Molecular Sciences, 24(8), 7503. https://doi.org/10.3390/ijms24087503.

5.1.7. Treatment of Endometriosis

Endometriosis necessitates long-term management because it is a chronic and progressive disease. It is crucial to take into account each patient's unique characteristics when determining the best course of action, especially with regard to their age and desire for children. Endometriosis can be treated medically or surgically, but there is no cure because the condition frequently returns. The objectives of therapy include managing pain, enhancing fertility, making the most use of medical interventions, and avoiding recurrent surgeries (Figure 5.4).

5.1.7.1. Medical Treatment of Endometriosis

- **Nonsteroidal Anti-inflammatory Drugs:** NSAIDs block the action of COX-1 and COX-2 enzymes, which prevents arachidonic acid from being converted to prostaglandins, which are the starting point for pain related to endometriosis. When it comes to treating women's pain brought on by primary dysmenorrhea, NSAIDs seem to be the only treatment option that doesn't interfere with fertility preservation. Women who use NSAIDs, however, should be aware that these medications can have unforeseen side effects, particularly in the nervous, cardiovascular, and gastrointestinal systems.
- **Progestins:** When algic symptoms are present, monotherapy with progestins ought to be the first line of treatment. Progestins have anti-inflammatory and proapoptotic effects, causing atrophy of the eutopic and ectopic endometrium. In two-thirds of patients, their use is linked to improved pain and quality of life; in the remaining one-third, progesterone resistance may result in nonresponse. Consequently, the likelihood of a postoperative endometrioma recurrence is decreased by these substances. Progestins can be given intrauterine, subcutaneously, intramuscularly, or orally.

The use of two 19-nortestosterone derivatives, dienogest and norethisterone acetate (NETA), at oral doses of 2 mg and 5.0 mg per day, respectively, is supported by evidence. While dienogest is antiandrogenic, NETA exhibits androgenic activity in addition to its stronger progestogenic effects. An alternate course of treatment might involve 150 mg intramuscular injections of medroxyprogesterone acetate (DMPA) every three to six months. Women who cannot tolerate systemic progestins should give special consideration to the levonorgestrel intrauterine system.

- **Danazol:** Danazol, a 17α-ethynyl testosterone derivative, has potent anti-estrogenic properties and inhibits gonadotropin release. Although it works well to treat pain associated with endometriosis, its use is restricted by androgenic side effects like weight gain, seborrhea, hypertrichosis, and an increase in low-density lipoprotein (LDL) levels. When used vaginally, danazol 200 mg per day has been shown to have good efficacy and tolerability.
- **Gonadotropin-Releasing Hormone (GnRH) Agonists:** Progestins and estrogen-progestins, such as goserelin, leuprolide, naparelin, buserelin, and triptorelin, are useful in the treatment of pain. These substances attach to GnRH receptors, which at first stimulate the pituitary gland and encourage the release of hormones. Prolonged and continuous exposure to these substances leads to hypoestrogenism and downregulation of the pituitary-ovarian axis. Significant side effects such as osteopenia, vaginal dryness, and hot flushes are caused by the hypoestrogenic state. In fact, because GnRH agonists may have detrimental effects on bone growth, adolescents should refrain from using them.

These side effects are lessened when estro-progestins are added to add-back therapy, usually in combination with norethindrone, without compromising the effectiveness of pain relief.

Only a maximum of six months of continuous use of GnRH agonists is authorized; however, add-back therapy may allow for longer usage.

- **GnRH Antagonist:** These substances have the advantage over GnRH agonists in that they block the GnRH receptor right away without first stimulating the hypothalamic-pituitary-gonadal axis (flare up). The FDA recently approved Elagolix, an oral GnRH antagonist, for the treatment of endometriosis.
- **Aromatase Inhibitors:** Aromatase catalyzes the conversion of testosterone and androstenedione to estradiol and estrone, respectively. It is present in endometriotic lesions and the eutopic endometrium of women with endometriosis. Aromatase inhibitors (AIs) cause hypoestrogenism by preventing the ovaries and the periphery from producing estrogen, so their use needs to be accompanied by add-back therapy. Off-label use of AIs is recommended, particularly for women who are refractory to other medical or surgical treatments due to severe pain.

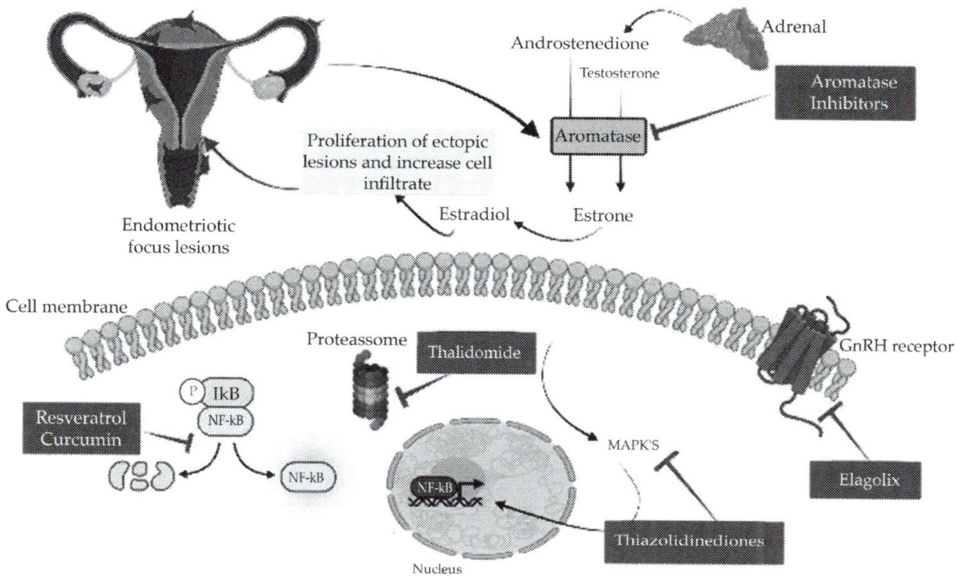

Figure 5.4. *Mechanisms of action of the main medical treatments of endometriosis.*

Source: *França PRdC, Lontra ACP, & Fernandes PD. (2022). Endometriosis: A disease with few direct treatment options. Molecules, 27(13), 4034. https://doi.org/10.3390/molecules27134034.*

5.1.7.2. Surgical Treatment

Because ovarian localizations have a high rate of relapse after surgery (10% per year for the first 5 years), clinicians now have a much more conservative attitude than they did in the past, especially in young women. Correct diagnosis and radiological staging of the illness are prerequisites for undergoing surgery. It is also important to anticipate potential surgical complications and conduct the proper preoperative counseling with the patient.

5.1.7.2.1. Surgical Treatment of Endometrioma

Compared to drainage and electrocoagulation, ovarian cystectomy has a lower risk of endometrioma recurrence, dysmenorrhea, dyspareunia, and non-menstrual pelvic pain.

Furthermore, endometrioma capsule excision appears to increase the rate of spontaneous pregnancies relative to other procedures. Clinicians should, however, advise endometrioma-affected women about the potential loss of the ovary and the possibility of decreased ovarian function following surgery.

5.1.7.2.2. Surgical Treatment of Deep Endometriosis

Technically speaking, treating deep endometriosis surgically is more challenging than treating ovarian lesions because it occasionally calls for knowledge of extragenital interventions (intestinal, urological). As such, the multidisciplinary approach is the most appropriate in certain cases of advanced pathology involving different anatomical districts.

Surgery has limited indications and should only be considered as a backup option if medical therapy fails or is contraindicated due to its complexity, the average patient's young age, the potential desire for progeny, the high rate of recurrence, and the consequent need for additional interventions. For instance, if the symptoms are severe enough to impair quality of life, radical bilateral hysterectomy and adnexectomy may be necessary in perimenopausal women who have finished their reproductive cycle.

Neuroablation, specifically presacral neurectomy (PSN) and uterine nerve ablation (UNA), is a potential treatment option for deep endometriosis.

Understanding anatomy is essential to comprehending these surgical techniques. Both the parasympathetic and sympathetic nervous systems innervate the pelvic organs.

Sympathetic fibers that originate from T10 to L1 are responsible for transmitting pain to the corpus, cervix, and proximal fallopian tubes. These fibers pass partially through the presacral nerves and partially through the uterosacral ligaments. Through the nervi erigentes, or pelvic splanchnic nerve, which runs from S2 to S4, the lateral pelvis transmits pain. The vesical, middle rectal, and uterovaginal plexuses split from the inferior hypogastric plexus, which is formed by the presacral nerve's division into the hypogastric nerve.

The purpose of these two surgical methods varies, but they both aim to cut off the nerve fibers that carry pain signals.

Interrupting pain signaling via the inferior hypogastric plexus is the aim of UNA. Although vaginal methods have been reported, laparoscopic procedures such as LUNAs are the most frequently used for this procedure. The uterosacral ligaments are divided as close to the cervix as is practical. Surgeons can perform this technique with a very short learning curve.

PSN is a fairly complex intervention with a lengthy learning curve and a higher risk of complications. It involves removing all of the presacral nerve fibers in the interiliac triangle and interrupting a greater number of cervical nerve fibers, which results in a greater reduction of pain. While PSN has demonstrated genuine effectiveness when performed by skilled surgeons, it is important to be aware that it is a challenging procedure that carries some risk and is potentially associated with post-operative complications. Multiple authors have demonstrated that UNA was not very effective in reducing painful symptoms, so guidelines suggest avoiding this procedure (de Ziegler et al., 2010; Ahn et al., 2015; Clemenza et al., 2018; Agarwal et al., 2019).

5.2. Infertility

This medical condition is distinct in that it affects the patient and their partner as a couple. This section will examine the assessment, management, and treatment of female infertility, even though male infertility is an essential component of any infertility discussion. To comprehend infertility, one must grasp normal fecundability or the likelihood of becoming pregnant in a single menstrual cycle. The healthcare team will be better able to refer patients and educate them about this medical condition if they have a basic understanding of it.

The fecundability rate has been repeatedly established by the research community, and this has helped determine normal pregnancy rates to aid in the diagnosis of infertility. According to the largest study, 85% of women would become pregnant in a year. The results of this study indicate that during the first three months of unprotected sexual activity, fecundability is 25%, and for the next nine months, it drops to 15%. The American Society of Reproductive Medicine (ASRM) has used this research to help determine when a couple should get evaluated for infertility. When a woman under 35 years old fails to conceive after 12 months of unprotected sexual relations or therapeutic donor insemination, or after 6 months for women over 35, the American Society of Reproductive Medicine (ASRM) advises beginning an evaluation for infertility.

5.2.1. Etiology

To ascertain the distribution of genders and the causes of infertility, the World Health Organization (WHO) conducted a sizable international study. Infertility in women accounted for 37% of cases of infertility in couples; infertility in men accounted for 35% of cases; and male factor infertility accounted for 8% of cases. According to the same study, the following are the most frequently identified causes of female infertility.

- Ovulatory disorders – 25%
- Endometriosis – 15%
- Pelvic adhesions – 12%
- Tubal blockage – 11%
- Other tubal/uterine abnormalities – 11%
- Hyperprolactinemia – 7%

5.2.2. Epidemiology

The prevalence of infertility declined with the woman's age in a National Survey of Family Growth study that involved 12,000 interviews with American women. An increasing number of women experience infertility as they age. The percentage of infertile women aged 15 to 34 ranged from 7.3% to 9.1%. Among women between the ages of 35 and 39, the percentage of infertile women rose to 25%. Finally, a woman's chance of becoming infertile was 30% if she was between the ages of 40 and 44. The Middle East, North Africa, and Eastern Europe have the highest rates of infertility in the world. 11% of women with a prior live birth were unable to have another 1, and 2% of women between the ages of 20 and 44 were never able to conceive.

5.2.3. Pathophysiology

5.2.3.1. Anovulation

25% of female infertility cases are known

to be caused by ovulatory disorders. Infertility arises from oligo-ovulation or anovulation, as there is no monthly release of oocytes. Pregnancy cannot occur if there is no oocyte present for fertilization. The World Health Organization separated ovulatory disorders into four classes: to aid in further classification and treatment.

1. Hypogonadotropic hypogonadal anovulation: i.e., hypothalamic amenorrhea
2. Normogonadotropic normoestrogenic anovulation: i.e., polycystic ovarian syndrome (PCOS)
3. Hypergonadotropic hypoestrogenic anovulation: i.e., premature ovarian failure
4. Hyperprolactinemic anovulation: i.e., pituitary adenoma

Functional hypothalamic amenorrhea (FHA), also known as hypothalamic amenorrhea, is linked to eating disorders and excessive exercise because it lowers hypothalamic GnRH secretion. Reduced calorie intake, weight loss related to it, or excessive exercise raise cortisol levels, which suppress GnRH. The anterior pituitary gland releases less gonadotropins, follicle-stimulating hormone (FSH), and luteinizing hormone (LH) when there is less or no pulsatility of GnRH. Anovulation, low estrogen levels, and aberrant follicle growth are the outcomes of these two deficiencies. Although the levels of FSH and LH will fluctuate between normal and low, the hormone ratio will resemble that of a prepubertal female, with FSH being higher than LH.

PCOS represents the most prevalent form of normogonadotropic normoestrogenic anovulation. PCOS affects 8% of all females of reproductive age and accounts for 80–85% of all anovulatory patients. The Rotterdam criteria, which require the presence of at least two of the three listed below in the absence of other pathological causes, can be used to diagnose PCOS.

- Oligoovulation/anovulation
- Clinical signs of hyperandrogenism and/or serological elevations of androgens
- Polycystic ovaries demonstrated with ultrasound

The category of ovarian resistance and premature ovarian insufficiency related to the age of females is called hypergonadotropic hypoestrogenic anovulation. As previously indicated, a woman's age has an impact on her fertility; this is because a well-researched phenomenon shows a progressive decrease in the quantity and quality of the patient's oocytes. At 20 weeks of gestation, the female fetus has about 6 million follicles in total. There are roughly 1 million follicles in a newborn. 300,000 follicles are left at the start of puberty. Throughout a woman's life, her rate of follicle loss persists and starts to accelerate in her mid-thirties. Reduced follicular quantity is also related to external factors. The most well-known and extensively studied is smoking cigarettes. The quantity of follicles and fecundability are inversely correlated with cigarette smoking. Cigarette smoking is also linked to early menopause (age less than 40); among ever-smokers, early menopause increases by more than 30%.

Overall fertility also depends on the quality of the ovaries. Meiotic nondisjunction is linked to oocyte quality loss throughout a woman's life, which causes aneuploidy. This is believed to be connected to changes in the granulosa cells brought on by aging and lifelong damage accumulation. Meiotic nondisjunction events and the resulting aneuploid or chromosomally aberrant oocytes and embryos are significantly more common in older women.

Hypergonadotropic hypogonadism before the age of 40 is known as primary ovarian insufficiency, or POI. The absence of folliculogenesis, a drop in estrogen, oocyte loss, and infertility are the hallmarks of this illness. Turner syndrome, or monosomy of the sex chromosomes resulting in a 45X karyotype, is the most frequent cause of POI.

Prolactinemia is one of the main causes of infertility in women, according to the WHO; however, according to guidelines released by the ASRM recently, prolactin does not necessarily need to be part of the initial workup. Prolactin suppresses the release of GnRH from the hypothalamus, which lowers LH levels and causes anovulation, amenorrhea, or oligomenorrhea. The luteal phase is shortened when prolactin serum levels between 20 and 50 ng/mL result in insufficient progesterone release from the corpus luteum. Prolactinemia is regarded as a cause of luteal phase defects, which result in infertility, despite this being a contentious statement. Atypical feedback on the hypothalamic-pituitary-ovarian axis results in amenorrhea or oligomenorrhea when prolactin levels range from 50 to 100 ng/mL. A concentration higher than 100 ng/mL is most frequently linked to pituitary adenomas and is linked to overt hypogonadism and amenorrhea.

5.2.3.2. Endometriosis

Endometrial tissue outside the uterus is known as endometriosis. The histological identification of endometrial glands and/or stroma outside the uterus serves as the basis for the diagnosis. Endometriosis affects 10 to 15% of women in their reproductive years and is most commonly found in the pelvis, though it can spread throughout the entire abdomen. 40 to 50% of women who have endometriosis will become infertile. The American Society of Reproductive Medicine has classified endometriosis into four stages: stage I is minimal, and stage IV is severe. Infertility is a known side effect of endometriosis, but the pathophysiology is assumed to vary depending on the stage. Infertility is thought to be linked to inflammation in stages I and II, with increased production of macrophages, natural killer cells, prostaglandins, and cytokines. Inflammation affects tubal and ovarian function, which leads to poor implantation, fertilization, and follicular development. Pelvic adhesions and/or masses that alter pelvic anatomy are linked to stages III and IV; these conditions will inevitably affect sperm motility, oocyte release, and tubal motility. Furthermore, it is thought that advanced endometriosis hinders folliculogenesis, which lowers the likelihood of fertilization.

5.2.3.3. Pelvic/Tubal Adhesions

A significant percentage of female infertility is caused by uterine and tubal abnormalities, as well as pelvic and tubal adhesions. Pelvic/tubal adhesions are primarily caused by infectious processes within the abdomen; pelvic inflammatory disease (PID) is the most common infectious process that affects infertility. Chlamydia trachomatis is the microorganism associated with the highest risk of infertility when combined with PID. The likelihood of pregnancy is inversely correlated with the presence of positive chlamydia antibodies, which affects one in four women with tubal factor infertility. The probability of infertility is influenced by the quantity and intensity of PID episodes. According to one study, the rates of pregnancy after one episode of PID were 89%, 77%, and 46%, respectively, after two and three episodes. 90%, 82%, and 57% of live births had mild, moderate, or severe PID, respectively.

Acute and chronic inflammation can cause hydrosalpinges, a tubal abnormality that compromises the structural integrity of the fallopian tube. This injury causes tubal obstruction, which obstructs the fallopian tube's ability to distribute physiological fluid and causes fluid buildup. It is thought that hydrosalpinges reduce fertility by causing endometrial receptivity to be compromised, which makes an environment unfavorable for implantation. This is achieved through the retrograde flow of prostaglandins and toxins into the endometrium. Research has shown that if a patient has a hydrosalpinx, their chances of becoming pregnant are reduced by 50% during in-vitro fertilization.

5.2.3.4. Uterine Causes

Space-occupying lesions or decreased endometrial receptivity are linked to uterine causes of infertility. One meta-analysis on uterine leiomyomas (fibroids) showed that when compared to other infertile controls, only submucosal or intracavitary fibroids affected implantation and pregnancy rates. Infertility is also linked to congenital uterine abnormalities (CUA), despite their rarity. Uterine septums are most frequently observed and are linked to repeated miscarriages. It is interesting to note that a study found that both infertile and fertile people had the same prevalence of CUA. Though approximately 8% of female causes of infertility are thought to be caused by CUAs, CUAs are also found in 25% of women who experience late first- or second-trimester miscarriages.

5.2.4. History and Physical

Women who have had an unsuccessful pregnancy should have their infertility evaluated after 12 months of regular, unprotected sexual activity, or 6 months if they are older than 35. While the focus of this section is on female infertility, it is important to keep in mind that a male infertility evaluation is also necessary and ought to be started at the same time. Before having an insemination, women who intend to use donor sperm should undergo the same examination for female infertility. The following is a summary of the important events in the history of the infertile woman.

- Duration of infertility
- Obstetrical history
- Menstrual history, including molimina
- Medical, surgical, and gynecological history to include a history of sexually transmitted infections
- Sexual history to include coital frequency and timing
  - Focusing on the male partner, which includes issues with erection and ejaculation
- Social and lifestyle history to include cigarettes, alcohol, and illicit drug use, exercise, and diet, occupation
- Family history, screening for genetic issues, history of venous thrombotic events, recurrent pregnancy loss, and infertility

The physical exam should include the following:

- Vital signs and BMI
- Thyroid evaluation
- Breast exam for galactorrhea
- Signs of androgen excess: dermatological and external genitalia exam
- The appearance of abnormal vaginal or cervical anatomy
- Pelvic masses or tenderness
- Uterine enlargement or irregularity
- Transvaginal ultrasonography is often done at the bedside as part of the initial physical exam

5.2.5. Evaluation

The five diagnostic evaluation categories are:

i. Semen analysis

ii. Assessment of ovarian function and reserve

iii. Assessment of the uterine cavity

iv. Assessment of the fallopian tubes

v. Endocrinological serum studies

It is beyond the purview of this review to evaluate and interpret a semen analysis; that being said, the significance of this test in the preliminary assessment before treatment initiation cannot be overstated.

The menstrual cycle history can be used as a basic tool for ovarian function assessment. Women who experience molimina (excessive tiredness, bloating, or tenderness in the breasts) in addition to regular, regular cycles and menstrual flow are most likely ovulating. Indirect proof of ovulation, a mid-cycle LH surge is detected by at-home urinary LH predictor kits, which also assist in determining the fertile window. Progesterone serum levels on cycle day 21, or more precisely, mid-luteal phase progesterone levels, can also be used to identify ovulation. One week before menstruation is the recommended time to take the lab test. A progesterone lab value of more than 3 ng/mL indicates ovulation. A more intrusive, precise, and probably superfluous method of detecting ovulation would be to use daily ultrasounds to track the development and demise of a follicle.

The two most popular tests for ovarian reserve assessment—anti-mullerian hormone (AMH) and cycle day 3 FSH and estradiol—will be the only ones covered in this review out of the many available tests.

According to the theory behind day 3 FSH and estradiol, women with healthy ovarian reserves produce enough ovarian hormones from small follicles early on to keep FSH at a low level. Numerous examples found in the literature suggest that the most crucial thing to do is to find women who have fewer follicles than normal. These women produce fewer hormones, which leads to a lack of inhibition and an increase in FSH. Less than 10 IU/mL is probably indicative of a normal ovarian reserve; 10 to 20 IU/mL is considered intermediate, and more than 20 IU/mL indicates a poor ovarian reserve and consequently a poor prognosis for spontaneous ovulation. The pregnancy rates per natural menstrual cycle, which correlate with the FSH levels above, are 32%, 17 to 19%, and 3%, according to one study. When the third day's estradiol level is less than 80 pg/mL, the ovarian reserve is deemed sufficient. Pregnancy rates were lowest for values above 80 pg/mL and 0% for values over 100 pg/mL.

Antral and preantral follicles produce the hormone AMH, which is a measure of ovarian function that can be taken at any point during a woman's cycle. Over the course of a woman's natural reproductive life, her AMH levels will progressively drop until they are undetectable at menopause. An effective predictor of the exogenous gonadotropin response appears to be AMH levels.

- <0.5 ng/mL predicts difficulty getting more than 3 follicles to grow
- <1.0 ng/mL shows limited egg supply that may require more aggressive ovulation induction protocols
- 1.0 to 3.5 ng/mL shows normal values
- >3.5 shows ample supply and may require mild induction to prevent ovarian hyperstimulation syndrome.

It is crucial to keep in mind that while the ovarian reserve tests that are currently accessible are accurate in identifying problems with ovulation induction, they cannot be used to diagnose live births or disqualify patients from in vitro fertilization (IVF) treatment.

Antral follicle counts are a reliable indicator of ovarian reserve and ovarian response to stimulation. They are calculated using transvaginal ultrasound to count the number of follicles in the ovaries that are less than 9 mm in size during the early follicular phase.

5.2.5.1. Tubal Evaluation

When assessing tubal patency, laparoscopy combined with chromopertubation is the gold standard. Although the hysterosalpingogram (HSG) has a higher specificity and is less invasive, laparoscopy is still recommended as the first diagnostic test for suspected pelvic adhesions, endometriosis, or other pelvic pathologies. It is more frequently used as the first evaluation for tubal patency and abnormalities. The HSG has poor predictability for intrauterine and tubal adhesions, but it is most effective at detecting abnormalities in cases of proximal occlusion, followed by distal occlusions. With oil-soluble media, the HSG also increases the rates of pregnancy and live births. Pregnancy and live birth rates rose following HSG in comparison to controls, according to a meta-analysis (OR 2.98, 95% CI 1.05–6.37).

5.2.5.2. Uterine Cavity

Hysteroscopy is the gold standard for evaluating the uterine cavity because it offers the chance for prompt surgical correction and direct visualization of intrauterine pathology. Saline infusion sonography (SIS) is a less invasive method that is more frequently used, even though hysteroscopy is still the gold standard. With or without 3-D model rendering, the SIS is a suitable screening tool before infertility treatment because it is extremely sensitive and specific for all intrauterine abnormalities.

5.2.6. Treatment and Management

5.2.6.1. Lifestyle Changes

Body mass index (BMI) extremes are often associated with infertility and ovulatory dysfunction in women. Women who have a BMI below 17 kg/m^2, a history of vigorous exercise, or eating disorders are more susceptible to hypogonadotropic hypogonadism, which results in pituitary gonadotropin secretions that are deceased. In Europe, women who do not respond to treatment can receive pulsatile GnRH therapy. In the United States, ovulation is induced by controlled ovarian stimulation using exogenous gonadotropins. One study showed how crucial behavioral modifications are for triggering ovulation. 87% of the women who underwent individual-directed therapy to address behavioral issues or energy deficiencies went back to their normal ovarian function, which helped to normalize their abnormal BMI.

Losing weight alone can improve ovulation in women with anovulation and a BMI greater than 27 kg/m^2. According to numerous studies, 50–100% of women will experience normal ovulation again in less than a year after losing 10% of their body weight. One study found that obese women who received counseling and weight-loss interventions before infertility treatment did not have higher rates of pregnancy or live births than obese women who received infertility treatment without weight-loss interventions, even though weight loss is important for many aspects of a patient's life. Thus, starting fertility treatment does not require a certain BMI.

5.2.6.2. Controlled Ovarian Hyperstimulation

Clomiphene citrate (CC) is the first-line treatment for infertility of unknown origin and is prescribed by the majority of healthcare professionals. With its estrogen antagonist and agonist properties, clomiphene is a selective estrogen receptor modulator (SERM) that eventually increases the anterior pituitary's release of gonadotropin. When it comes to treating WHO classes 2 and 3, clomiphene is ineffective, while it works well for classes 1 and 3. Doses of clomiphene are administered starting on cycle days 2, 3, 4, or 5 and continuing for five days in a row. It is suggested that the couple start having sex five days after the last pill and continue every other day for a week. However, clomiphene plus intrauterine insemination (IUI) may improve the chances of getting pregnant. Between cycle days 2 and 5, there is minimal variation in the outcomes of ovulation, pregnancy, or live birth with respect to the day the medication is initiated.

Letrozole is another medication that is frequently taken orally to induce ovulation. As an aromatase inhibitor, letrozole stops testosterone and androstenedione from converting into estrone and estradiol, hence preventing the production of estrogen. Letrozole is deemed off-label when used for ovulation induction; the FDA has approved it for extended adjuvant treatment of breast cancer. Nonetheless, a plethora of scientific research and numerous committee rulings bolster the effectiveness and safety of using it to induce ovulation. Letrozole, which is similar to clomiphene, is dosed starting at 2.5, 5, or 7.5 mg/day on cycle days 3, 4, 5, 6, and 7, with sexual activity every other day 5 days after finishing the medication. Letrozole, rather than clomiphene, ought to be the first-line treatment for women with PCOS, according to ACOG. Letrozole has the following advantages over clomiphene:

- Higher rate of monofollicular development and a corresponding decrease in twin gestations
- Shorter half-life
- No antiestrogenic effects on the endometrium and central nervous system
- Lower estradiol levels, which is a benefit for women with breast cancer undergoing IVF

In the future, letrozole may take the place of clomiphene as the first-line treatment due to its superior benefit profile.

When treating anovulatory disorders classified as WHO Class 1, 2, or 3, gonadotropin therapy is a more intensive medical regimen. Gonadotropins are helpful as a backup course of treatment for women who experience infertility despite undergoing several cycles of clomiphene. One study found that using gonadotropins increased the live birth rate more than continuing to use clomiphene. Various dosing regimens are employed based on the infertility treatment chosen and the preferences of the provider. These procedures are not covered in this review. It is crucial to talk about the need for close observation when taking more invasive and potent gonadotropins, though. Every two to three days during the late follicular phase, transvaginal ultrasounds are used to monitor follicular growth and assess mature follicles. A mature follicle has a diameter of more than 18 mm and an estradiol concentration of more than 200 pg/mL. Recombinant HCG 250 mg subcutaneous injection or 10,000 U intramuscular injection of urine-derived HCG is administered to induce ovulation after a mature follicle has been detected. 24-36 hours after the trigger shot is administered, an IUI takes place. All ovarian induction agents can be used in conjunction with IUIs, and using IUI in conjunction with medication is recommended to increase the likelihood of conception. The benefits of letting a natural LH surge versus an HCG trigger before IUI are not well supported by data. The selection of a treatment plan should be based on patient convenience, hospital staffing constraints, and cost, as indicated by a 2010 meta-analysis that found no conclusive evidence to support one treatment option over another.

5.2.6.3. Tubal and Pelvic Adhesions

The first-line treatment for bilateral tubal factor infertility is in vitro fertilization (IVF). Reconstructive tubal ligation increases the risk of an ectopic pregnancy and has poorer pregnancy outcomes. To improve the likelihood of IVF pregnancy, women with severe tubal disease—including those with hydrosalpinx—are advised to undergo a bilateral salpingectomy. Fimbrioplasty is a viable option for women with mild distal tubal disease to enable multiple pregnancies without the need for IVF. A small study found that for mild tubal disease, the pregnancy rate was comparable to that of IVF; however, the risk of an ectopic pregnancy was 15% as opposed to 0.7% with IVF treatment.

An important tubal factor population consists of patients who have undergone bilateral salpingectomy or tubal ligation for contraception in the past. It is imperative that healthcare providers always talk to women who want tubal ligation about the possibility of regret. The patient's age, the type of ligation used, and the available tubal length all affect the likelihood of becoming pregnant following tubal reanastomosis. The best candidates are younger women with tubal lengths greater than 4 cm who have had a ring or clip; their pregnancy rates are comparable to those of in vitro fertilization. However, compared to IVF, the time to pregnancy after tubal surgery is much longer.

5.2.6.4. Uterine Abnormalities

The impact of leiomyomas on the rates of live births and infertility is not well-established. It is advised that before conducting additional research on fibroids, the patient undergoes a thorough infertility workup. The location of fibroids is the most crucial factor. Impaired implantation and a higher incidence of miscarriage are the outcomes of fibroids pressing against the endometrium and distorting the uterine cavity. Pregnancy rates have been demonstrated to be lower in women with submucosal or submucosal-intramural fibroids that cause uterine cavity distortion. The rate of pregnancy and live births rises when these fibroids are removed. Operative hysteroscopy is the first-line treatment for removing the most harmful fibroids. Although they can lead to infertility, other uterine pathologies such as uterine synechiae and septa are more frequently associated with recurrent pregnancy loss. Women with both synechiae and septa have significantly less pregnancy loss after operative hysteroscopy. Infertility has also been demonstrated to be caused by asymptomatic polyps. According to one study, performing a polypectomy on asymptomatic infertile women before IUI increased the likelihood of getting pregnant from 28% to 63%.

5.2.6.5. IVF Procedures

The best course of treatment for infertility will not be covered in this section; instead, an overview of IVF procedures will be covered. The first step is usually controlled ovarian hyperstimulation using injectable gonadotropins. 36 hours following an HCG injection, also known as a trigger shot, an expert will conduct an oocyte retrieval and transvaginal ultrasound-guided needle aspiration. Following retrieval, normal sperm is transferred to the dish for insemination and the oocytes are placed in a special medium. Intracytoplasmic sperm injection (ICSI) is used if there are aberrant sperm. During the ICSI process, a single spermatozoon is inserted straight into the cytoplasm of the egg. Upon fertilization, the embryo is evaluated and assigned a grade. On either Day 3 or Day 5, the embryos are then transferred. An additional IVF procedure called preimplantation genetic testing (PGT) aids in the detection of balanced translocation or known genetic mutations in the parents. PGT can also be used to identify aneuploidy from all 23 chromosome pairs, including monosomies and trisomies. In addition to having a known parental carrier for a balanced translocation or genetic mutation, PGT is probably advantageous in cases of unexplained infertility, repeated IVF failures with high-grade embryos, and advanced maternal age.

5.2.7. Differential Diagnosis

A very complicated condition, infertility has a big impact on the couple as a whole. It is critical to keep in mind that infertility can have several causes, which it frequently does. Infertility can have a wide differential diagnosis, and a complete workup is necessary to make sure no dangerous disease process is overlooked. The manuscript will concentrate on the differential diagnosis of PCOS because of its high prevalence in the infertile population and the expansive nature of this discussion.

The differential diagnosis for patients with suspected PCOS includes:

- Androgen producing ovarian tumors
- Adrenal tumors
- Nonclassic congenital adrenal hyperplasia
- Cushing syndrome
- Prolactinemia disorders
- Thyroid disorders

To evaluate a virilizing ovarian or adrenal tumor or nonclassical congenital adrenal hyperplasia (CAH), the investigation of PCOS should include total testosterone, DHEA-S, and 17-hydroxyprogesterone. There is a suggestion that since a mildly elevated DHEA-S level does not impact management, DHEA-S should only be administered to women who have experienced severe virilization. Thyroid-stimulating hormone and prolactin should also be measured.

- The upper limit of normal for female testosterone is 45 to 60 ng/dL.
- A testosterone value greater than 150 ng/dL warrants investigation for ovarian and adrenal androgen-secreting tumors.
- DHEA-S of greater than 500 to 700 mcg/dL warrants further investigation of an adrenal tumor.
- A fasting 17-hydroxyprogesterone greater than 200 ng/dL collected during the follicular phase warrants an ACTH stimulation test, and a value greater than 500 ng/dL is diagnostic for nonclassical congenital adrenal hyperplasia.

5.2.8. Prognosis

The pregnancy rates per cycle for each of the treatment modalities will be discussed in this section. The data is consistent for known causes of infertility but primarily comes from the evaluation of infertility that cannot be explained. IVF success rates can differ significantly depending on many different factors. The subsequent pregnancy rates were gathered through a retrospective examination of 45 distinct studies:

- No treatment: 1.3% to 3.8%
- IUI alone: 4%
- Clomiphene citrate (CC) alone: 5.6%
- CC with IUI: 8.3%
- Gonadotropins alone: 7.7%
- Gonadotropins with IUI: 17.1%
- IVF: 20.7%

For women for whom IVF is not an option and who have not been successful with CC plus IUI, letrozole alone or in combination with IUI can produce similar pregnancy rates to those of CC plus IUI.

A 2009 study indicated that rather than starting gonadotropins plus IUI before IVF, women who failed CC plus IUI should proceed directly to IVF. As a result of this study, getting pregnant took less time, required fewer treatment cycles, and cost less money overall for each delivery.

According to the aforementioned research, doctors can treat infertility with clomiphene alone as a first line of treatment. That's no longer the case. A randomized control trial conducted in 2008 revealed that expectant management had a higher live birth rate (17%) than clomiphene alone (14%). While there is a benefit to patient satisfaction over expectant management, as this section did demonstrate, most women in both groups were happy with their care. The ASRM committee opinion, released in light of this study, recommended against using clomiphene in conjunction with timed intercourse as a first-line treatment for infertility that cannot be explained.

5.2.9. Complications

Ectopic pregnancy, ovarian hyperstimulation syndrome, and multiples are the three main side effects of infertility treatments.

5.2.9.1. Multiple Gestations

Since the beginning of artificial reproductive technologies, the possibility of multiple births has been a concern. Within the U. S. 32% of pregnancies obtained through ART were multiples, compared to 3.4% of births that occurred naturally. The chances of singleton, twin, or higher-order pregnancies with IVF fresh embryo transfer were 62%, 29%, and 3%, respectively, in 2009, according to the CDC. When compared to gonadotropins, the oral ovarian induction agent's letrozole and clomiphene have a lower risk of multiple gestations, with percentages of twins, triplets, and quadruplets of 7%, 0.5%, and 0.3%, respectively. A gonadotropin's chance of multiple gestations—including triplets—is 13%. At the moment, patients with a good prognosis are being strongly encouraged to use elective single embryo transfer (eSET) by the ASRM and CDC. The rates of twins and triplets decreased to less than 1% with the use of eSET. Furthermore, because of the high risk of multiples, there is ongoing discussion about whether gonadotropins should be used for ovulation induction outside of an IVF protocol. The use of gonadotropins in conjunction with IUI will probably continue to decline as the number of IVF procedures rises.

5.2.9.2. Ectopic Pregnancy

Another risk associated with treatment for infertile patients is ectopic pregnancy, which calls for intensive counseling. Patients with infertility have a two- to three-fold increase in ectopic pregnancies. This is believed to be linked to a high rate of infertility caused by tubal factors. The greatest risk of an ectopic pregnancy is following tubal surgery to address infertility caused by tubal factors. After tubal reconstructive surgery, the rate of ectopic pregnancy is about 9%, but some reports put it as high as 30%. Although fresh embryo transfers carry a higher risk of ectopic pregnancy than frozen embryo transfers, the overall rate of ectopic pregnancies using IVF is only about 1.3%. However, in a large study comparing the ovulation induction agents: clomiphene, letrozole, and gonadotropins had ectopic pregnancy rates of 4%, 6%, and 8%, respectively. It appears that there is no increase in ectopic pregnancies with the use of ovulation induction agents combined with IUI versus natural conception.

5.2.9.3. Ovarian Hyperstimulation Syndrome (OHSS)

Acute respiratory distress syndrome, electrolyte imbalances, cardiac arrhythmias, sepsis, nausea, vomiting, enlarged ovaries, third-spacing of fluids, renal failure, and venous thrombosis are just a few of the many signs and symptoms that can arise from this iatrogenic complication of controlled ovarian hyperstimulation. The following complications can lead to mortality if severe OHSS is not treated and closely watched. Golan and colleagues have classified the various stages of OHSS. 1989. A fluid shift into the third space is the result of increased capillary permeability, which is the underlying pathophysiological feature. Patients with more than 20 mature follicles who also receive an HCG trigger shot are the women most at risk of developing OHSS. With IVF, the incidence of moderate and severe OHSS varies from 6% to 1%, respectively. This manuscript does not address the diagnosis, prevention, or treatment of OHSS.

5.2.10. Deterrence and Patient Education

If a woman is unable to conceive after a year of unprotected timed sexual activity, or six months if she is older than 35, she should see her healthcare provider for a referral to an infertility subspecialist. It is crucial to clarify that male and female factors, as well as a combination of the two, can lead to infertility. This is crucial to keep in mind because the majority of infertile couples seek care from the female partner's physician, possibly undervaluing the role played by the male partner. The available treatments and drugs for female infertility have been thoroughly researched and their risk profiles are well established. The patient must be informed of the possibility of OHSS, multiple gestations, and ectopic pregnancy. The patient must also be aware of the chances of becoming pregnant with each treatment cycle for each modality. It is important to fully understand the possibility of not being able to conceive, even with IVF, before investing a significant amount of money in infertility treatment.

5.2.11. Enhancing Healthcare Team Outcomes

All members of the healthcare team should view infertility as a disease process because it is a devastating diagnosis. According to the author, conducting an immediate and comprehensive investigation into both partners is the best way to help the patient cope with the interpersonal, social, emotional, and physical stresses associated with infertility. Referral to a fertility subspecialist can be made after completing the simple evaluation. This will improve and speed up the specialist's ability to start treatments and follow-up research. A known cause of anovulation may be corrected with the use of either letrozole or clomiphene plus timed intercourse alone; however, this should not delay the referral to a subspecialist. When counseling infertile couples, primary care physicians should be realistic about the likelihood of conception and the potential for difficulties. Finally, while not exhaustive, this manuscript offers a solid foundation of knowledge to enable one to feel at ease when discussing a patient's family planning objectives, starting an assessment, and going over available treatments.

5.3. Sexually Transmitted Diseases

Sexually transmitted diseases (STDs), also known as STIs, are infections that are spread from one person to another during intercourse. Usually, they are transferred during anal, oral, or vaginal sex. However, on occasion, they may spread by other forms of sexual contact with the anus, mouth, vagina, or penis. This is due to the fact that skin-to-skin contact can transmit certain STIs, such as herpes and HPV. Pregnant women may transfer certain sexually transmitted infections (STIs) to their unborn child either during or after pregnancy. Certain STIs can also spread through sharing needles, receiving blood transfusions, and breastfeeding.

5.3.1. STD Symptoms

If an STD starts with a symptomatic STI, you might first experience:

- pain or discomfort during sexual activity or urination
- sores, bumps, or rashes on or around the vagina, penis, testicles, anus, buttocks, thighs, or mouth
- unusual discharge or bleeding from the penis or vagina
- painful or swollen testicles
- itchiness in or around the vagina
- unexpected periods or bleeding after sexual activity

But keep in mind that not every STI causes symptoms. The symptoms of a STI that develops into an STD can differ. Some of these, like pain during urination, pain during sexual activity, and painful or irregular periods, might be comparable to those mentioned above. Other symptoms, however, can vary greatly depending on the STD. They might consist of:

- fever
- recurring pain
- fatigue
- memory loss
- changes to vision or hearing
- nausea
- weight loss
- lumps or swellings

5.3.2. Underlying STD Causes

A STI is the source of all STDs. Usually, these infections are spread through intercourse, including anal, vaginal, and oral sex, as well as through bodily fluids or skin contact. Some of them even go away on their own, and some of them never develop into diseases, especially if they are treated. However, a STI will develop into an STD if the pathogens that caused the infection manage to harm the body's cells and interfere with its normal processes.

5.3.3. Types of STDs

There are fewer STDs, even though the list of STIs is rather long. They range from certain types of cancer brought on by the human papillomavirus (HPV) to pelvic inflammatory disease (PID), which is brought on by STIs like chlamydia and gonorrhea. The primary STDs to be mindful of are listed below.

5.3.3.1. Pelvic Inflammatory Disease

Common STIs like gonorrhea, chlamydiasis, and trichomoniasis can cause PID if untreated. However, not every case of PID is brought on by a STI because other bacterial infections can also be the cause. Based on information provided by the Centers for Disease Control and Prevention (CDC), approximately 2.5 million women in the US have a history of PID diagnoses. Despite being categorized as a disease, this infection of the female reproductive system affects some individuals without any symptoms.

Those who do have symptoms may experience:

- pelvic or lower abdominal pain
- pain during penetrative vaginal sex or when urinating
- irregular, heavy, or painful vaginal bleeding
- unusual vaginal discharge
- nausea
- high temperature

PID can be effectively treated with antibiotics if it is identified early enough. They will not, however, address any potential scarring on the fallopian tubes. One in ten PID patients experience infertility as a result of this scarring, which has been related to an increased risk of an ectopic pregnancy.

5.3.3.2. Tertiary Syphilis

Syphilis is a relatively uncommon infection, and its early stages are classified as STIs. One or more tiny, circular sores on the mouth, anus, or genitalia are the initial signs of the infection. Syphilis will enter the latent phase, which has no symptoms if treatment is not received. But from this point on, about 25% of individuals will develop tertiary syphilis, which can develop anywhere from 10 to 30 years after the initial infection. This illness may have detrimental effects on the body's organ systems, including:

- loss of vision
- loss of hearing
- memory loss
- mental health conditions
- infections of the brain or spinal cord
- heart disease

The less harm that syphilis causes, the earlier it is identified and treated. Penicillin injections can't undo the damage that has already been done, even though they are usually used to treat tertiary syphilis and eradicate the bacteria from the body. Naturally, additional drugs and treatments might be needed if the illness affects vital organs like the heart.

5.3.3.3. Cancer

While certain HPV strains typically do not cause illness, other strains can result in aberrant alterations to cells. Cancer may result from this, including:

- oral cancer
- cervical cancer
- vulvar cancer
- penile cancer
- anal cancer

The National Cancer Institute states that HPV 16 and HPV 18 are the primary causes of HPV-related cancer cases in the United States. Nearly all cervical cancers, over 90% of anal cancers, 75% of vaginal cancers, and more than 60% of penile cancers are caused by HPV. The location of these cancers in the body determines their symptoms. Pain, bleeding, and lumps can occur frequently. Early detection makes it frequently easier to treat cancer with radiation, chemotherapy, or surgery. There are screening tests available to identify HPV-related alterations in precancerous cells.

5.3.3.4. Genital Warts

Genital warts are a condition that can be brought on by certain low-risk HPV strains. Every year, more than 350,000 people get these skin-colored or white pimples on their genitalia or anus. Although treatable, the underlying virus may persist, making a cure impossible. (Occasionally, HPV goes away on its own). Genital warts can also spontaneously disappear, but they can also recur. You have the choice of freezing, burning them off, or using a chemical cream or liquid to get rid of them.

5.3.3.5. AIDS

HIV can weaken the immune system, raise the chance of catching other viruses or bacteria, and raise the risk of getting some cancers. Many HIV-positive individuals now lead long, healthy lives thanks to modern treatments. However, AIDS, which makes the body susceptible to dangerous infections and illnesses, can result from the virus if treatment is not received. AIDS patients may go through:

- rapid weight loss
- extreme fatigue
- sores
- infections

- neurologic disorders
- cancers

5.3.4. STDs and Pregnancy

There isn't an AIDS cure. Furthermore, the life expectancy without treatment is approximately three years because of the range of diseases that can be acquired as a result of a severely compromised immune system.

An unborn child may contract syphilis, which could lead to a dangerous infection, miscarriage, or stillbirth.

While very rare, genital warts can also be passed on to a baby.

PID can impact subsequent pregnancies, increasing the likelihood of an ectopic pregnancy and contributing to infertility in 1 in 10 cases.

Here's what else to consider if you're pregnant:

- Get screened for STIs, including HIV and syphilis, to avoid complications by ensuring any infection can be detected and treated.
- Speak with a healthcare professional if you have an STD. They may need to check that a medication is safe for you to use or delay treatment where necessary.
- Note that a cesarean delivery may be needed —particularly if genital warts make it difficult for the vagina to stretch.

5.3.5. STD Diagnosis

Healthcare providers will need to perform certain tests and examinations because it is difficult for them to diagnose an STD solely based on symptoms. The following could apply, depending on the suspected STD:

- physical examinations
- swabs of bodily fluids
- blood tests
- specialist procedures, such as keyhole surgery or a colposcopy

5.3.6. STD Treatment Options

STDs can affect the body in a variety of ways. Depending on the condition, there are several treatment options, such as:

- antibiotics
- other oral or topical medications
- surgery
- laser

It might also be suggested that you change your way of living, like not having sex until the course of treatment is finished.

Keep in mind that, with the majority of STDs, any harm already done by the illness cannot be reversed. Furthermore, some STDs, like AIDS and genital warts, cannot be cured.

5.3.7. Tips for STD Prevention

Preventing STIs is the best way to avoid an STD. And staying away from sexual contact is the only surefire way to do that. However, there are steps you can take to make sex safer and lower your chance of getting a STI:

- Have an open discussion about sexual history with a new partner before engaging in any sexual activity, and decide what you're comfortable with.
- Get tested regularly for STIs, especially if you have a new partner or multiple partners. Ask any partners to do the same.
- Use a condom properly during vaginal, anal, and oral sex to help prevent STIs that spread through

fluids. Dental dams can also provide protection during oral sex.

- Consider getting vaccinated for HPV and hepatitis B.
- If you're at a higher risk of contracting HIV, think about taking PrEP medication every day.

5.4. Uterine Fibroids

Leiomyomas, another name for uterine fibroids, are growths consisting of muscle and tissue that develop in or on the uterine wall. These growths are the most common noncancerous tumors in women and individuals assigned female at birth (AFAB), and they are typically benign (not cancerous).

Numerous symptoms, including pain and heavy, irregular vaginal bleeding, can be brought on by uterine fibroids. There are situations when a person has fibroids but is unaware of them. Usually, fibroids are treated based on your symptoms.

Fibroids can grow in clusters or as a single nodule, or single growth. Fibroid clusters can vary in diameter from 1 millimeter to over 20 centimeters (8 inches) or even larger. In contrast, fibroids range in size from a seed's size to that of a watermelon. The development of these growths may occur on the exterior of your uterus, inside its main cavity, or within its wall.

Uterine fibroids can be classified into various types based on their location and mode of attachment. Particular varieties of uterine fibroids consist of:

- **Intramural Fibroids**: These fibroids are embedded into the muscular wall of your uterus. They're the most common type.
- **Submucosal Fibroids**: These fibroids grow under the inner lining of your uterus.
- **Subserosal Fibroids**: This type of fibroid grows under the lining of the outer surface of your uterus. They can become quite large and grow into your pelvis.
- **Pedunculated Fibroids**: The least common type, these fibroids attach to your uterus with a stalk or stem. They're often described as mushroom-like because they have a stalk and then a wider top.

5.4.1. Epidemiology

The most prevalent benign tumors in fertile women are called uterine fibroids. Various series report their prevalence between 5 and 70% of women, with 70% of women between the ages of 40 and 60 having at least one fibroid found. In addition, fibroids are the primary cause of hysterectomy, which has a significant negative effect on a fertile woman's health and quality of life.

Risk factors commonly associated with the condition include age, genetics, race (black women are younger when diagnosed and more likely to have severe symptoms and undergo hysterectomy), obesity, late menopause, early menarche, prolonged and early use of contraceptives, diets high in red meat, alcohol, and caffeine, and so on). On the other hand, protective factors would include pregnancy, the use of progestin-only injectable contraceptives, and consumption of fruit, vegetables, low-fat dairy products, and tobacco.

5.4.2. Etiopathogenesis

The exact genetic mutations that have been linked to the development of fibroid formations notwithstanding, the causes of uterine fibroids remain a mystery. Leiomyoma frequently exhibits chromosomal rearrangements, paracentric inversions, and translocations. Furthermore, fibroid formation may also be influenced by genetic mutations affecting the gene or genes regulating growth factors and myometrial proliferation.

There are several known risk factors for the development of fibroids. Fibroids are primarily hormone-dependent tumors associated with an environment of progesterone and estrogen. The smooth uterine muscle, which is made up of fibroblasts and smooth muscle cells, is where fibroids first appear. As a result, they are categorized as a clonal illness brought on by a malfunction in the hormone receptors. Progesterone and progesterone receptors (PR) are also necessary for the growth of fibroid tissue and cellular proliferation. In contrast to the surrounding myometrium, fibroids exhibit higher concentrations of PR-A and PR-B. Therefore, progesterone and its receptors may be useful targets for preventing the growth of fibroids.

Additionally, extracellular matrix (ECM) constituents like collagen, fibronectin, laminins, and proteoglycans are found in higher concentrations in fibroids. These proteins cause the integrin-Rho/p38 MAPK/ERK pathway, which in turn causes gene expression to be upregulated, cell proliferation to increase, apoptosis to decrease, and an altered extracellular matrix (ECM). However, other factors that have been linked to ECM function, remodeling, and accumulation (fibrosis) include matrix metalloproteinases (MMPs), growth factors (TGF-β, activin-A, and PDGF), cytokines (TNF-α), steroid hormones (progesterone and estrogen), and microRNAs (miR-29 family, miR-200c, and miR-93/106b). Activin-A and TGF-βs (1 and 3) are two growth factors that may direct myofibroblast differentiation during the fibrosis process.

Numerous research works have proposed the role of miRNAs in ECM regulation. These miRNAs cause RNA degradation and/or directly inhibit the translation of proteins, which accumulate extracellular matrix and form uterine fibroids. Specifically, uterine leiomyoma expresses the miRNA miR-29 family at lower levels than the myometrium. The development of potential present and future treatment options will be aided by medical treatments that target ECM. Several substances have actually been investigated as medical treatments that target extracellular matrix (ECM) in uterine leiomyoma. These include gonadotropin-releasing hormone (GnRH) agonists (leuprolide acetate), GnRH antagonists (cetrorelix acetate), selective progesterone receptor modulators (ulipristal acetate and asoprisnil), and anti-progestins (mifepristone).

5.4.3. Symptoms of Uterine Fibroids

20 to 50% of women have fibroids-related symptoms, which can include AUB, pelvic pain, compressive symptoms, or reproductive issues. Pelvic pressure, bowel dysfunction, frequency and urgency of urination, retention of urine, low back pain, constipation, and dyspareunia are other less common symptoms. Still, the majority of fibroids don't cause any symptoms.

5.4.4. Diagnosis

The primary methods for diagnosing uterine fibroids are magnetic resonance imaging (MRI), ultrasound, pelvic exam, and anamnesis. A thorough examination of the menstrual pattern—which is typically heavy and prolonged—and its correlation—if any—with the existence of anemia syndrome and pelvic pain may help to clarify the diagnosis. A pelvic examination can also be used to assess the size, shape, and mobility of the uterus because women who have fibroids have enlarged, irregular uterine contours. When it comes to identifying the size, quantity, and location of uterine fibroids, transvaginal ultrasonography is thought to be the gold standard for diagnosis. An endocavitary study is made possible by the combined 2D/3D approach, which also defines the differential diagnosis of adenomyosis. Additionally, ultrasound provides information about the features of the endometrium and ovaries. The gold standard for studying the endometrial cavity is hysteroscopy, which makes it possible to diagnose and treat submucosal fibroids (FIGO 0–2).

When there are large uterine volumes or fibroids, MRI can be a valuable tool for differential diagnosis of adenomyosis. It also gives precise information about the number, location, and size of the fibroids.

5.4.5. Treatment

The majority of fibroids won't cause any symptoms, so all that's needed is expectant management rather than treatment.

The patient's age, desired uterine preservation, and symptoms should all be taken into consideration when treating fibroids. The management will be contingent upon the patient's symptoms, which will include bleeding, pain, compressive symptoms (vesico-rectal, voiding symptoms, ureteral compression, risk of ureterohydronephrosis), and reproductive history. The patient's age, desire to preserve her uterus, and desire to become pregnant in the future are also considered. Submucosal fibroids and future gestational desire are indications for treatment, even in asymptomatic patients. However, the fibroid's size by itself does not suggest a course of action. Medical and surgical treatment are the two main approaches to treating fibroids; these will be discussed in more detail below.

5.4.5.1. Medical Treatment

Combination oral contraceptives, levonorgestrel intrauterine devices (LNG-IUDs), progestins, gonadotropin-releasing hormone (GnRH) agonists, androgenic steroids, and selective progesterone receptor modulators (SPRMs) are among the hormonal treatments used to treat uterine fibroids.

Studies showing that the use of combined oral contraceptives prevents the formation of fibroids but does not reduce their size are available. Oral contraceptives are helpful for pelvic pain, bleeding, and changes in ovulation that are linked to fibroids, but they are not effective in controlling the size of the tumor or compressive symptomatology.

For AUB, controlling heavy menstrual bleeding (HMB), treating anemia, and providing contraception, LNG-IUD is recommended. Due to cavity distortion, there is a relative contraindication in submucosal fibroids because women with fibroids may have higher expulsion rates from LNG-IUDs. Progestin-containing medications also lessen the amount of bleeding brought on by endometrial atrophy.

One useful medical intervention for uterine fibroids is the use of GnRH agonists. They are beneficial in preventing blood loss (amenorrhea), which makes the presurgical anemic syndrome treatable. Furthermore, they have the potential to reduce tumor size by 50–70%, which could facilitate vaginal or laparoscopic surgery or allow for a different type of abdominal approach incision. Its side effects (hypoestrogenism) restrict its use to six months, and the year after stopping it usually sees the uterine volume return to normal. They cause reversible climacteric symptomatology and only when treatments are received for longer than 12 months do they raise the risk of osteoporosis.

The most popular is leuprolide acetate, which the US Food and Drug Administration (FDA) has approved for use in treating women's fibroids and anemia before surgery. It should be mentioned that if it is used before a myomectomy, it interferes with the cleavage plane and does not facilitate surgery. Therefore, it is only recommended in the aforementioned situations: pre-hysteroscopic resection of submucosal fibroids, restoration of hematological parameters in cases of severe anemia, and large volume less invasive surgery. For perimenopausal women, it would be a reasonable course of treatment to manage symptoms without resorting to surgery.

Danazol and gestrinone are examples of androgenic steroids. While they manage anemia linked to HMB, danazol does not lessen the volume of fibroids. Both of them have virilization-related side effects, and their limited effectiveness and/or side effects prevent their widespread use.

SPRM are substances that attach to progesterone receptors and alter transcription in a particular tissue type in a way that is favorable (e.g., progesterone, a pure agonist) or adverse (e.g., mifepristone, antagonistic pure) meaning. Both isoforms of PR are overexpressed in uterine fibroids.

- PG receptors in the myometrium and fibroid are reduced by mifepristone, also known as RU-486. It is comparable to GnRH agonists in that it lessens menstrual bleeding and can cause amenorrhea in up to 70% of cases. The FDA does not, however, support its use for fibroids due to the high daily doses needed and the documented cases of endometrial hyperplasia that go along with it.
- The EMA has authorized Ulipristal acetate (UPA) for use at a dose of 5 mg per day since 2012. It is currently approved for use as a single course of treatment before fibroids surgery for women with moderate-to-severe symptoms, as an intermittent treatment for women for whom surgery is not appropriate, and as preoperative treatment in patients with these conditions. In one week, UPA causes amenorrhea in 75% of patients and returns menstrual bleeding to normal in 90% of patients. It also similar to the analogs shrinks fibroids by about 30%, causing apoptosis and preventing cell division. This effect lasts for six months after treatment ends, and the proliferative phase of the estradiol levels results in fewer side effects. Menstruation and ovulation resume one month after treatment ends, and UPA restores quality of life test scores to levels seen in healthy women. The physiological alterations linked to progesterone receptors on the endometrium, known as Progesterone Associated Endometrial Changes, or PAECs, are reversible two months after the conclusion of treatment and do not indicate the need for additional testing or diagnosis. These offer the initial choice for uterine fibroids' long-term pharmacologic management.

Additionally, non-hormonal medical treatments, such as NSAIDs and anti-fibrinolytic drugs, are used, particularly for pain management. In contrast to AUB in a normal uterus, there is less data to support these medical interventions in the presence of uterine fibroids. Uterine fibroid-associated HMB can be successfully treated with tranexamic acid (Amchafibrin), an anti-fibrinolytic agent that the FDA approved in 2009 for this purpose.

NSAIDs lessen idiopathic AUB and the discomfort connected to dysmenorrhea, whether or not it is related to fibroids.

5.4.5.2. Surgical Treatment

For symptomatic patients (with bleeding and/or pelvic discomfort) who have been fully informed of the benefits, risks, and alternatives and do not wish to preserve their fertility, a hysterectomy is thought to be the definitive course of treatment. Additionally, it is linked to high patient satisfaction levels. Uterine fibroids are the most frequent cause of hysterectomy indications (uterine fibroids account for one out of every four hysterectomies performed). The most suitable methods are vaginal and laparoscopic procedures, provided they are technically possible.

For symptomatic women who want to keep their uterus because they want to have children or because they personally prefer to do so, a myomectomy is the recommended course of treatment. Compared to a hysterectomy, this procedure results in greater blood loss; the 5-year risk of recurrence is roughly 50–60%, according to ultrasound. In the following five to ten years, up to 10 to 25% of women who have myomectomy surgery will require a hysterectomy (particularly those with large uterine volumes and multiple fibroids). Patients should always be made aware of the possibility that a hysterectomy may be required in the extremely unlikely event that complications during myomectomy (1%) arise.

Regarding the overall quantity and size of fibroids and the surgical technique used to remove them, there are no set restrictions; instead, the method selected will be determined by the particulars of each case, the surgeon's experience, and the clinical judgment. According to the American Association of Gynecologic Laparoscopists, hysteroscopic myomectomy, also known as hysteroscopic resection, is the first-line surgical treatment for symptomatic fibroids type 0–1, type 2 up to 4 cm, and asymptomatic patients with reproductive desire.

5.4.5.3. Nonsurgical Alternatives

An alternative for premenopausal women with bleeding fibroids (single or multiple; subserosal pedunculated and fibroids >10 cm excluded) in which surgery is contraindicated or refused is selective uterine artery embolization (UAE). Women who would like to maintain their fertility should not have this procedure done. It necessitates an endometrial biopsy, MRI-arteriography, and ultrasound pre-embolization study. Under anesthesia, the femoral artery is used to gain access, and microparticles are then injected to obstruct both uterine arteries. Reducing the blood flow to the fibroids is intended to induce an infarction and eventually cause the fibroids to shrink. Although it is not a permanent cure in many cases, it is an effective treatment that reduces bleeding in 80–85% of cases and pain in 70–80% of patients. 10% of patients may need a hysterectomy, 3% may need a myomectomy, and 2% may need a new UAE at the five-year follow-up.

Serious complications include hemorrhage, persistent pain, expulsion of fibroids (especially submucous fibroids), bleeding after embolization (due to infection and uterine necrosis), and a mortality rate of approximately 0.3% associated with it.

With well-defined safety margins, coagulative necrosis is caused by a controlled temperature increase in magnetic resonance-guided focused ultrasound surgery (MRgFUS), which destroys the fibroids. As a result, fibroids become smaller and lose perfusion, which lessens symptoms. The fibroids are not gone entirely and will always be there. High-resolution ultrasound (USgFUS) or magnetic resonance imaging (MRI) can be used for image monitoring (MRgFUS, magnetic resonance-guided focused ultrasound surgery). It is recommended for premenopausal women who have finished gestational desire to control fibroid symptoms. It does not require anesthesia, but it does require a preoperative MRI study. Note that the majority of research is based on treating a maximum of four fibroids.

This minimally invasive therapy may not be recommended in fibroids >10 cm, hypervascularized fibroids, abdominal scars, and the presence of fixed intestinal adhesions, but it may be limited in cases of severe adenomyosis, ≥5 fibroids, intolerance to gadolinium, and fibroids presenting hyperintense signal in T2.

Very minor complications include fever, minor blood loss, grade I–II skin burns, and mild pain. No hysterectomies, ovarian lesions, or transfusions have been reported. Recurrences at the 24-month follow-up are associated with the treated area: approximately 15% of the total fibroid volume may require a myomectomy if the treated area accounts for more than 20% of the total.

Using a percutaneous radiofrequency handpiece with a deployable electrode array and a laparoscopic ultrasound probe to identify fibroids, the laparoscopic radiofrequency volumetric thermal ablation (RFVTA) technique is carried out. Upon removal, the insertion tract coagulates and the fibroids are ablated. The FDA approved it in 2012 for women who wanted a quick recovery (less blood loss during surgery and a shorter hospital stay). Although the evidence is currently limited, encouraging outcomes in terms of symptom control and enhanced quality of life have been documented. For symptomatic uterine myomas, transvaginal radiofrequency myolysis guided by ultrasound may be a practical, safe, and effective treatment. The myoma size and AUB of patients treated with this technique were reduced, and the Uterine Fibroids Symptom and Health-related Quality-of-life Questionnaire showed a significant clinical improvement. For uterine myoma with symptoms, laparoscopic cryomyolysis is a reliable and secure substitute procedure. It has been demonstrated to reduce fibroid size and alleviate symptoms, particularly AUB, at a 12-month follow-up (de Ziegler et al., 2010; Ahn et al., 2015; Clemenza et al., 2018; Agarwal et al., 2019).

A Closer Look

Uterine Fibroids and Reproduction

Pathophysiology of Uterine Fibroid-Related Infertility

Several mechanisms of action have been proposed to explain the impact of myomas on fertility. Changes in the anatomy of the endometrium may lead to obstruction of the fallopian tubes or endometrial cavity distortion. In the same line, functional changes such as increased uterine contractility may alter sperm progression. Also, abnormal blood supply due to fibroids may alter fertility, and chronic inflammation may play a role in altering the myometrial environment hindering implantation. Histological alterations, such as elongation/distortion of the glands, hyperplasia, polyposis, and ectasia may also impair implantation. Finally, an abnormal hormonal environment and fibroids' paracrine effects on the endometrium may also impact fertility. Cells involved in endometrial decidualization, such as macrophages and uterine natural killer cells, are also reduced in women with uterine fibroids, negatively affecting implantation. Molecular mechanisms underlying the effect for fibroids on fertility are unclear; however, uterine fibroids reduce endometrial HOXA-10 and HOXA-11 expression, which are factors that mediate stromal cell proliferation during implantation. Also, cytokines involved in implantation and early embryonic development are reduced in women with submucosal fibroids.

Uterine Fibroid-Related Infertility

When considering the type of fibroid and its impact on infertility, subserosal fibroids do not seem to have a significant effect on reproductive outcomes. Thus, there is no evidence of benefit on fertility when myomectomy is performed to remove subserosal fibroids.

In contrast, the effect of intramural fibroids on fertility is controversial, and it is still a matter of debate. Intramural fibroids have been associated with a negative effect on implantation, pregnancy/life birth, and spontaneous miscarriage. Sunkara et al. reported a significant decrease in pregnancy rates and in live birth in women presenting intramural fibroids undergoing IVF treatment. Additionally, it should be taken into account that number and size of intramural fibroids also play a role in infertility. When considering fibroid size, pieces of evidence point out that intramural fibroids ≥4 cm may also negatively influence fertility.

Regarding submucous fibroids, these have been clearly associated with a detrimental effect on implantation, pregnancy/life birth, and spontaneous miscarriage. Hence, benefits on fertility should be expected when fibroids are removed. In this line, evidence reported higher spontaneous pregnancy rates in women who undergo myomectomy versus non-myomectomized patients at 12 months after surgery. When patients underwent a myomectomy prior to IVF, higher pregnancy rates were observed compared to the non-myomectomized group. Additionally, surgery is a potential source of damage and must be taken into account. Surgery not only involves morbidity risk but also implies myometrial trauma, suturing and scar healing, and the potential development of defective functional myometrium and adhesions. Also, intrauterine adhesions correlate with a decrease in reproductive outcomes. Due to the increased uterine rupture risk involved in surgery, it is recommended to postpone future conception to 6 months after myomectomy.

During pregnancy, uterine fibroids have been associated with an increased risk of spontaneous miscarriage rates, complications, and adverse pregnancy outcomes. Fibroids adjacent to the placenta are prone to bleeding in early pregnancy and spontaneous miscarriage. In contrast, no difference is observed in preterm delivery rates among women with fibroids. Fibroid treatment may improve pregnancy outcome, although large randomized clinical trials are needed to support the limited data available. Also, timely treatment is crucial, since women who receive treatment early are more likely to have successful outcomes compared to women with long-duration infertility. In these women, the prognosis is worse irrespective of treatment

Following myomectomy is reported to cause a decrease in the miscarriage rate. Moreover, in women who underwent myomectomy for submucosal myomas, clinical pregnancy, live birth, and spontaneous abortion rates normalize over time, compared to infertile women without fibroids

After MRgFUS Surgery a high rate of pregnancies and deliveries has been reported; however, data are still preliminary. To note, the miscarriage rate reported after the procedure was 28%. UAE is not a treatment of first choice for women with infertility, since an increased risk of negative pregnancy outcome may be present following the procedure; however, it has not been adequately studied.

UPA is a novel and effective treatment used for fibroid reduction that shows feasible and safe conception, but also high miscarriage rates. Thus, the presence of fibroids impacts pregnancy rates, since pregnancy rates after myomectomy are higher than after reductive therapies (de Ziegler et al., 2010; Ahn et al., 2015; Clemenza et al., 2018; Agarwal et al., 2019).

Summary

- Reproductive health refers to the condition of male and female reproductive systems during all life stages. These systems are made of organs and hormone-producing glands, including the pituitary gland in the brain. Ovaries in females and testicles in males are reproductive organs, or gonads, that maintain the health of their respective systems. They also function as glands because they produce and release hormones.
- In women, numerous conditions can affect the reproductive system, such as cancer, uterine fibroids, endometriosis, ovarian cysts, infertility, and sexually transmitted diseases (STDs) and more.
- Endometriosis is a chronic benign disease characterized by the presence and proliferation of endometrial tissue outside the uterine cavity. The predominant location of endometriosis is the pelvic cavity, and the ovary is the most commonly affected organ; however endometrial tissue can be also found outside of the pelvis. Typically the disease interests women in their reproductive period and affects fertility and quality of life.
- Pain is the most common endometriosis symptom. However, not everyone with endometriosis experiences pain the same way.
- Infertility is a medical condition that can cause psychological, physical, mental, spiritual, and medical detriments to the patient. The unique quality of this medical condition involves affecting both the patient and the patient's partner as a couple.
- Sexually transmitted infections (STIs), or sexually transmitted diseases (STDs), are infections that are passed from one person to another through sexual contact. They are usually spread during vaginal, oral, or anal sex. But sometimes they can spread through other sexual contact involving the penis, vagina, mouth, or anus. This is because some STIs, like herpes and HPV, are spread by skin-to-skin contact.
- Gonorrhea, chlamydia, and trichomoniasis are common STIs that can lead to PID if left untreated. However, not all cases of PID are caused by an STI, as other bacterial infections can play a role.
- HIV can damage the immune system and increase the risk of contracting other viruses or bacteria and developing certain cancers. With today's treatments, many people with HIV live long, healthy lives. But if left untreated, the virus can lead to AIDS, where the body becomes vulnerable to serious infections and illnesses.
- Uterine fibroids (also called leiomyomas) are growths made of muscle and tissue that form in or on the wall of your uterus. These growths are usually not cancerous (benign) and are the most common noncancerous tumors in women and people assigned female at birth (AFAB).
- Uterine fibroids can cause a variety of symptoms like pain and heavy, irregular vaginal bleeding. Sometimes, a person has no symptoms and is unaware they have fibroids. Treatment for fibroids typically depends on your symptoms.

References

1. Agarwal, S. K., Chapron, C., Giudice, L. C., Laufer, M. R., Leyland, N., Missmer, S. A., Singh, S. S., & Taylor, H. S. (2019). Clinical diagnosis of endometriosis: A call to action. *American Journal of Obstetrics and Gynecology, 220*(4), 354.e1–354.e12. https://doi.org/10.1016/j.ajog.2018.12.039.
2. Ahn, S. H., Monsanto, S. P., Miller, C., Singh, S. S., Thomas, R., & Tayade, C. (2015). Pathophysiology and immune dysfunction in endometriosis. *BioMed Research International, 2015*, 795976. https://doi.org/10.1155/2015/795976.
3. Bourgioti, C., Preza, O., Panourgias, E., Chatoupis, K., Antoniou, A., Nikolaidou, M. E., & Moulopoulos, L. A. (2017). MR imaging of endometriosis: Spectrum of disease. *Diagnostic and Interventional Imaging, 98*(11), 751–767. https://doi.org/10.1016/j.diii.2017.06.010.
4. Clemenza, S., Sorbi, F., Noci, I., Capezzuoli, T., Turrini, I., Carriero, C., Buffi, N., Fambrini, M., & Petraglia, F. (2018). From pathogenesis to clinical practice: Emerging medical treatments for endometriosis. *Best Practice & Research Clinical Obstetrics & Gynaecology, 51*, 92–101. https://doi.org/10.1016/j.bpobgyn.2018.07.010.
5. de Ziegler, D., Borghese, B., & Chapron, C. (2010). Endometriosis and infertility: Pathophysiology and management. *The Lancet, 376*(9742), 730–738. https://doi.org/10.1016/S0140-6736(10)60490-4.
6. Dovey, S., & Sanfilippo, J. (2010). Endometriosis and the adolescent. *Clinical Obstetrics and Gynecology, 53*(2), 420–428. https://doi.org/10.1097/GRF.0b013e3181db7bdb.
7. Dunselman, G. A., Vermeulen, N., Becker, C., et al. (2014). ESHRE guideline: Management of women with endometriosis. *Human Reproduction, 29*(3), 400–412. https://doi.org/10.1093/humrep/det457.
8. González-Foruria, I., Santulli, P., Chouzenoux, S., Carmona, F., Chapron, C., & Batteux, F. (2017). Dysregulation of the ADAM17/Notch signaling pathways in endometriosis: From oxidative stress to fibrosis. *Molecular Human Reproduction, 23*(7), 488–499. https://doi.org/10.1093/molehr/gax027.
9. Haas, D., Shebl, O., Shamiyeh, A., & Oppelt, P. (2013). The rASRM score and the Enzian classification for endometriosis: Their strengths and weaknesses. *Acta Obstetricia et Gynecologica Scandinavica, 92*(1), 3–7. https://doi.org/10.1111/aogs.12008.
10. Hufnagel, D., Li, F., Cosar, E., Krikun, G., & Taylor, H. S. (2015). The role of stem cells in the etiology and pathophysiology of endometriosis. *Seminars in Reproductive Medicine, 33*(5), 333–340. https://doi.org/10.1055/s-0035-1567816.
11. Johnson, N. P., Hummelshoj, L., Adamson, G. D., Keckstein, J., Taylor, H. S., Abrao, M. S., Bush, D., Kiesel, L., Tamimi, R., Sharpe-Timms, K. L., Rombauts, L., & Giudice, L. C. (2017). World endometriosis society consensus on the classification of endometriosis. *Human Reproduction, 32*(2), 315–324. https://doi.org/10.1093/humrep/dew293.
12. Machairiotis, N., Stylianaki, A., Dryllis, G., Zarogoulidis, P., Kouroutou, P., Tsiamis, N., Katsikogiannis, N., Sarika, E., Courcoutsakis, N., Tsiouda, T., Gschwendtner, A., Zarogoulidis, K., Sakkas, L., Baliaka, A., & Machairiotis, C. (2013). Extra pelvic endometriosis: A rare entity or an under diagnosed condition? *Diagnostic Pathology, 8*, 194. https://doi.org/10.1186/1746-1596-8-194.

13. Muzii, L., Bianchi, A., Bellati, F., Cristi, E., Pernice, M., Zullo, M. A., Angioli, R., & Panici, P. B. (2007). Histologic analysis of endometriomas: What the surgeon needs to know. *Fertility and Sterility, 87*(2), 362–366. https://doi.org/10.1016/j.fertnstert.2006.06.040.

14. Novembri, R., Borges, L. E., Carrarelli, P., Rocha, A. L., De Pascalis, F., Florio, P., & Petraglia, F. (2011). Impaired CRH and urocortin expression and function in eutopic endometrium of women with endometriosis. *Journal of Clinical Endocrinology & Metabolism, 96*(4), 1145–1150. https://doi.org/10.1210/jc.2010-2121.

15. Parazzini, F., Esposito, G., Tozzi, L., Noli, S., & Bianchi, S. (2017). Epidemiology of endometriosis and its comorbidities. *European Journal of Obstetrics & Gynecology and Reproductive Biology, 209*, 3–7. https://doi.org/10.1016/j.ejogrb.2016.04.021.

16. Proctor, M., Latthe, P., Farquhar, C., Khan, K., & Johnson, N. (2005). Surgical interruption of pelvic nerve pathways for primary and secondary dysmenorrhea. *Cochrane Database of Systematic Reviews, 2005*(4), CD001896. https://doi.org/10.1002/14651858.CD001896.pub.

17. Tosti, C., Biscione, A., Morgante, G., Bifulco, G., Luisi, S., & Petraglia, F. (2017). Hormonal therapy for endometriosis: From molecular research to bedside. *European Journal of Obstetrics & Gynecology and Reproductive Biology, 209*, 61–66. https://doi.org/10.1016/j.ejogrb.2016.12.032.

18. Tosti, C., Pinzauti, S., Santulli, P., Chapron, C., & Petraglia, F. (2015). Pathogenetic mechanisms of deep infiltrating endometriosis. *Reproductive Sciences, 22*(9), 1053–1059. https://doi.org/10.1177/1933719115584444.

19. Vercellini, P., Buggio, L., Berlanda, N., Barbara, G., Somigliana, E., & Bosari, S. (2016). Estrogen-progestins and progestins for the management of endometriosis. *Fertility and Sterility, 106*(7), 1552–1571. https://doi.org/10.1016/j.fertnstert.2016.09.005.

20. Vercellini, P., Viganò, P., Somigliana, E., & Fedele, L. (2014). Endometriosis: Pathogenesis and treatment. *Nature Reviews Endocrinology, 10*(5), 261–275. https://doi.org/10.1038/nrendo.2013.255.

21. Vilos, G. A., Allaire, C., Laberge, P.-Y., Leyland, N., Vilos, A. G., Murji, A., & et al. (2015). The management of uterine leiomyomas. *Journal of Obstetrics and Gynaecology Canada, 37*(2), 157–178. https://doi.org/10.1016/S1701-2163(15)30338-8.

22. Wilbur, M. A., Shih, I. M., Segars, J. H., & Fader, A. N. (2017). Cancer implications for patients with endometriosis. *Seminars in Reproductive Medicine, 35*(1), 110–116. https://doi.org/10.1055/s-0036-1597126.

23. Zupi, E., Centini, G., Sabbioni, L., Lazzeri, L., Argay, I. M., & Petraglia, F. (2016). Nonsurgical alternatives for uterine fibroids. *Best Practice & Research Clinical Obstetrics & Gynecology, 34*, 122–131. https://doi.org/10.1016/j.bpobgyn.2015.11.014.

Chapter

SYMPTOMS OF STOMACH AND DIGESTIVE DISEASES

6

Contents

Introduction

Stomach and digestive diseases encompass a wide range of conditions that affect the gastrointestinal tract, resulting in diverse symptoms that can significantly impact an individual's health and well-being. Abdominal pain is a common symptom across many digestive disorders, varying from mild discomfort to severe cramping or sharp pains. Bloating and distension often accompany abdominal pain, contributing to feelings of discomfort and fullness. Nausea and vomiting may occur due to various causes, including inflammation, infection, or obstruction within the digestive system. Diarrhea and constipation represent opposite ends of the spectrum of bowel movement changes and can result from conditions such as gastroenteritis, irritable bowel syndrome (IBS), or bowel obstruction. Changes in appetite or weight, such as unintended weight loss or gain, may indicate underlying digestive issues, including malabsorption disorders or malignancies. Heartburn, characterized by a burning sensation in the chest or throat, is a hallmark symptom of gastroesophageal reflux disease (GERD), often exacerbated by lying down or consuming certain foods. Indigestion, or dyspepsia, encompasses a range of symptoms, including upper abdominal discomfort, fullness, and bloating, often occurring after meals. Excessive gas, belching, and flatulence can result from the fermentation of undigested food by gut bacteria or swallowing excess air. More serious conditions, such as gastritis, peptic ulcers, and gastrointestinal bleeding, may present with symptoms such as persistent abdominal pain, black or bloody stools, or vomiting blood. Inflammatory bowel diseases (IBD), including Crohn's disease and ulcerative colitis, are chronic conditions characterized by inflammation of the gastrointestinal tract, leading to symptoms such as diarrhea, abdominal pain, rectal bleeding, fatigue, and weight loss. Irritable bowel syndrome (IBS) is a functional gastrointestinal disorder characterized by abdominal pain or discomfort, along with changes in bowel habits, without evidence of structural abnormalities. Extra-intestinal symptoms, such as joint pain, skin rashes, or eye inflammation, may occur in some digestive disorders, including celiac disease, inflammatory bowel disease (IBD), and autoimmune gastritis. Prompt evaluation by a healthcare professional is crucial for diagnosing and managing stomach and digestive diseases, as early intervention can help alleviate symptoms, prevent complications, and improve quality of life. Treatment approaches may include dietary modifications, medication therapy, lifestyle changes, and, in some cases, surgical intervention, tailored to address the underlying cause of the condition and alleviate symptoms effectively.

Orientation and Directional Terms

Term	Definition	Illustration
Gastroesophageal Reflux Disease (GERD)	Gastroesophageal reflux disease (GERD) is a common condition in which the stomach contents move up into the esophagus.	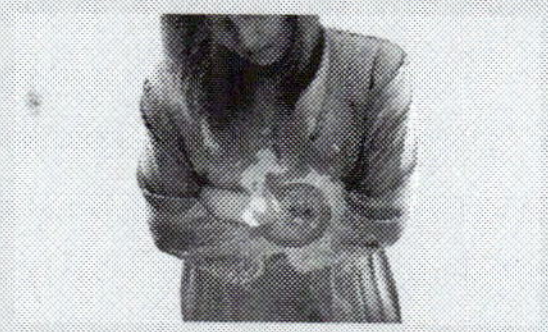
Irritable Bowel Syndrome (IBS)	Irritable bowel syndrome (IBS) is a common condition characterized by abdominal discomfort associated with altered bowel movements and is currently diagnosed according to the new Rome IV criteria.	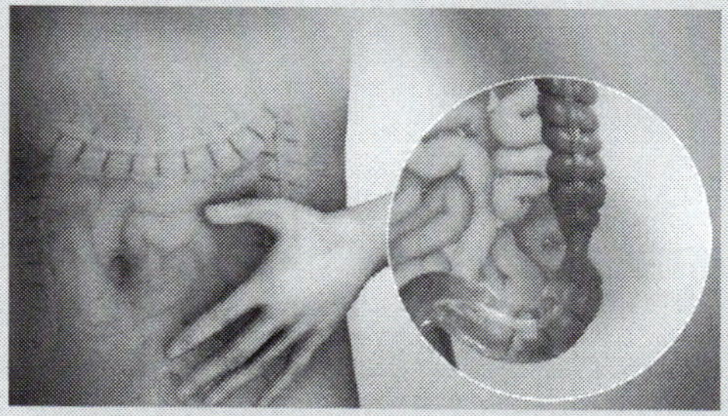
Crohn's Disease	Crohn's disease is a type of inflammatory bowel disease (IBD). It causes swelling of the tissues (inflammation) in your digestive tract, which can lead to abdominal pain, severe diarrhea, fatigue, weight loss and malnutrition.	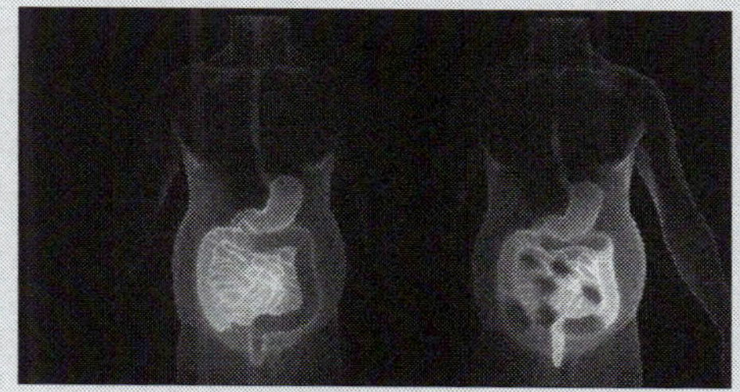
Anal Fissure	Anal fissure is a small tear in the thin, moist tissue that lines the anus. The anus is the muscular opening at the end of the digestive tract where stool exits the body. Common causes of an anal fissure include constipation and straining or passing hard or large stools during a bowel movement.	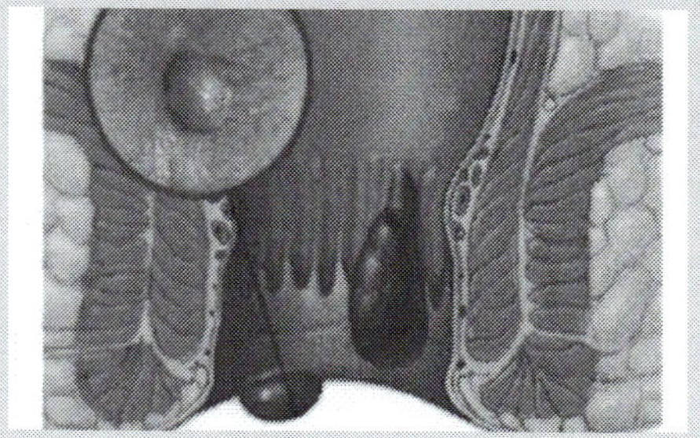
Lower Esophageal Sphincter (LES)	Lower esophageal sphincter (LES) is a high-pressure zone located where the esophagus meets the stomach and protects the esophagus from the reflux of gastric contents. The LES is composed of intrinsic and extrinsic components.	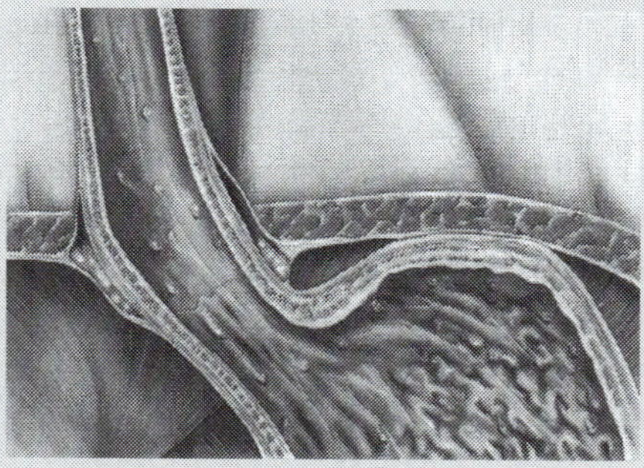

6.1. Rectal Bleeding

The passage of bright red blood from the rectum or anus is referred to as rectal bleeding or hematochezia. The severity can vary, from minor bleeding that fills the toilet bowl to substantial bleeding that leaves tiny amounts of blood on toilet paper or in the stool. Hemorrhoids, anal fissures, constipation, and inflammatory bowel disorders like ulcerative colitis or Crohn's disease are some of the conditions that can result in rectal bleeding. Colorectal cancer, diverticulosis, colorectal polyps, and gastrointestinal infections are further possible causes. Even though rectal bleeding might not always point to a dangerous underlying illness, it should be examined right away by a medical expert to ascertain the cause and the best course of action. Sometimes symptoms like weakness, weariness, bowel habit changes, abdominal pain, or inadvertent weight loss accompany rectal bleeding. These symptoms could point to a more serious issue that needs to be looked into further. The management of rectal bleeding is contingent upon the underlying cause and may involve dietary adjustments, medication, minimally invasive procedures, or surgery, as determined by a medical professional. Effective management of rectal bleeding and the avoidance of possible complications depend on early diagnosis and intervention (Figure 6.1).

- **How Does Rectal Bleeding Appear?:** You might see or experience rectal bleeding in a few different ways, including:
    - o Noticing fresh blood on your toilet paper when you wipe.
    - o Seeing blood in the bowl of the toilet after you use the bathroom. The water in the bowl might look like it is been dyed red.
    - o Seeing bright red, dark red or tarry black poop in the toilet.

Rectal bleeding is the term used to describe bleeding that originates from the butthole, but it can actually originate from anywhere in your gastrointestinal (GI) tract. All gastrointestinal bleeding exits through the same route, which runs through your stomach, small intestine, colon, rectum, and anus.

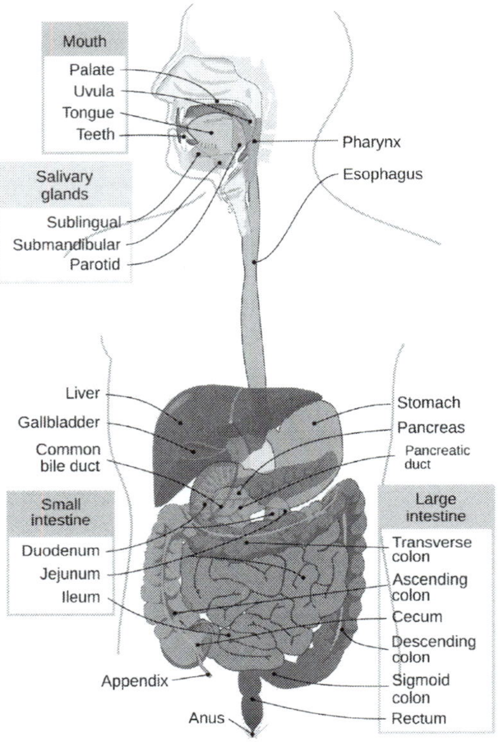

Figure 6.1. *The tract.*

By Mariana Ruiz, Jmarchn – Own work, Public Domain, https://commons.wikimedia.org/w/index.php?curid=2898771.

- **What Does Blood in Stool Look Like?:** There are various ways that blood can appear in your stool. Blood clots, bright red streaks of blood, or a mixture of blood and mucus could be visible in your poop. Additionally, your stool may appear tarry, dark, and black. The color of the blood you see may be a clue to where it is coming from:

- Bright red blood in your stool usually means the bleeding is lower in your colon, rectum or anus.
- Dark red or maroon blood can mean that you have bleeding higher up in your colon or your small intestine.
- Melena (black stool) often points to bleeding in your stomach, such as a bleeding stomach ulcer.

Rectal bleeding occasionally hides from view and is only detectable under a microscope. We refer to this as occult bleeding. If you have a fecal occult blood test, which is a laboratory test performed on a stool sample, you might find this kind of blood in your stool. It is a colorectal cancer screening test.

- **Is Blood in Your Stool Serious?:** Not always, but it is possible. Consultation with a healthcare provider is advised whenever you experience rectal bleeding or blood in your stool. While in certain cases minor conditions may not require treatment, in others they may. Additionally, rectal bleeding may indicate a more serious ailment that requires medical attention.
- **Is Bright Red Blood in My Stool Worse Than Darker Blood?:** The presence of bright red blood in your stool may be more concerning as it indicates bleeding that is ongoing. Darker blood typically indicates past bleeding that has stopped. However, darker blood in your stool can be misinterpreted. It simply indicates that the bleeding is coming from a higher place, not necessarily that it has stopped. It takes longer for bleeding from your upper gastrointestinal tract to leave your body and exit your nose. The chemicals used in digestion cause it to gradually darken as it moves. The blood is bright red and comes from below. It might be the result of something fairly innocuous, like a flesh wound. There is less chance that an upper GI bleed will be innocuous.
- **When Should You Worry About Blood in Your Stool?:** Consulting a healthcare professional regarding blood in your stool is always beneficial, particularly if:
    - **You Don't Know Why it is Happening:** Rectal bleeding can occasionally be connected to a medical condition you already know you have. If you have bleeding when you have diarrhea, constipation, or a chronic bowel illness, you may not be very surprised. However, it is more unexpected and worrisome if blood in your stool is the first indication of any gastrointestinal ailment.
    - **It is Painful:** Pain is always a warning sign that your body needs to be attended to. Take note of the pain's location. It might be a new wound if it is in your rectum or anus. Lower abdominal pain may indicate colitis, an inflammatory condition affecting the lining of the colon that can have a variety of causes. It could be your stomach if you have black stools and upper abdominal pain.

- **It is Heavy or Frequent:** Heavy or frequent bleeding is more likely to lead to serious blood loss, including anemia and, in rare cases, hypovolemic shock. If you have sudden severe bleeding, or if you've had consistent bleeding for several days, seek healthcare right away. If you have a sudden drop in blood pressure and feel lightheaded or like you're fainting, go to the emergency room (ER).
- **It is Been Going on for a Week or Longer:** Long-term rectal bleeding requires medical attention, even if you're not bleeding heavily or experiencing any pain. Over time, slow bleeding can still result in a large loss of blood. Above all, it is an indication of a non-improving condition. In addition to causing blood in your stool, that condition might be causing other harm.

6.1.1. Causes Of Rectal Bleeding

Hematochezia can occur for a variety of reasons, including rectal bleeding or blood in the stool. These causes range from common and benign conditions to uncommon and severe conditions that require emergency care. Other symptoms may occasionally provide hints as to the underlying cause.

Common causes of rectal bleeding include:

- **Hemorrhoids:** Veins inside your rectum or anus that are enlarged are called hemorrhoids, or piles. They are the most frequent cause of rectal bleeding and are extremely common. These veins protrude near the skin's surface, and occasionally the skin bursts and the veins bleed. They aren't sincere. Usually, they have to do with pressure or straining, such as when lifting heavy objects, pregnant, or trying to urinate.
- **Anal Fissure:** A tear in the anal canal lining is called an anal fissure. It frequently occurs after straining to pass a hard stool, much like a hemorrhoid. Hemorrhoids can be mistaken for anal fissures. They are related to constipation and have the potential to result in bleeding and anal pain. There may be more pain in a fissure. While either can mend on its own, fissures occasionally require medical attention.
- **Inflammatory Bowel Disease (IBD):** The small and large intestine linings become chronically inflamed when you have inflammatory bowel disease (IBD). Your small intestine is primarily affected by Crohn's disease, whereas your large intestine is primarily affected by ulcerative colitis. In addition to chronic diarrhea and abdominal pain, inflammatory bowel disease (IBD) can also result in bleeding.
- **Diverticulitis:** The colon, usually near the lower end near the rectum, is where diverticulitis develops. It arises from the infection and inflammation of diverticula, which are tiny pockets in the inner lining of your colon. These pockets can become more prone to rupturing due to inflammation, which weakens the blood vessels within. Urinary tract bleeding may occur if this occurs.

Other possible causes include:

- **Infectious Colitis:** Certain bacterial infections, such as *E. coli* and *C. difficile*, which can result in hemorrhagic colitis, or colon bleeding. Usually, this manifests as bloody diarrhea. If you have an infection, you'll know it, and it usually goes away on its own. But antibiotics might be required for some infections. Make contact with your healthcare provider if your illness persists for more than a few days.
- **Sexually Transmitted Infections (STIs):** Certain common STIs can cause inflammation and bleeding in your anal or rectal lining, including gonorrhea, chlamydia and syphilis. Herpes causes sores that may bleed and human papillomavirus (HPV) causes anal warts that may bleed a little. Most STIs need specific treatment, so it is important to get diagnosed and inform sexual contacts. In many countries, it is mandatory to report STIs.
- **Peptic Ulcer Disease:** The top of your small intestine, the duodenum, is where peptic ulcers occur. They develop when the lining of the stomach is worn down by stomach acid, resulting in open sores. An ulcer can bleed and produce a burning or gnawing type of stomach pain. Blood in your upper gastrointestinal tract may appear dark, black, and tarry because it takes longer to drain.
- **Colon Polyps and Colorectal Cancer:** A polyp may resemble a mushroom that is protruding from your colon's side. Larger polyps may bleed, and they are frequently seen. They can develop into cancer at times, and malignant polyps bleed more frequently than non-cancerous ones. To rule out colon cancer, your healthcare provider might want to perform a colonoscopy to look into any unexplained rectal bleeding.

6.1.2. Treatment for Rectal Bleeding

Treatment for rectal bleeding depends on the underlying cause and severity of the condition. Here are some common approaches:

- **Hemorrhoids:** For mild cases of rectal bleeding due to hemorrhoids, over-the-counter remedies such as topical creams, ointments, or suppositories containing hydrocortisone or witch hazel may help reduce inflammation and discomfort. Increasing fiber intake, staying hydrated, and avoiding straining during bowel movements can also alleviate symptoms. In more severe cases, minimally invasive procedures such as rubber band ligation or infrared coagulation may be performed to shrink or remove hemorrhoids.
- **Anal Fissures:** Treatment for anal fissures often involves measures to promote healing and reduce pain, such as using topical ointments containing calcium channel blockers or nitroglycerin to relax the anal sphincter and improve blood flow to the area. Sitz baths, which involve soaking the anal area in warm water, can also provide relief and promote healing. In refractory

cases, surgical intervention may be necessary to repair the fissure or reduce sphincter pressure.

- **Inflammatory Bowel Disease (IBD):** Managing rectal bleeding associated with inflammatory bowel disease (such as Crohn's disease or ulcerative colitis) typically involves a combination of medications to reduce inflammation and suppress the immune system, such as corticosteroids, immunomodulators, or biologic therapies. In addition to medication, dietary modifications, stress management techniques, and lifestyle changes may help manage symptoms and reduce flare-ups.
- **Colorectal Polyps or Cancer:** Treatment for rectal bleeding caused by colorectal polyps or cancer depends on the stage and extent of the disease. Options may include surgical removal of polyps or tumors, chemotherapy, radiation therapy, or a combination of treatments. Early detection through regular screening, such as colonoscopy, is crucial for identifying and treating colorectal cancer at its earliest stages.
- **Gastrointestinal Bleeding:** Treatment for gastrointestinal bleeding causing rectal bleeding may involve hospitalization for monitoring and supportive care, along with interventions such as endoscopy to identify and treat the source of bleeding, blood transfusions to replace lost blood, and medication to reduce stomach acid and promote healing of ulcers.
- **Anemia:** If rectal bleeding leads to iron deficiency anemia, treatment may involve iron supplementation, dietary changes to increase iron intake, and addressing the underlying cause of the bleeding to prevent further loss of blood and nutrients.

It is important for individuals experiencing rectal bleeding to seek medical evaluation and appropriate treatment to determine the underlying cause and prevent potential complications. Treatment should be tailored to the individual's specific condition, medical history, and overall health (Walsh et al., 2018).

6.2. Gastroesophageal Reflux Disease (GERD)

The chronic upper gastrointestinal illness known as gastroesophageal reflux disease (GERD) or gastro-oesophageal reflux disease (GORD) is characterized by a persistent and regular reflux of stomach contents into the esophagus, which can lead to symptoms and/or complications. There are two types of GERD: non-erosive GERD (no lesions visible in the esophageal mucosa) and erosive GERD (presence of esophageal mucosal breaks at endoscopy). There are two categories of GERD symptoms: extraesophageal and esophageal symptoms. The two most common esophageal symptoms are regurgitation and heartburn. Regurgitation is the feeling of an acidic substance flowing into the mouth or hypopharynx, while heartburn is the burning sensation in the retrosternal area. Symptoms of extra-esophageal reflux include cough, dysphagia, sore throat, and disturbed sleep.

Additional conditions referred to as "atypical manifestations," or "extra esophageal manifestations," can be broadly categorized into three categories: breathing manifestations, thoracic atypical pain, and manifestations in the oral cavity and otorhino-laryngea region. GERD can occur in people without heartburn symptoms, so those who have asthma, a dry cough, or trouble swallowing could also have this digestive illness. When a patient exhibits one of the following hallmark symptoms, upper gastrointestinal endoscopy confirms that the patient has gastroesophageal reflux disease (GERD): (i) painful reflux and/or heartburn more than twice a week; (ii) erosions of the esophagus near the junction with the stomach; and (iii) abnormal 24-hour esophageal pH monitoring values.

Nowadays GERD is considered a chronic entity that must be treated correctly. This is important considering that permanent acid reflux can induce esophageal complications such as esophagitis (i.e., inflammation of the esophageal mucosa), hemorrhage, Barrett's esophagus, and adenocarcinoma in the esophagus (Figure 6.2).

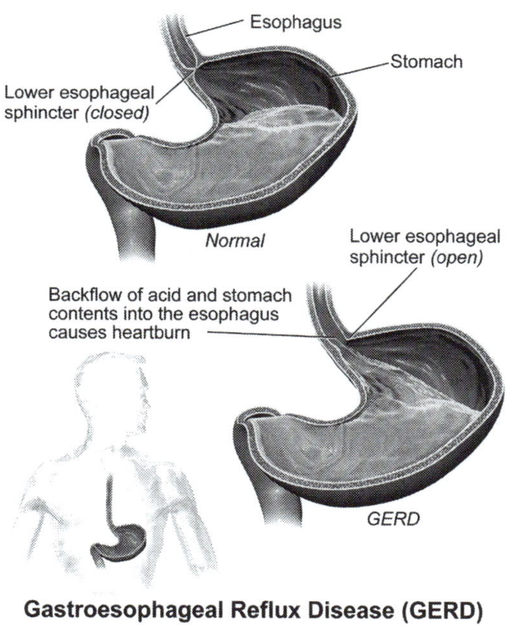

Figure 6.2. *Gastroesophageal reflux disease (GERD).*

By BruceBlaus – Own work, CC BY-SA 4.0, https://commons.wikimedia.org/w/index.php?curid=44923646.

6.2.1. GERD Causes

The stomach and esophagus are referred to as "gastroesophageal." Reflux is the verb for return or flow back. The term "gastric reflux" refers to the reflux of stomach contents into the esophagus. Your LES opens to let food enter your stomach during normal digestion. Subsequently, it shuts to prevent food particles and stomach acid from returning to your esophagus. When the LES is weak or relaxes when it shouldn't, it can lead to gastroesophageal reflux disease. This permits the contents of the stomach to ascend into the esophagus.

Several factors can contribute to GERD:

1. **Hiatal Hernia:** This occurs when the upper part of the stomach moves up into the chest through a small opening in the diaphragm (hiatus). Hiatal hernias can weaken the lower esophageal sphincter (LES), allowing acid to reflux into the esophagus.
2. **Weak Lower Esophageal Sphincter (LES):** The LES is a ring of muscle at the junction of the esophagus and stomach. Normally, it acts as a valve to prevent stomach acid from backing up into the esophagus. If it weakens or relaxes abnormally, acid can reflux.
3. **Dietary Factors:** Certain foods and beverages can trigger or worsen GERD symptoms. These may include spicy foods, fatty foods, citrus fruits, tomatoes, chocolate, caffeine, and alcohol.
4. **Obesity:** Excess weight, particularly around the abdomen, can put pressure on the stomach and LES, increasing the risk of acid reflux.
5. **Pregnancy:** Hormonal changes and the growing uterus can put pressure

on the stomach, leading to GERD symptoms during pregnancy.

6. **Smoking:** Smoking weakens the LES and can also stimulate acid production in the stomach, making reflux more likely.
7. **Certain Medications:** Some medications can relax the LES or irritate the esophagus, leading to GERD symptoms. These may include certain asthma medications, calcium channel blockers, antihistamines, painkillers, and sedatives.
8. **Delayed Stomach Emptying (Gastroparesis):** When the stomach takes longer than normal to empty its contents, there's a higher chance of reflux.
9. **Connective Tissue Disorders:** Conditions like scleroderma and Ehlers-Danlos syndrome can weaken the connective tissues throughout the body, including those in the LES.
10. **Smaller Factors:** Other factors that may contribute to GERD include stress, lack of sleep, certain medical conditions like diabetes, and genetic predisposition.

Managing GERD typically involves lifestyle changes, such as dietary modifications, weight loss, avoiding triggers, and medications to reduce acid production or strengthen the LES. In severe cases, surgery may be recommended to strengthen the LES or repair a hiatal hernia.

6.2.2. Risk Factors for GERD

More than 60 million American adults experience heartburn monthly, with over 15 million experiencing it daily, including many pregnant women. Recent research has found that gastroesophageal reflux disease (GERD) is more common in infants and children than previously believed, leading to frequent vomiting and respiratory issues like coughing. Some medical professionals believe that a hiatal hernia may contribute to GERD by weakening the lower esophageal sphincter (LES). A hiatal hernia occurs when the upper portion of the stomach protrudes into the chest through a small opening in the diaphragm known as the diaphragmatic hiatus. Studies suggest that this opening in the diaphragm plays a role in supporting the lower esophagus.

Many people who have a hiatal hernia do not experience reflux or heartburn. However, stomach contents may reflux more readily into the esophagus if you have a hiatal hernia. A hiatal hernia can develop as a result of vomiting, coughing, straining, or abrupt physical activity that increases abdominal pressure. A small one is present in many otherwise healthy adults over 50. All ages are affected by hiatal hernias, despite the fact that they typically occur in middle age. Most of the time, hiatal hernias heal on their own. However, it might be required if the hernia is at risk of being twisted into a strangulation or severing the blood supply. If you have one and severe GERD or esophagitis (esophageal inflammation), you might also need to treat it. Your physician might operate to reduce the size of the hernia or avoid strangulation.

Several other things can make it more likely that you'll have GERD:

- Being overweight or obese
- Pregnancy
- Delayed emptying of the stomach (gastroparesis)
- Diseases of connective tissue such as rheumatoid arthritis, scleroderma, or lupus

Diet and lifestyle choices may make acid reflux worse if you already have it:

- Smoking

- Certain foods and drinks, including chocolate and fatty or fried foods, coffee, and alcohol
- Large meals
- Eating too soon before bed
- Certain medications, including aspirin

6.2.3. GERD Symptoms

Acid reflux disease, also known as heartburn, is the most typical GERD symptom. Usually, it feels like a searing pain in your chest that travels up to your neck and throat from behind your breastbone. A lot of people report feeling as though food is returning to their mouths, leaving behind an acidic or bitter taste. Heartburn can cause pressure, burning, or pain that lasts for up to two hours. Usually, it gets worse after eating. Additionally, bending over or lying down can cause heartburn. Many people find that standing up straight or taking an antacid that removes acid from the esophagus helps them feel better.

There are distinctions between the pain of heartburn and that of heart disease or a heart attack, which is sometimes the case. Pain from heart disease may get worse with exercise and get better with rest. Physical activity has a lower correlation with heartburn pain. You can't tell the difference, though, so if you experience any chest pain, get medical attention straight away.

Besides pain, you may also have

- Nausea
- Bad breath
- Trouble breathing
- A hard time swallowing
- Vomiting
- Wearing away of tooth enamel
- A lump in your throat

If you have acid reflux at night, you may also have:

- A lingering cough
- Laryngitis
- Asthma that comes on suddenly or gets worse
- Sleep problems

6.2.4. GERD Treatment and Home Remedies

The goal of GERD treatment is to reduce reflux or the harm that refluxed materials cause to the lining of the esophagus.

Your doctor may recommend over-the-counter or prescription medications to treat your symptoms.

- **Antacids:** These medications can help prevent heartburn by neutralizing stomach and esophageal acid. A lot of people discover that over-the-counter antacids offer fleeting or incomplete relief. For certain people, combining an antacid with a foaming agent is helpful. Scientists believe that these substances create a foam layer over the stomach to prevent acid reflux. However, prolonged use of antacids can result in adverse effects such as magnesium accumulation, diarrhea, and altered calcium metabolism, which is a change in how the body breaks down and uses calcium. A high magnesium intake can be dangerous for those with renal disease. See your doctor if you require antacids for a period longer than two weeks.
- **H2 Blockers:** In cases of persistent reflux and heartburn, the physician might suggest drugs that lower stomach acid. Among these medications are H2 blockers, which

assist in preventing the stomach's production of acid. Cimetidine (Tagamet), famotidine (Pepcid), and nizatidine are examples of H2 blockers. Acid pumps, also known as proton pump inhibitors (PPIs), are medications that obstruct a protein required for the production of stomach acid. PPIs consist of pantoprazole (Protonix), rabeprazole (Aciphex), omeprazole (Prilosec), lansoprazole (Prevacid), esomeprazole (Nexium), and dexlansoprazole (Dexilant).

- **Prokinetics:** While rare, prokinetic drugs can accelerate stomach emptying, reducing leftover acid and alleviating symptoms such as bloating, nausea, and vomiting. However, these medications can also cause severe side effects, limiting their use to only those who can tolerate them for a short duration. Examples of prokinetics include domperidone and metoclopramide (Clopra, Maxolon, Metozolv, Reglan).

6.2.5. Diet and Lifestyle Changes

Doctors advise you to modify your lifestyle in a few ways to help reduce your GERD symptoms.

- **Avoid Foods and Beverages Triggers:** Foods like chocolate, peppermint, fatty foods, caffeine, and alcoholic beverages should be avoided as they can relax the LES. Citrus fruits and juices, tomato products, and pepper are among the foods and drinks that should be avoided if they cause symptoms due to their potential to irritate a damaged esophageal lining.
- **Eat Smaller Servings:** Reducing the size of meals may also aid in symptom management. Additionally, eating meals two to three hours before going to bed allows your stomach to partially empty and reduce acid production.
- **Eat Slowly:** Take your time at every meal.
- **Chew Your Food Thoroughly:** It may help you remember to do this if you set your fork down after you take a bite. Pick it up again only when you've completely chewed and swallowed that bite.
- **Stop Smoking:** Cigarette smoking weakens the LES. Stopping smoking is important to reduce GERD symptoms.
- **Elevate Your Head:** Gravity can reduce the amount that refluxes into your esophagus when you sleep on a specially made wedge or raise the head of your bed on 6-inch blocks. Avoid using pillows as self-support. That only makes the stomach feel more compressed.
- **Stay at a Healthy Weight:** Symptoms are frequently made worse by obesity. When they lose weight, many overweight people experience relief.
- **Wear Loose Clothes:** Clothes that squeeze your waist put pressure on your belly and the lower part of your esophagus.
- **Acupuncture:** In one study, acupuncture treatment more effectively and durably stopped reflux in the test group than PPIs. Although larger studies are necessary to verify this, preliminary findings are encouraging.

6.2.6. Severe GERD Diagnosis

You might require testing to get a more accurate diagnosis if you have severe, chronic reflux disease or if treatment doesn't improve your symptoms. Your doctor may use one or more procedures to do this:

- **Endoscopy:** To check for tissue irritation or inflammation (esophagitis), your doctor may insert an endoscope—a tiny, lighted tube with a tiny video camera—into your esophagus. A small tissue sample may be removed for additional testing (biopsy) if the results are unusual or dubious.
- **Upper GI Series:** One of your doctor's initial tests might be this one. This type of X-ray displays your stomach, duodenum, and upper portion of your small intestine. It can help rule out other conditions, like peptic ulcers, but it provides limited information about potential reflux.
- **Esophageal Manometry and Impedance Study:** This test checks for low pressure in your esophagus. It can also show defects in how your esophageal muscles contract.
- **pH Testing:** Your doctor may use this test to measure the acid levels in your esophagus if a definitive diagnosis is difficult to make. It monitors your esophageal acid production during meals, physical activity, and sleep. This is a more useful tool now that longer-termpH tracking has been done using newer methods.

6.2.7. Surgery for Severe GERD

You might require GERD surgery if your symptoms cannot be controlled with medicine, you have a hiatal hernia, and you require frequent high doses of PPIs. However, you ought to exhaust all alternative therapies first.

- **Fundoplication**: Your lower esophageal pressure will rise as a result of this operation. Your stomach's upper region will be wound around the LES by the doctor. In order to stop reflux, this tightens the muscle and increases the pressure in your lower esophagus. They will either perform open surgery or use a laparoscope, which is a device that pokes tiny holes in the abdomen.
- **Transoral Incisionless Fundoplication (TIF)**: In a more recent version of the procedure, the stomach is wrapped around the LES with plastic fasteners using an endoscope, and a tiny tube with a camera. Compared to a standard fundoplication, it is less invasive.
- **Stretta Procedure**: Your LES will be reshaped by your doctor using low-radiofrequency heat and a tiny tube that is inserted down your esophagus.
- **LINX Surgery**: Your esophageal-gastric junction is bandaged by your physician with magnetic titanium beads. The beads' magnetic pull keeps it just tight enough to prevent reflux but loose enough to allow food to pass through into the stomach.

6.2.8. GERD Complications

Sometimes GERD leads to serious complications:

- **Esophageal Ulcer**: Your esophagus is eroded by stomach acid until an open sore appears. These sores may bleed and are frequently painful. They could make swallowing difficult.
- **Esophageal Stricture**: Scar tissue forms and the lower portion of your esophagus is damaged by stomach acid. The accumulation of scar tissue causes the esophagus to narrow, making it difficult to swallow food.
- **Barrett's Esophagus**: Acid reflux modifies the esophageal lining's cellular composition. The lining thickens and becomes crimson. This illness is associated with an increased risk of esophageal cancer.
- **Lung Problems**: Reflux can irritate and hurt your throat if it reaches the back. It can then enter the lungs through perspiration from there. You might get hoarse if this occurs. You might also be experiencing persistent coughing and chest congestion. You run the risk of developing pneumonia, bronchitis, and asthma if your lungs become inflamed (El-Serag et al., 2014; NIDDK, 2015).

6.3. Helicobacter Pylori Infection

Helicobacter pylori (*H. pylori*) is a type of bacteria that infects your stomach. It can damage the tissue in your stomach and the first part of your small intestine (the duodenum). Pain and inflammation may result from this. It may also occasionally result in excruciating lesions in your upper digestive tract known as peptic ulcers. *H. pylori* is widespread. It is possessed by many. The majority of those who have it won't experience any symptoms or ulcers. However, ulcers are mostly caused by it. The stomach lining that guards your stomach is attacked by *H. pylori*. Urease is an enzyme produced by the bacteria. This enzyme lowers the acidity of the stomach acids. It also thins the lining of your stomach. Therefore, the risk of damage to your stomach cells from strong digestive fluids like acid and pepsin is increased. That may result in duodenal or stomach sores or ulcers.

Helicobacter pylori infections can be asymptomatic for up to a lifetime or cause damage to the linings of the stomach and duodenum through inflammatory reactions brought on by a variety of mechanisms linked to multiple virulence factors. *H. pylori*-induced gastritis, an inflammation of the stomach lining that was added to the ICD11 list of diseases, can be initially caused by colonization. Untreated, this will develop into chronic gastritis. Peptic ulcers (duodenal or gastric) and stomach lining atrophy can result from chronic gastritis. These alterations could be interpreted as phases in Correa's cascade, the process by which gastric cancer develops. *H. pylori* has been connected to extragastric complications such as anemia from iron or vitamin B12 deficiency, diabetes, cardiovascular disease, and some neurological disorders.

Peptic ulcers are the result of inflammation that enables the digestive enzyme pepsin and stomach acid to overcome the mucous membranes' defenses. The acidity of the stomach influences the *H. pylori* colonization site, which in turn determines the ulcer's location. *H. pylori* colonizes in the duodenum's pyloric antrum (exit) of individuals who produce a lot of acid in order to evade the fundus, which is the stomach's entrance and home to parietal cells that secrete acid. G cells exhibit a comparatively elevated expression of PD-L1, which shields these cells from immune destruction brought on by *H. pylori*. *H. pylori* has the ability to colonize the remainder of the stomach in individuals who produce normal or decreased levels of acid. The hormone gastrin is secreted by G cells in the antrum as a result of an inflammatory response brought on by bacteria colonizing close to the pyloric antrum. This hormone then passes through the bloodstream to parietal cells in the fundus. In addition to increasing the amount of acid that the parietal cells secrete into the stomach lumen, glutathione also gradually increases the number of parietal cells. The duodenum is harmed by the elevated acid load, which may ultimately result in ulcer development.

Class I carcinogen *Helicobacter pylori* has been linked to gastric mucosa-associated lymphoid tissue (MALT) lymphomas and gastric cancer. Diffuse large B-cell lymphoma of the stomach is a rare but potentially fatal condition. Approximately 89% of stomach cancers are caused by *H. pylori* infection, which is also connected to the development of 55% of cancer cases globally. While data from various countries varies, in general, 1–3% of individuals with *Helicobacter pylori* infection go on to develop gastric cancer during their lifetime, compared to 0.13% of those without the infection. As of 2018, gastric cancer caused by *H. pylori* ranked third globally in terms of cancer-related death. Upon final diagnosis, gastric cancer is frequently fairly advanced due to its typical lack of symptoms. Upon initial diagnosis, over 50% of patients with gastric cancer have metastases to lymph nodes.

Chronic inflammation that is a feature of cancer development is characterized by infiltration of neutrophils and macrophages to the gastric epithelium, which favors the accumulation of pro-inflammatory cytokines, reactive oxygen species (ROS) and reactive nitrogen species (RNS) that cause DNA damage. The oxidative DNA damage and levels of oxidative stress can be indicated by a biomarker, 8-oxo-dG. Other damage to DNA includes double-strand breaks.

H. pylori gastritis-induced mucosal damage is more frequently observed in conjunction with small gastric and colorectal polyps, which are adenomas. Over time, larger polyps may develop into malignant ones. As of 2020, causality remained to be established despite a slight correlation between *H. pylori* and the emergence of colorectal cancers (Figure 6.3).

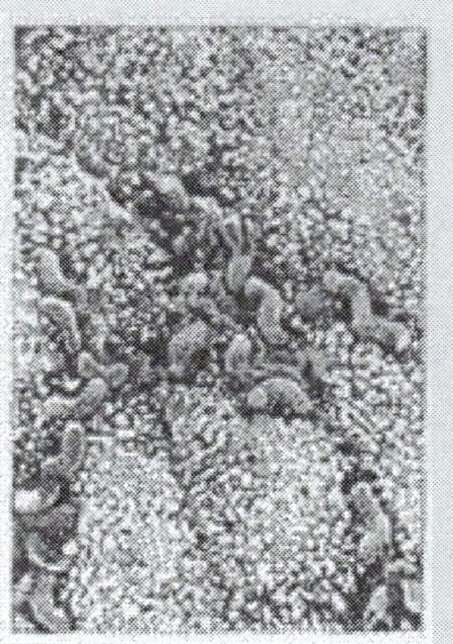

Figure 6.3. *Helicobacter pylori infection treatment.*

By Helicobacter_pylori.jpg: USGov-HHS-NIHderivative work: F. Lamiot (talk) – Helicobacter_pylori.jpg, Public Domain, https://commons.wikimedia.org/w/index.php?curid=9580156.

6.3.1. Signs and Symptoms

The majority of *H. pylori* infected individuals never show any symptoms or complications, but they do carry a 10–20% risk of peptic ulcers or a 0.5–2% risk of stomach cancer. Acute gastritis caused by *H. pylori* can manifest as stomach pain, nausea, and persistent dyspepsia (indigestion), which can occasionally be accompanied by anxiety and depression. The same symptoms apply if the gastritis progresses to chronic gastritis, or an ulcer; these include indigestion, pain in the stomach or abdomen, nausea, bloating, belching, morning hunger, feeling full too soon, and occasionally vomiting, heartburn, bad breath, and weight loss. Severe signs and symptoms of ulcer complications include black or tarry stool, which indicates bleeding into the stomach or duodenum; vomit that is either red or coffee-ground in color; severe or persistent abdominal pain; dizziness; and a rapid heartbeat. Bleeding is the most frequent side effect. Hemostasis was more important in *H. pylori*-related cases, frequently necessitating gastric resection. Extended bleeding can result in anemia, which can make you weak and exhausted. While inflammation of the corpus may result in a gastric ulcer, inflammation of the pyloric antrum, which connects the stomach to the duodenum, is more likely to cause duodenal ulcers. Constipation, vomiting, diarrhea, nausea, and unexplained weight loss are all possible side effects of stomach cancer. Adenomas known as gastric polyps are typically benign and asymptomatic, but they can also cause dyspepsia, heartburn, stomach bleeding, and, in rare cases, blockage of the gastric outlet. Larger polyps might have developed into cancer. Rectal bleeding, anemia, constipation, diarrhea, weight loss, and abdominal pain can all be related to colorectal polyps.

6.3.2. Pathophysiology

A pathogen can successfully colonize a host by avoiding the host's immune response thanks to virulence factors. The various components of virulence include the exotoxins CagA and VacA, as well as the urease, adhesins, and serine protease HtrA (high temperature requirement A) that it produces. More advanced results are linked to the presence of VacA and CagA. One oncoprotein linked to the emergence of stomach cancer is called CagA.

The DNA repair machinery's epigenetically decreased efficiency is linked to *H. pylori* infection, which promotes the development of mutations, genomic instability, and gastric carcinogenesis. Research indicates that the expression of two DNA repair proteins, PMS2 and ERCC1, was significantly decreased when the *H. pylori* infection developed into dyspepsia. About 20% of those with the infection experience dyspepsia. The DNA repair proteins MLH1, MGMT, and MRE11 all exhibit epigenetically decreased protein expression. Reduced DNA repair is probably a major contributor to the development of gastric carcinogenesis because it increases the risk of carcinogenic mutations when DNA damage is elevated. The methylation of CpG sites in gene promoters and the altered expression of several microRNAs are the causes of these epigenetic changes brought on by *H. pylori*. There are two related theories as to how *H. pylori* might cause cancer. A possible mechanism could be the higher generation of free radicals in the vicinity of *H. pylori*, coupled with a higher rate of host cell mutation. The other mechanism, referred to as a perigenetic pathway, focuses on enhancing the phenotype of the transformed host cell through modifications in cell proteins, including adhesion proteins. Tumor necrosis factor (TNF), also referred to as tumor necrosis factor alpha (TNFα), and/or interleukin 6 (IL-6) have been shown to cause inflammation and elevated levels of TNF locally. The perigenetic mechanism proposed here states that inflammation-associated signaling molecules, like TNF, can modify gastric epithelial cell adhesion and cause mutated epithelial cells to disperse and migrate without requiring additional mutations in tumor suppressor genes, like those encoding cell adhesion proteins.

6.3.2.1. Flagellum

The flagellum of *Helicobacter pylori* is the first virulence factor that permits colonization. *H. pylori* has a high motility because it possesses two to seven flagella at the same polar location.

The two copolymerized flagellins, FlaA and FlaB, which are encoded by the genes flaA and flaB, make up the approximately 3-micrometer-long flagellar filaments. The major flagellin FlaA makes up the remainder of the flagellum, while the minor flagellin FlaB is found in the proximal region. The flagella are shielded from the acidity of the stomach by a continuation of the outer membrane of the bacterium. The sheath is also where the outer membrane vesicles that shield the bacterium from bacteriophages originate.

The proton motive force produced by urease-driven hydrolysis powers flagella motility by enabling chemotactic movements in the direction of the less acidic pH gradient of the mucosa. *H. pylori* can infiltrate the mucosa, the underlying epithelial cell layer, and the gastric pits where they colonize and thrive in the gastric glands after reaching the mucosa. On rare occasions, the bacteria are discovered inside the epithelial cells. The bacteria use quorum sensing to form a biofilm, which promotes more persistent colonization. *H. pylori* can evade the effects of antibiotics and host-immune reactions within the layers of the biofilm.

6.3.2.2. Urease

Apart from avoiding regions with low pH (high acidity) through chemotaxis, *H. pylori* also balances the acid in its surroundings by generating significant quantities of urease, an enzyme that converts urea in the stomach to ammonia and carbonic acid. These create an area that is neutralized around *H. pylori*by reacting with the strong acids in the surrounding environment. One of the rare species of bacteria known to possess a specially arranged urea cycle is Helicobacter pylori. 10% of the cell is made up of nitrogen, which requires balance. Any surplus is held in reserve and released during the urea cycle. Arginase is an essential enzyme in the pathophysiology of *Helicobacter pylori* and the last stage of the urea cycle. The enzyme urease converts ornithine and urea produced by arginase into carbonic acid and ammonia. The most prevalent protein in the bacterium is urease, which makes up 10–15% of the protein content overall. Its expression is necessary for both sustaining chronic infection and establishing initial colonization during the conversion of urea to carbonic acid and ammonia. Ammonia lowers stomach acidity, which facilitates the bacterial establishment on a local level. Through its consumption of arginine, which macrophages use to produce nitric oxide, which has potent antimicrobial properties, arginase facilitates the persistence of infection. Epithelial cells are poisoned by the ammonia generated to maintain pH balance.

6.3.2.3. Adhesins

H. pylori needs to adhere to the epithelial cells in order to resist being washed away by the mucus's continual regrowth and movement. Bacterial adhesins, which are virulence factors, are proteins found on their outer membrane that provide them with adhesion. Blood group antigen binding adhesin, or BabA, plays a major role in early colonization, while SabA plays a role in persistence. BabA binds to the epithelium's glycans and mucins. Furthermore, the Lewis B antigen that is present on the surface of epithelial cells is bound by BabA, which is encoded by the *babA2* gene. BabA adherence is acid-sensitive and can be completely undone by lowering pH. According to some theories, BabA's acid responsiveness permits both adherence and a successful escape from an unfavorable environment, like a low pH that is detrimental to the organism. Increased sialyl-Lewis X antigen expression on the stomach mucosa is bound by SabA.

6.3.2.4. Cholesterol Glucoside

Cholesterol glucoside is a sterol glucoside that is inserted into the outer membrane of the stomach gland cells by *H. pylori*after it has been glycosylated from the cholesterol within them.

This cholesterol glucoside, which is uncommon in other bacteria, is crucial for immunological evasion, morphology, and membrane stability. This is caused by the enzyme cholesteryl α-glucosyltransferase (αCgT), also known as Cgt, which is encoded by the HP0421 gene. Disruption of the cholesterol-rich lipid rafts in the epithelial cells is one of the main effects of Cgt's depletion of host cholesterol. Since lipid rafts are involved in cell signaling, their disruption lowers interferon-gamma, which in turn lowers the immune inflammatory response. The type IV secretion system is also responsible for the selective secretion of Cgt, which helps to create gastric niches that are favorable to the pathogen. Its absence has been demonstrated to increase bacteria's susceptibility to environmental stressors and to interactions mediated by CagA.

6.3.2.5. Catalase

As an initial line of defense for the immune system, colonization triggers a strong anti-inflammatory reaction. Antibodies are generated when phagocytic leukocytes and monocytes enter the infection site. The phagocytes' ability to function is hindered by the organism's ability to stick to their surface. The phagocyte produces and releases oxygen metabolites into the surrounding area in response to this. Because of the activity of catalase during its attachment to the surface of phagocytic cells, *H. pylori* can withstand this response. Hydrogen peroxide is broken down by catalase into oxygen and water, shielding the bacteria from harm. It has been demonstrated that catalase virtually totally inhibits the phagocytic oxidative response. It is encoded by the katA gene.

6.3.2.6. Tip

Tumor necrosis factor is induced by TNF-inducing protein alpha (Tipα), a carcinogenic protein specific to *H. pylori* that is encoded by HP0596. When tipα reaches gastric cancer cells, it binds to nucleolin on the cell surface and causes vimentin to be expressed. Vimentin plays a crucial role in the epithelial-mesenchymal transition that occurs as tumors grow.

6.3.2.7. CagA

The oncoprotein *H. pylori* is virulent due in large part to a factor called CagA (cytotoxin-associated antigen A), which is encoded by the cagA gene. Gastric cancer, MALT lymphomas, and ulcers have all been linked to bacterial strains carrying the cagA gene. A comparatively lengthy (1186 amino acid) protein is encoded by the cagA gene. About 30 genes make up the cag pathogenicity island (PAI), some of which code for an intricate type IV secretion system. The island may have been acquired by horizontal transfer from another bacterial species, as indicated by the low GC-content of the cag PAI in comparison to the rest of the Helicobacter genome. Another important player in the pathophysiology of H is the serine protease HtrA. pylori. The HtrA protein is required for both the translocation of CagA and the bacterium's ability to migrate across the epithelium of the host cells.

The cag pathogenicity island genes, which are present in between 50 and 70% of *H. pylori*strains in Western nations, may enhance the virulence of the bacteria. Compared to those infected with strains lacking the island, Westerners infected with strains carrying the cag PAI have a stronger inflammatory response in the stomach and are more likely to develop peptic ulcers or stomach cancer. The type IV secretion system expressed by the cag PAI injects peptidoglycan, an agent that causes inflammation, into the stomach epithelial cells once *H. pylori* has attached to them. The cytoplasmic pattern recognition receptor (immune sensor) Nod1 recognizes the injected peptidoglycan and triggers the production of pro-inflammatory cytokines. Additionally, the stomach's epithelial cells are injected with the cag PAI-encoded protein CagA by the type-IV secretion apparatus. This causes disruptions to various cellular processes, including cell polarity, intracellular signaling, adhesion to neighboring cells, and the cytoskeleton. A host cell membrane-associated tyrosine kinase (TK) phosphorylates the CagA protein on tyrosine residues once it has entered the cell. Protein tyrosine phosphatase/protooncogene Shp2 is then allosterically activated by CagA. These proteins give off a strong signal to the immune system that an invasion is occurring and are directly toxic to the stomach lining cells. Neutrophils and macrophages settle in the tissue as a result of the bacterial invasion to combat the bacteria. Epidermal growth factor receptor (EGFR), a membrane protein with a TK domain, has been demonstrated to be activated by pathogenic strains of Helicobacter pylori. Pathogenesis may be aided by altered signal transduction and gene expression in host epithelial cells following *H. pylori*-induced EGFR activation. Independent of protein tyrosine phosphorylation, it has also been proposed that the C-terminal region of the CagA protein (amino acids 873–1002) can control host cell gene transcription. The variations amongst H strains are quite substantial. pylori, and the individual's strain of infection can determine the result.

6.3.2.8. VacA

The vacA gene encodes VacA, which is a significant virulence factor known as vacciolating cytotoxin auto transporter. Although this gene is present in all *H. pylori* strains, only 50% of them are able to produce the cytotoxin that is encoded. VacA has four primary subtypes: s1/m1, s1/m2, s2/m1, and s2/m2. It is established that s1/m1 and s1/m2 raise the risk of stomach cancer. An oligomeric protein complex called VacA causes the epithelial cells to gradually vacuolate, which ultimately results in the cells' death. Because the vacuolation damages the TRPML1 calcium channel cell membrane, it has also been linked to the promotion of intracellular reservoirs of *H. pylori*. It has been demonstrated that VacA upregulates COX2, which in turn upregulates prostaglandin synthesis, indicating a robust inflammatory response by host cells.

6.3.2.9. Outer Membrane Proteins and Vesicles

Proteins found on the outer membrane that belong to five families are encoded by about 4% of the genome. The bacterial adhesins belong to the largest family. Porins, iron transporters, flagellum-associated proteins, and proteins with unknown functions make up the other four families. The phospholipids and lipopolysaccharide (LPS) that make up the outer membrane are similar to those of other common gram-negative bacteria. Lewis blood group antigens on the stomach epithelium may resemble the fucosylated O-antigen of lipopolysaccharides (LPS). *H. pylori* produces outer membrane blebs that pinch off to form outer membrane vesicles, which offer a different way for virulence factors like CagA to be delivered. It is well known that the Helicobacter cysteine-rich protein HcpA causes inflammation by inducing an immunological response. DupA, a virulence factor of Helicobacter pylori, is linked to the development of duodenal ulcers.

6.3.2.10. Mechanisms of Tolerance

H. pylori must withstand not only the severe gastric acidity in the stomach but also the continuous phagocytic attack, which releases reactive oxygen species, and the sweeping of mucus by continuous peristalsis. Different mechanisms of tolerance have evolved as a result of their need to survive, allowing them to persist. Bacterial response mechanisms are triggered by stress and are controlled by proteins that are produced by regulator genes. Its genome may contain potentially fatal mutagenic DNA adducts caused by oxidative stress. Transformation-mediated recombinational repair, which aids in successful colonization, supports surviving this DNA damage. Interaction of the mechanisms can lead to an overall response to multiple stressors. Overcoming the effects of antibiotics can also be aided by the mechanisms of persistence and tolerance.

An effective sustained colonization response is the formation of a biofilm. Layers of aggregated bacteria form a biofilm. Cells in the deep layers are nutritionally deprived and enter the coccoid dormant-like state. Some of these cells will be antibiotic resistant and may remain in the host as persister cells. Following eradication the persister cells can cause a recurrence of the infection.

Transformation appears to be a component of an adaptation for DNA repair, meaning that DNA is transferred from one bacterial cell to another through the intervening medium. *H. pylori* can change by nature. *H. pylori* remains competent throughout logarithmic growth, in contrast to many other organisms that are only competent under specific environmental circumstances, such as starvation. Genetic programs are encoded in all organisms to respond to stressful situations, including those that damage DNA. Homologous recombination is necessary for *H. pylori* double-strand breaks (DSBs) to heal. RecA is loaded onto single-strand DNA (ssDNA) by the AddAB helicase-nuclease complex, which resects double-strand breaks (DSBs) and mediates strand exchange, resulting in homologous recombination and repair. It appears that *H. pylori* is either exposed to double-strand DNA damage in the stomach that needs to be repaired or requires some other recombination-mediated event, as evidenced by the requirement of RecA plus AddAB for effective gastric colonization. In particular, DNA damage in *H.pylori* increases natural transformation, and a relationship has been found between the DNA uptake and the DNA damage response, indicating that natural competence plays a role in the bacteria's persistence in its human host and accounts for the majority of clinical isolates' ability to retain competence. Compared to other bacteria, *H. pylori* exhibits significantly higher rates of recombination and mutation. It is possible to find genetically distinct strains in distinct stomach regions as well as within the same host.

Because it resolves what are known as Holliday junctions, the RuvC protein is crucial to the recombinational repair process. RuvC-deficient *H. pylori* mutants show decreased survival in macrophages, increased susceptibility to oxidative stress and DNA-damaging agents, and an inability to successfully infect mice. In a similar vein, RecN protein is crucial for *H. pylori* DSB repair. The weakened capacity of *H. pylori* recN mutant to colonize mouse stomachs emphasizes the significance of recombinational DNA repair for the survival of *H. pylori* within its host.

6.3.3. Causes of H. pylori Infection

H. pylori bacteria are most likely passed directly from person to person. This tends to happen during childhood. The infection remains throughout life if not treated.

It is not clear how the bacteria are passed from one person to another. The bacteria may spread from:

- Mouth-to-mouth contact
- GI tract illness (particularly when vomiting occurs)
- Contact with stool (fecal material)
- Contaminated food and water

The bacteria may trigger ulcers in the following ways:

- *H. pylori* enters the mucus layer of the stomach and attaches to the stomach lining.

- *H. pylori* cause the stomach to produce more stomach acid. This damages the stomach lining, leading to ulcers in some people.

Besides ulcers, *H. pylori* bacteria can also cause chronic inflammation in the stomach (gastritis) or the upper part of the small intestine (duodenitis).

H. pylori can also sometimes lead to stomach cancer or a rare type of stomach lymphoma.

6.3.4. Diagnosing Helicobacter pylori (H. pylori)

Colonization using *H. pylori* is a condition linked to several stomach illnesses rather than a disease in and of itself. Testing is advised for patients with peptic ulcer disease, low-grade gastric MALT lymphoma, first-degree relatives with gastric cancer, following endoscopic resection of early-stage gastric cancer, and in some cases of dyspepsia. Long-term use of aspirin or other non-steroidal anti-inflammatory drugs, iron deficiency anemia that cannot be explained, and immune thrombocytopenic purpura are additional signs that warrant testing for *H. pylori*. There are numerous non-invasive and invasive testing techniques available.

Stool tests, urea breath tests, and serological antibody tests are non-invasive methods for diagnosing *H. pylori* infection. Carbon-13, or radioactive carbon-14, is used in carbon urea breath tests to produce labeled carbon dioxide that can be found in the breath. *H. pylori* can be diagnosed with high sensitivity and specificity using carbon urea breath tests. Antibiotics and proton-pump inhibitors should be stopped for at least 30 days before undergoing infection tests or eradication, since both treatments impede the growth of *H. pylori* and could produce erroneous negative results. It is advised to undergo testing to verify eradication at least 30 days following the conclusion of *H. pylori* infection treatment. Testing for stool antigens or *H. pylori* breathalyzers are both appropriate methods to verify eradication. IgG antibodies and other *H. pylori* serologic tests are not advised as measures of eradication because the antibodies can persist elevated for years following successful treatment of the infection. An invasive method to check for *H. pylori* infection is an endoscopic biopsy. Multiple samples are advised because a biopsy may miss low-level infections. A histological examination from two sites following endoscopic biopsy, in conjunction with either a rapid urease test or microbial culture, is the most accurate method for detecting *H. pylori* infection. In general, unless there are particular reasons to do so, repeating endoscopy is not advised to confirm *H. pylori* eradication.

6.3.5. Prevention of H. pylori

Antibiotic-based therapy regimens are advised to eradicate the bacteria when infection is suspected to prevent the development of diseases related to *H. pylori*. If effective, the disease's progression is stopped. Regardless of the presence of *H. pylori*, first-line therapy is advised if low-grade gastric MALT lymphoma is diagnosed. Antibiotic-based treatment plans are not suggested, though, if a severe case of atrophic gastritis with gastric lesions is reached because these lesions frequently cannot be reversed and will eventually lead to gastric cancer. It is recommended that an eradication program be followed if the cancer is managed to be treated to stop an infection from recurring or to lessen a metachronous cancer recurrence. Alternative treatments are obviously needed because *H. pylori* is a major cause of certain diseases, especially cancers, and because its resistance to antibiotic therapy is constantly growing. It would also be possible to prevent the development of gastric ulcers with a vaccine that targets the development of gastric cancer, including MALT lymphoma. The primary objectives are to develop a vaccine that would be therapeutic in the future and prophylactic for use in children. Complex host-immune responses and the extreme genomic diversity displayed by *H. pylori* present challenges to this.

6.3.6. Treatment of H. pylori

6.3.6.1. Gastritis

In accordance with the Maastricht Consensus Reports, Helicobacter pylori-induced gastritis (*H. pylori* gastritis) is now included in ICD11 and is classified as such. At the beginning, the infection usually only affects the stomach's upper mucosal layers. The *H. pylori* strain's cytotoxicity is correlated with the severity of chronic inflammation. When mucous glands are lost, atrophic gastritis will develop from a non-atrophic one due to increased cytotoxicity. Peptic ulcers and gastric adenocarcinoma both have this ailment as a precursor. A triple-drug therapy consisting of amoxicillin, clarithromycin, and a proton-pump inhibitor given for 14–21 days is often considered first-line treatment. Various antibiotic plus proton-pump inhibitor drug regimens are used to eradicate the infection and thereby successfully treat the disorder (Matsuo et al., 2017; FitzGerald & Smith, 2021).

6.3.6.2. Peptic Ulcers

The standard protocol is to remove *H. pylori* from the stomach and let the ulcer heal if it is found in a patient with a peptic ulcer. The typical first-line treatment consists of a 14-day triple therapy that includes the antibiotics clarithromycin and amoxicillin along with an acid-suppressive medication, usually a proton-pump inhibitor like omeprazole or a less common potassium-competitive acid blocker like vonoprazan. Because they inhibit the bacterium's P-type ATPase or urease, proton pump inhibitors may have a direct bacteriostatic effect on *H. pylori*. Over time, modifications to the triple therapy have been developed, such as substituting metronidazole for amoxicillin in cases of penicillin allergy or employing a different proton pump inhibitor, such as pantoprazole or rabeprazole. Alternatives are advised in regions where clarithromycin resistance is more prevalent. Such therapy has transformed the management of peptic ulcers and opened the door to the illness's cure. Before, the only options were to use proton pump inhibitors, H2-antagonists, or antacids alone to control symptoms. The subsequent decreased risk of duodenal or gastric ulcer recurrence is linked to the eradication of *H. pylori*.

6.3.6.3. Antibiotic Resistance

The primary reason for initial treatment failure is an increase in antibiotic resistance. Resistance-associated factors include biofilm formation, efflux pumps, and mutations. Clarithromycin is one of the primary antibiotics used in eradication treatments; however, since strains of the antibiotic are now well-established and resistant to it, other options for treatment must be taken into account. Additionally, multidrug resistance has grown. The goal of next-generation sequencing is to pinpoint early, specific antibiotic resistances so that more effective treatments can be targeted.

In 2018, the WHO listed *H. pylori* as a high-priority pathogen for the research and discovery of new drugs and treatments. The increasing antibiotic resistance encountered has spurred interest in developing alternative therapies using several plant compounds. Plant compounds have fewer side effects than synthetic drugs. Most plant extracts contain a complex mix of components that may not act on their own as antimicrobials but can work together with antibiotics to enhance treatment and work towards overcoming resistance. Plant compounds have a different mechanism of action that has proved useful in fighting antimicrobial resistance. Various compounds can act for example by inhibiting enzymes such as urease, and adhesions to the mucous membrane. Sulfur-containing compounds from plants with high concentrations of polysulfides, coumarins, and terpenes have all been shown to be effective against *H. pylori*. Other treatments or more antibiotic rounds may be employed. A quadruple therapy comprising a proton pump inhibitor, bismuth, tetracycline, and nitroimidazole for 10–14 days is advised as the first line of treatment for patients with any history of exposure to macrolides or penicillin allergies. One suggested treatment option for *H. pylori* strains resistant to clarithromycin is to include levofloxacin in the regimen.

It has been demonstrated that using probiotic yogurts that contain lactic acid bacteria, Bifidobacteria, and Lactobacillus suppresses *H. pylori* infection and increases eradication rates. Butyrate, which functions as a prebiotic and strengthens the mucosal immune barrier, is produced by certain commensal intestinal bacteria, which are a component of the gut microbiota. By using them as probiotics, you may be able to counteract the dysbiosis of the gut caused by antibiotic use. It has been demonstrated that certain probiotic strains balance the dysbiosis of the gut and exhibit bactericidal and bacteriostatic action against *H. pylori*. Saliva and dental plaque contain *H. pylori*. Since oral-oral transmission is one of its known modes of transmission, the dental plaque may serve as a bacterial reservoir. Therefore, scaling and root planing, also known as periodontal therapy, has been recommended as an extra treatment to increase eradication rates; however, further research is required.

6.3.6.4. Stomach Cancer

Helicobacter pylori is a risk factor for gastric adenocarcinomas. Treatment is highly aggressive with even localized disease being treated sequentially with chemotherapy and radiotherapy before surgical resection. Since this cancer, once developed, is independent of *H. pylori* infection, eradication regimens are not used.

6.3.6.5. Gastric MALT lymphoma and DLBCL

Malignancies of mucosa-associated lymphoid tissue are known as MALT lymphomas. 70 to 95% of cases of early gastric MALTomas caused by *H. pylori* can be successfully treated with one or more eradication programs. After the pathogen is eradicated, 50–80% of patients experience a remission and long-term clinical control of their lymphoma within 3–28 months. These localized cases have also been successfully treated with radiation therapy to the stomach and surrounding (peri-gastric) lymph nodes. Those without symptoms who have non-localized (i.e., systemic Ann Arbor stages III and IV) disease have been treated with watchful waiting or, if symptomatic, with rituximab, an immunotherapy medication, administered for four weeks in combination with chlorambucil, a chemotherapy medication, for six to twelve months. At five years, 58% of these patients achieve a progression-free survival rate. Patients in the frail stage III/IV have responded well to treatment with either rituximab or cyclophosphamide, a chemotherapy drug, by itself. *H. pylori*-positive MALT lymphomas of the rectum have been successfully treated with antibiotic-proton pump inhibitor eradication therapy and localized radiation therapy; however, radiation therapy has produced marginally better results and is thus recommended as the disease's preferred treatment. However, rituximab is frequently used in conjunction with different chemotherapy medications as the preferred course of treatment for patients with systemic involvement.

Seldom can a MALT lymphoma progress into the more aggressive diffuse large B-cell lymphoma (DLBCL). In cases where an *H. pylori* infection is linked to this, the DLBCL is less severe and more treatable. Sometimes, *H. pylori* eradication programs have been effective in treating them when they are stomach-specific. More advanced types have been successfully treated with immunotherapy, local radiotherapy, or more conventional chemotherapy (CHOP) if the patient is unresponsive or exhibiting deterioration.

6.3.7. Prognosis

Most people have *Helicobacter pylori* colonizing their stomachs for decades, which causes chronic gastritis, a persistent stomach inflammation. Most infected individuals never experience symptoms, but 10-15% go on to develop duodenal and stomach ulcers as well as a 1-2% lifetime risk of gastric cancer. A diet high in salt is conducive to the growth of *H. pylori*, which is thought to be an environmental risk factor for its link to gastric cancer. Consuming a lot of salt promotes colonization, inflammation, the expression of *H. pylori* virulence factors, and the exacerbation of chronic gastritis. Intriguingly, it has been discovered that kimchi extracts—a salted probiotic food—prevent the development of stomach cancer linked to *H. pylori*. If therapy is not received, the *H. pylori* infection typically lasts a lifetime. The stomach mucosa of the elderly may become less hospitable to colonization and more atrophic, potentially leading to the disappearance of infection. Studies on young children up to the age of two have revealed that infections in this age range can be temporary.

Even after being eradicated, *H. pylori* can resurface in a person. Either the original strain (recrudescence) or a different strain (reinfection) may be to blame for this recurrence. The global per-person annual rates of recurrence, reinfection, and recrudescence are 4.3%, 3.1%, and 2.2%, respectively, according to a 2017 meta-analysis. What the primary risk factors are is unknown. An increasing body of research indicates that *H. pylori* plays a significant role in disease prevention. The incidence of Barrett's esophagus, esophageal cancer, and acid reflux disease has been sharply increasing concurrently with a decline in *H. pylori*. In the year 1996, Martin J. Blaser promoted the theory that *H. pylori* regulates stomach acidity, which has a positive impact. The idea is not widely accepted because multiple randomized controlled trials did not show that the symptoms of acid reflux disease worsened after *H. pylori* was eradicated. Blaser has nevertheless reiterated his belief that *H. pylori* is a component of the typical stomach microbiota. He hypothesizes that the recent rise in the incidence of multiple diseases, such as type 2 diabetes, obesity, and asthma, is due to modifications in gastric physiology brought about by the loss of *H. pylori*. Recent research by his group has demonstrated a link between *H. pylori* colonization and a decreased incidence of childhood asthma (Matsuo et al., 2017; FitzGerald & Smith, 2021).

6.4. Irritable Bowel Syndrome (IBS)

Your digestive system is impacted by a collection of symptoms known as irritable bowel syndrome (IBS). It is a gastrointestinal disease or condition that affects your intestines, that is common but uncomfortable. Abdominal pain and cramping are among the symptoms that people with IBS encounter. Additionally, frequent constipation, diarrhea, or both may be symptoms of IBS. Irritable bowel syndrome (IBS) does not lead to gastrointestinal (GI) tract tissue damage or raise the risk of more serious illnesses like colon cancer. Rather, it is a chronic (long-term) illness that most people can control with dietary adjustments, behavioral therapy, medication, and routine changes (Figure 6.4).

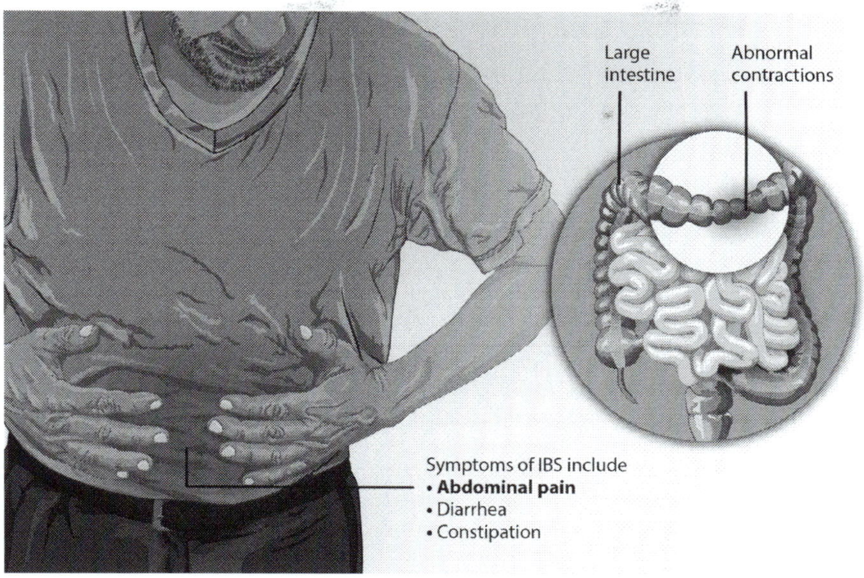

Figure 6.4. *Irritable bowel syndrome (IBS).*

https://upload.wikimedia.org/wikipedia/commons/c/c4/Depiction_of_a_person_suffering_from_Irritable_Bowel_Syndrome_%28IBS%29.png.

6.4.1. Types of IBS

Based on the appearance of your stools (poop) on days when your symptoms flare up, researchers classify IBS patients. The majority of IBS sufferers experience irregular bowel movements occasionally and regular ones on other days. The abnormal days define the kind of IBS you have.

- IBS with constipation (IBS-C): Most of your poop is hard and lumpy.
- IBS with diarrhea (IBS-D): Most of your poop is loose and watery.
- IBS with mixed bowel habits (IBS-M): You have both hard and lumpy bowel movements and loose and watery movements.

The differences are important. Certain treatments only work for specific types of IBS.

6.4.2. Symptoms of Irritable Bowel Syndrome (IBS)

Irritable Bowel Syndrome (IBS) is a chronic gastrointestinal disorder characterized by a combination of symptoms that can vary from person to person. The most common symptoms of IBS include:

1. **Abdominal Pain and Discomfort**: This is one of the hallmark symptoms of IBS. The pain or discomfort is typically located in the lower abdomen and may vary in intensity. It is often relieved by passing gas or having a bowel movement.
2. **Altered Bowel Habits**: Individuals with IBS may experience changes in bowel habits, including:

- **Diarrhea:** Some people with IBS experience frequent loose or watery stools.

- **Constipation:** Others may have infrequent bowel movements or difficulty passing stools.
- **Mixed Bowel Habits:** Some individuals may alternate between episodes of diarrhea and constipation.

3. **Bloating and Gas**: Many people with IBS experience bloating and increased gas production, which can contribute to discomfort and abdominal distention.
4. **Abnormal Stool Characteristics**: Stool characteristics may vary in individuals with IBS. Stools may be harder or softer than usual, and they may appear lumpy, loose, or pellet-like.
5. **Mucus in Stool**: Some individuals with IBS may notice the presence of mucus in their stools.
6. **Feeling of Incomplete Bowel Movements**: People with IBS may feel like they haven't completely emptied their bowels after a bowel movement.
7. **Abdominal Cramping**: Cramping or spasms in the abdomen are common in individuals with IBS, especially during bowel movements.
8. **Symptoms Related to Eating**: Symptoms of IBS may be triggered or worsened by certain foods or eating patterns. Some individuals may experience symptoms after eating certain trigger foods, large meals, or fatty or spicy foods.
9. **Fatigue and Sleep Disturbances**: Chronic symptoms of IBS can lead to fatigue and sleep disturbances, impacting overall quality of life.

It is important to note that symptoms of IBS can vary in severity and may come and go over time. Additionally, the exact cause of IBS is not fully understood, but factors such as abnormal gastrointestinal motility, visceral hypersensitivity, inflammation, changes in gut microbiota, and psychological factors may play a role in its development. If you experience symptoms suggestive of IBS, it is essential to consult a healthcare professional for proper evaluation and management.

6.4.3. Causes of IBS

The exact cause of Irritable Bowel Syndrome (IBS) is not fully understood, but it is believed to involve a combination of various factors, including:

- **Abnormal Gastrointestinal Motility**: Dysfunction in the movement of the digestive system, including both increased and decreased motility, may contribute to the symptoms of IBS. This can lead to alterations in bowel habits such as diarrhea, constipation, or alternating between the two.
- **Visceral Hypersensitivity**: Some individuals with IBS have increased sensitivity to pain or discomfort originating from the internal organs of the digestive system (viscera). Even normal intestinal contractions or gas can cause significant discomfort in these individuals.
- **Intestinal Inflammation**: Low-grade inflammation or immune system dysfunction in the intestines may play a role in some cases of IBS, particularly those with symptoms resembling inflammatory bowel diseases (IBD) such as Crohn's disease or ulcerative colitis.

- **Altered Gut Microbiota**: Imbalance or dysbiosis in the composition of gut bacteria (microbiota) has been observed in some individuals with IBS. Changes in the microbiota may influence intestinal function, immune response, and symptom development in IBS.
- **Intestinal Permeability (Leaky Gut)**: Increased permeability of the intestinal lining, often referred to as "leaky gut," may allow substances to pass through the intestinal barrier and trigger immune responses, inflammation, and symptoms associated with IBS.
- **Food Intolerances and Sensitivities**: Certain foods or dietary components may trigger or exacerbate symptoms of IBS in susceptible individuals. Common triggers include high-fat foods, spicy foods, dairy products, gluten-containing foods, and fermentable carbohydrates (FODMAPs).
- **Psychological Factors**: Emotional stress, anxiety, depression, and other psychological factors can influence the severity and frequency of IBS symptoms. The gut-brain axis, which involves bidirectional communication between the gut and the brain, plays a significant role in the development and exacerbation of IBS symptoms.
- **Genetic Predisposition**: There may be a genetic component to IBS, as it tends to run in families. However, specific genetic factors contributing to IBS susceptibility are still being investigated.
- **Infectious Triggers**: In some cases, gastrointestinal infections (e.g., gastroenteritis) caused by bacteria, viruses, or parasites may trigger the onset of IBS symptoms, particularly in individuals with post-infectious IBS (PI-IBS).
- **Hormonal Changes**: Fluctuations in hormone levels, particularly in women during menstruation or hormonal changes associated with menopause, may influence IBS symptoms.

IBS is a complex and heterogeneous condition, and the underlying mechanisms may vary from person to person. Additionally, multiple factors often interact to contribute to the development and persistence of IBS symptoms. Treatment of IBS typically involves a multidisciplinary approach targeting symptom management, dietary modifications, stress reduction, and, in some cases, medication or behavioral therapies.

6.4.4. Diagnosis of IBS

IBS cannot be conclusively diagnosed with a test. A thorough medical history, physical examination, and testing to rule out other illnesses like celiac disease and inflammatory bowel disease (IBD) are likely to be the first things your healthcare provider does. After other conditions have been ruled out, your provider is likely to use one of these sets of diagnostic criteria for IBS:

- **Rome Criteria:** These requirements include having experienced stomach discomfort and pain on average one day per week for the previous three months. Additionally, this needs to happen in conjunction with at least two of the following: altered stool consistency, decreased frequency of defecation, or pain and discomfort associated with it.

- **Type of IBS:** Based on your symptoms, there are four types of IBS for treatment purposes: mixed, constipation-predominant, diarrhea-predominant, and unclassified.

Your provider will also likely assess whether you have other symptoms that might suggest another, more serious, condition. These include:

- Onset of symptoms after age 50
- Weight loss
- Rectal bleeding
- Fever
- Nausea or recurrent vomiting
- Belly pain, especially if it is not related to a bowel movement, or occurs at night
- Diarrhea that is ongoing or awakens you from sleep
- Anemia related to low iron

If you have these symptoms, or if an initial treatment for IBS doesn't work, you'll likely need additional tests.

6.4.4.1. Additional Tests

In order to check for infections, your provider might suggest a number of tests, including stool studies. Additionally, stool studies can determine whether your intestines are having problems absorbing nutrients. This condition is referred to as malabsorption. It might be advised to have more testing done to rule out alternative reasons for your symptoms.

Diagnostic procedures can include:

- **Colonoscopy:** Your provider uses a small, flexible tube to examine the entire length of the colon.
- **CT Scan:** This test produces images of your abdomen and pelvis that might rule out other causes of your symptoms, especially if you have belly pain.
- **Upper Endoscopy:** A long, flexible tube is inserted down your throat and into the esophagus, which is the tube connecting your mouth and stomach. A camera on the end of the tube allows your provider to view your upper digestive tract. During an endoscopy, a tissue sample (biopsy) may be collected. A sample of fluid may be collected to look for overgrowth of bacteria. An endoscopy may be recommended if celiac disease is suspected.

Laboratory tests can include:

- **Lactose Intolerance Tests:** Lactase is an enzyme you need to digest the sugar found in dairy products. If you don't produce lactase, you may have problems similar to those caused by IBS, including belly pain, gas and diarrhea. Your provider may order a breath test or ask you to remove milk and milk products from your diet for several weeks.
- **Breath Test for Bacterial Overgrowth:** A breath test also can determine if you have bacterial overgrowth in your small intestine. Bacterial overgrowth is more common among people who have had bowel surgery or who have diabetes or some other disease that slows down digestion.
- **Stool Tests:** Your stool might be examined for bacteria, parasites or the presence of bile acid. Bile acid is a digestive liquid produced in your liver.

6.4.5. Treatment of IBS

Treatment of IBS focuses on relieving symptoms so that you can live as symptom-free as possible. Mild symptoms can often be controlled by managing stress and by making changes in your diet and lifestyle. Try to:

- Avoid foods that trigger your symptoms
- Eat high-fiber foods
- Drink plenty of fluids
- Exercise regularly
- Get enough sleep

Your provider might suggest that you eliminate from your diet:

- **High-Gas Foods:** If you experience bloating or gas, you might avoid items such as carbonated and alcoholic beverages and certain foods that may lead to increased gas.
- **Gluten:** Research shows that some people with IBS report improvement in diarrhea symptoms if they stop eating gluten (wheat, barley and rye) even if they don't have celiac disease.
- **FODMAPs:** Some people are sensitive to certain carbohydrates such as fructose, fructans, lactose and others, known as FODMAPs — fermentable oligosaccharides, disaccharides, monosaccharides and polyols. FODMAPs are found in certain grains, vegetables, fruits and dairy products.

A dietitian can help you with these diet changes. If your problems are moderate or severe, your provider might suggest counseling — especially if you have depression or if stress tends to make your symptoms worse.

Based on your symptoms, medications may be recommended, including:

- **Fiber Supplements:** Constipation may be managed by taking a psyllium (Metamucil) supplement along with fluids.
- **Laxatives:** Your doctor might suggest over-the-counter laxatives like polyethylene glycol (Miralax) or magnesium hydroxide oral (Phillips' Milk of Magnesia) if fiber is ineffective in relieving constipation.
- **Anti-Diarrheal Medications:** Diarrhea can be controlled with over-the-counter medications like loperamide (Imodium A-D). A bile acid binder, such as cholestyramine (Prevalite), colestipol (Colestid), or colesevelam (Welchol), may also be prescribed by your doctor. Bloating can result from bile acid binders.
- **Anticholinergic Medications:** Medications like bentyl (dicyclomine) can ease the agony of spasms in the bowel. Those who experience episodes of diarrhea may occasionally be prescribed them. Though generally safe, these drugs may result in dry mouth, constipation, and blurred vision.
- **Tricyclic Antidepressants:** In addition to its ability to alleviate depression, this kind of medication blocks the activity of neurons that govern the intestines. This could lessen discomfort. Your doctor might recommend a lower-than-normal dosage of imipramine (Tofranil), desipramine (Norpramin), or nortriptyline (Pamelor) if you have diarrhea and stomach pain without depression. Some side

effects of the medication include dry mouth, blurred vision, dizziness, and sleepiness. These effects may be minimized if you take the medication right before bed.

- **SSRI Antidepressants:** If you suffer from pain and constipation along with depression, selective serotonin reuptake inhibitor (SSRI) antidepressants like paroxetine (Paxil) or fluoxetine (Prozac) may be able to help.
- **Pain Medications:** Pregabalin (Lyrica) or gabapentin (Neurontin) might ease severe pain or bloating.

6.4.6. Medications Specifically for IBS

Medications approved for certain people with IBS include:

- **Alosetron (Lotronex):** The purpose of Alosetron is to calm the colon and reduce the rate at which waste passes through the lower intestine. Only physicians who are enrolled in a specific program are authorized to prescribe it. Only severe cases of diarrhea-predominant IBS in female patients who have not responded to prior treatments should be treated with Alosetron. Men are not permitted to use it. Since alevetron has been associated with significant but uncommon side effects, it should only be taken into consideration in cases where other therapies have failed.
- **Eluxadoline (Viberzi):** By lessening intestinal fluid secretion and muscle contractions, eluxadoline helps alleviate diarrhea. It also aids in improving the rectum's muscular tone. Abdominal pain, nausea, and mild constipation are possible side effects. Additionally, pancreatitis—which can be severe and more common in some people—has been linked to eluxadoline.
- ***Rifaximin (Xifaxan)*:** This antibiotic can decrease bacterial overgrowth and diarrhea.
- ***Lubiprostone (Amitiza)*:** To aid in the passage of stool, lubiprostone can increase the amount of fluid secreted in your small intestine. It is generally prescribed only for women with severe symptoms who have not responded to other treatments. It is approved for women with constipation who have IBS.
- **Linaclotide (Linzess**): To facilitate the passage of stool, linaclotide can also enhance the small intestine's fluid secretion. Although linaclotide can cause diarrhea, it may be helpful to take the medication 30 to 60 minutes before eating.

6.5. Cyclic Vomiting Syndrome (CVS)

Vomiting is the forceful, involuntary release of stomach contents through the mouth and occasionally the nose. Food poisoning, gastroenteritis, pregnancy, motion sickness, hangovers, and brain tumors can all cause vomiting. Other conditions that can cause vomiting include high intracranial pressure, brain tumors, and radiation exposure. Nausea is the sensation of being about to throw up; it frequently comes on before vomiting but is not always the result of it. Vomit inhalation can occur as a result of alcohol impairment or anesthesia. Intravenous fluid may be necessary in severe cases where dehydration sets in. In certain cases, antiemetics are required to prevent nausea and vomiting. Self-induced vomiting, also known as purging disorder, is now recognized as a distinct eating disorder and can be a part of eating disorders like bulimia.

6.5.1. Symptoms and Causes of Cyclic Vomiting Syndrome (CVS)

Cyclic vomiting syndrome (CVS) involves sudden, repeated episodes of severe nausea and vomiting. Episodes often unfold like this:

- **Prodrome Phase:** You start feeling nauseated and sweaty in the minutes or hours leading up to the vomiting. For most people, the feeling starts in the early morning hours.
- **Vomiting Phase:** You vomit, sometimes several times an hour. Children with CVS may projectile vomit. The vomiting may last for a few hours or even a few days. The experience can feel so intense that you're unable to talk to others and need to stay in bed alone.
- **Recovery Phase:** The vomiting and nausea gradually improve.
- **Well Phase:** You return to feeling like yourself again.

Other signs and symptoms of CVS include:

- Abdominal pain.
- Diarrhea.
- Dizziness or vertigo.
- Drooling or spitting.
- Extreme thirst.
- Loss of appetite.
- Pale skin.
- Severe headaches and fatigue.
- Sensitivity to light or sound.
- Low-grade fever (up to 101 degrees Fahrenheit or 38.33 degrees Celsius).
- Retching (dry-heaving), where your vomiting reflex forces you to throw up, but nothing comes out.

6.5.1.1. Causes Cyclic Vomiting Syndrome (CVS)

There isn't a single known cause of CVS. Instead, several factors may play a role, including:

- **Issues with Your Brain-Gut Axis:** Problems with how your brain communicates with nerves in your gastrointestinal (GI) tract may lead to uncontrollable vomiting. Some scientists call CVS a brain-gut disorder.
- **Changes or Imbalances in Your Autonomic Nervous System:** Your autonomic nervous system controls involuntary activities, like your heartbeat, blood pressure and vomiting reflex. A glitch in the system can lead to vomiting episodes.
- **Migraine Headaches:** Migraine headaches appear in up to 80% of children and 25% of adults with CVS. A migraine is significantly more intense than just a bad headache. Like CVS, it usually begins with an uncomfortable feeling that an episode is about to start. Many people with CVS have a family history of migraines.
- **Abnormal Mitochondrial DNA:** Mitochondria power cells. The instructions that tell mitochondria

how to work (DNA) can become abnormal because of an illness, a genetic condition or exposure to drugs or toxins. The nerve cells in your gut require a lot of energy to work correctly. Problems with their power source (mitochondria) may cause uncontrollable vomiting.

6.5.1.2. Triggers Cyclic Vomiting Syndrome (CVS)

Certain conditions, events and emotional states can trigger a vomiting episode, including:

- Seasonal changes (symptoms are more common in fall and winter).
- Reactions to foods like chocolate, cheese, caffeine or MSG.
- Heightened positive emotions, like excitement (in children).
- Panic attacks, stress and anxiety (in adults).
- Allergies, sinus infections or the flu.
- Physical exhaustion.
- Prolonged fasting.
- Prolonged marijuana use.
- Menstrual periods.
- Motion sickness.

6.5.2. Diagnosis and Tests

Eliminating illnesses that produce comparable symptoms is a necessary step in the diagnosis of CVS. Your doctor will inquire about your past medical history, your family's medical history, and your pattern of nausea and vomiting.

There isn't a single test to diagnose CVS. Instead, your provider may order several tests to exclude other conditions that cause vomiting. Tests include:

- **Lab Tests (Blood and Urine Tests):** Lab tests check body fluids for signs of metabolic disorders, mitochondrial disease or problems with your organs that can cause CVS symptoms.
- **Imaging Tests:** Imaging tests can reveal issues with organs in your digestive and nervous systems that cause vomiting. You may need an abdominal ultrasound, a brain MRI (magnetic resonance imaging), CT scan (computed tomography scan) or X-rays called an upper GI series. You may need a gastric emptying test to see how food moves through your digestive system.
- **Upper Endoscopy:** This test can show problems in your esophagus, stomach or small intestine that may be causing your vomiting episodes.

6.5.2.1. Conditions for Cyclic Vomiting Syndrome

A CVS diagnosis involves ruling out common conditions that cause vomiting, including infections, acid reflux (GERD) and stomach ulcers. Your provider may also need to exclude:

- **Inflammation:** Swelling and irritation in your stomach (gastritis), pancreas (pancreatitis) or appendix (appendicitis).
- **Volvulus or Malrotation:** Twisting of your intestine.
- **Ureteropelvic (UPJ) Obstruction:** A blockage where your kidney attaches to your bladder.
- **Metabolic Disorders:** Conditions that involve problems with how your body turns food into energy.

6.5.3. Management and Treatment of Cyclic Vomiting Syndrome

The management and treatment of Cyclic Vomiting Syndrome (CVS) typically involve a combination of approaches aimed at preventing episodes, managing symptoms during episodes, and supporting overall health and well-being. Here are some common strategies used in the management of CVS:

1. **Identifying Triggers**: Work with a healthcare provider to identify potential triggers for CVS episodes, which may include stress, certain foods or beverages, hormonal changes, infections, and sleep disturbances. Keeping a detailed diary of symptoms and potential triggers can help identify patterns and triggers specific to individual cases.
2. **Lifestyle Modifications**: Making lifestyle changes to reduce stress and promote overall health may help prevent CVS episodes. This may include practicing stress-reduction techniques such as relaxation exercises, mindfulness meditation, and regular physical activity.
3. **Dietary Modifications**: Some individuals with CVS find that certain foods or dietary factors trigger or exacerbate symptoms. Working with a dietitian to identify and eliminate trigger foods from the diet may help prevent episodes. In some cases, a low-fat, low-acid, or low-FODMAP (fermentable oligosaccharides, disaccharides, monosaccharides, and polyols) diet may be recommended.
4. **Medications**: Several medications may be used to prevent CVS episodes or manage symptoms during episodes:
   - **Prophylactic Medications:** Certain medications, such as tricyclic antidepressants, cyproheptadine, and anticonvulsants (e.g., topiramate), may be prescribed to reduce the frequency and severity of CVS episodes.
   - **Antiemetic Medications:** Antiemetic drugs, such as ondansetron, promethazine, or metoclopramide, may be used to help control nausea and vomiting during episodes.
   - **Abortive Medications:** Medications such as triptans (commonly used for migraines) or benzodiazepines may be used to help abort or shorten the duration of CVS episodes in some cases.
5. **Fluid and Electrolyte Replacement**: During vomiting episodes, it is important to prevent dehydration and electrolyte imbalances by replacing fluids and electrolytes lost through vomiting. In severe cases, intravenous fluids may be necessary to rehydrate the body.
6. **Psychological Support**: Because stress and psychological factors can contribute to CVS, psychological support may be beneficial. Cognitive-behavioral therapy (CBT), biofeedback, relaxation techniques, and counseling may help individuals better cope with stress and manage symptoms.
7. **Supportive Care**: Providing supportive care during vomiting episodes is essential to prevent complications and improve comfort. This may include rest in a quiet,

darkened room, application of cool compresses to the forehead, and administration of antiemetic medications as prescribed.

8. **Monitoring and Follow-Up**: Regular monitoring by a healthcare provider is important to track symptoms, adjust treatment as needed, and address any concerns or complications that may arise. Follow-up appointments may also provide an opportunity to assess treatment response and make further recommendations.

It is important for individuals with CVS to work closely with a healthcare provider, typically a gastroenterologist or a specialist in functional gastrointestinal disorders, to develop a comprehensive management plan tailored to their specific needs and circumstances. While there is no cure for CVS, many individuals find that with proper management, they can reduce the frequency and severity of episodes and improve their quality of life (Matsuo et al., 2017; FitzGerald & Smith, 2021).

A Closer Look

Functional Dyspepsia

Functional Dyspepsia (FD) is a common gastrointestinal disorder characterized by chronic or recurrent upper abdominal discomfort or pain, often accompanied by symptoms such as early satiety, postprandial fullness, bloating, belching, and nausea. The term "functional" indicates that the symptoms are not related to any underlying structural or biochemical abnormalities but rather result from disturbances in gastrointestinal motility, sensation, or the interaction between the gut and the brain. The exact cause of FD is not well understood, but several factors may contribute to its development, including abnormalities in gastric emptying, impaired gastric accommodation, altered gut-brain axis function, visceral hypersensitivity, psychological factors, and dietary triggers. Diagnosis of FD is based on the presence of characteristic symptoms in the absence of any identifiable organic or structural abnormalities on diagnostic tests. The Rome criteria, which classify FD into subtypes based on predominant symptoms, are often used to aid in diagnosis. Management of FD typically involves a combination of lifestyle modifications, dietary changes, symptom-directed medications, and psychological interventions. Lifestyle modifications may include stress reduction techniques, regular physical activity, and avoidance of dietary triggers such as fatty or spicy foods, caffeine, and alcohol. Symptom-directed medications may include acid-suppressing drugs, prokinetic agents to improve gastric emptying, and medications to alleviate pain or discomfort. Psychological interventions such as cognitive-behavioral therapy (CBT), relaxation techniques, and mindfulness meditation may also be beneficial in managing symptoms. It is important for individuals with FD to work closely with a healthcare provider to develop a personalized management plan tailored to their specific symptoms and needs. While FD can be chronic and challenging to treat, many individuals find relief with appropriate management strategies, allowing them to improve their quality of life and minimize the impact of symptoms on daily activities. Regular follow-up with a healthcare provider is important to monitor symptom progression, adjust treatment as needed, and address any concerns or complications that may arise.

Summary

- Rectal bleeding, also known as hematochezia, is the passage of bright red blood from the rectum or anus. It can vary in severity, ranging from small amounts of blood on toilet tissue or in the stool to significant bleeding that fills the toilet bowl.
- An anal fissure is a tear in the lining of your anal canal. Like a hemorrhoid, it often happens after straining to pass a hard stool. Anal fissures are easily mistaken for hemorrhoids.
- Diverticulitis occurs in your colon, usually in the lower end, close to your rectum. It happens when little pockets in the inner lining of your colon — called diverticula — become infected and inflamed.
- Gastroesophageal reflux disease (GERD) or gastro-oesophageal reflux disease (GORD) is a chronic upper gastrointestinal disease in which stomach content persistently and regularly flows up into the esophagus, resulting in symptoms and/or complications.
- GERD treatment aims to cut down on the amount of reflux or lessen damage to the lining of the esophagus from refluxed materials.
- An infection with *Helicobacter pylori* can either have no symptoms even when lasting a lifetime, or can harm the stomach and duodenal linings by inflammatory responses induced by several mechanisms associated with a number of virulence factors.
- Peptic ulcers are a consequence of inflammation that allows stomach acid and the digestive enzyme pepsin to overwhelm the protective mechanisms of the mucous membranes. The location of colonization of *H. pylori*, which affects the location of the ulcer, depends on the acidity of the stomach.
- *Helicobacter pylori* is a class I carcinogen, and potential cancers include gastric mucosa-associated lymphoid tissue (MALT) lymphomas and gastric cancer. Less commonly, diffuse large B-cell lymphoma of the stomach is a risk.
- Most people infected with *H. pylori* never experience any symptoms or complications, but will have a 10% to 20% risk of developing peptic ulcers or a 0.5% to 2% risk of stomach cancer. *H. pylori* induced gastritis may present as acute gastritis with stomach ache, nausea, and ongoing dyspepsia (indigestion) that is sometimes accompanied by depression and anxiety.
- *H. pylori* infection is associated with epigenetically reduced efficiency of the DNA repair machinery, which favors the accumulation of mutations and genomic instability as well as gastric carcinogenesis.
- In addition to using chemotaxis to avoid areas of low pH (high acidity), *H. pylori* also neutralizes the acid in its environment by producing large amounts of urease, an enzyme that breaks down the urea present in the stomach to carbonic acid and ammonia.
- Phagocytic leukocytes and monocytes infiltrate the site of infection, and antibodies are produced. *H. pylori* is able to adhere to the surface of the phagocytes and impede their action. This is responded to by the phagocyte in the generation and release of oxygen metabolites into the surrounding space.

- TNF-inducing protein alpha (Tipα) is a carcinogenic protein encoded by HP0596 unique to *H. pylori* that induces the expression of tumor necrosis factor. Tipα enters gastric cancer cells where it binds to cell surface nucleolin, and induces the expression of vimentin.
- *Helicobacter pylori* is a risk factor for gastric adenocarcinomas. Treatment is highly aggressive with even localized disease being treated sequentially with chemotherapy and radiotherapy before surgical resection.
- Irritable bowel syndrome (IBS) is a group of symptoms that affect your digestive system. It is a common but uncomfortable gastrointestinal disease, or condition that affects your intestines. People with IBS experience symptoms that include abdominal pain and cramps.

References

1. Blaser, M. J. (2006). Who are we? Indigenous microbes and the ecology of human diseases. *EMBO Reports, 7*(10), 956–960.
2. Byles, J. E., Redman, S., Hennrikus, D., Sanson-Fisher, R. W., & Dickinson, J. (1992). Delay in consulting a medical practitioner about rectal bleeding. *Journal of Epidemiology & Community Health, 46*(3), 241–244.
3. Carroll, W. (2016). *Gastroenterology & Nutrition: Prepare for the MRCPCH. Key Articles from the Pediatrics & Child Health Journal*. Elsevier Health Sciences.
4. Chen, C. C., Liou, J. M., Lee, Y. C., Hong, T. C., El-Omar, E. M., & Wu, M. S. (2021). The interplay between *Helicobacter pylori* and gastrointestinal microbiota. *Gut Microbes, 13*(1), 1–22.
5. Clinical Practice Committee, American Gastroenterological Association. (2004). American gastroenterological association medical position statement: Diagnosis and treatment of hemorrhoids. *Gastroenterology, 126*(5), 1461–1462.
6. Crosland, A., & Jones, R. (1995). Rectal bleeding: Prevalence and consultation behavior. *BMJ, 311*(7003), 486–488.
7. Ellis, B. G., & Thompson, M. R. (2005). Factors identifying higher risk rectal bleeding in general practice. *British Journal of General Practice, 55*(521), 949–955.
8. El-Serag, H. B., Sweet, S., Winchester, C. C., & Dent, J. (2014). Update on the epidemiology of gastro-oesophageal reflux disease: A systematic review. *Gut, 63*(6), 871–880.
9. Eslick, G. D., Kalantar, J. S., & Talley, N. J. (2009). Rectal bleeding: Epidemiology, associated risk factors, and healthcare seeking behavior: A population-based study. *Colorectal Disease, 11*(9), 921–926.
10. Farrands, P. A., & Hardcastle, J. D. (1984). Colorectal screening by a self-completion questionnaire. *Gut, 25*(5), 445–447.
11. FitzGerald, R., & Smith, S. M. (2021). An overview of *Helicobacter pylori* infection. In *Helicobacter pylori* (Vol. 2283, pp. 1–14). Methods in Molecular Biology.
12. Fontem, R. F., & Eyvazzadeh, D. (2023). Internal hemorrhoid. In *StatPearls*. StatPearls Publishing. Retrieved from: https://www.ncbi.nlm.nih.gov/books/NBK470314/ (accessed on 16 July 2024).
13. Granderath, F. A., Kamolz, T., & Pointner, R. (2006). *Gastroesophageal Reflux Disease: Principles of Disease, Diagnosis, and Treatment*. Springer Science & Business Media.

14. Hershcovici, T., & Fass, R. (2011). Pharmacological management of GERD: Where does it stand now? *Trends in Pharmacological Sciences, 32*(4), 258–264.

15. Kewenter, J., Haglind, E., & Smith, L. (1989). Value of a risk questionnaire in screening for colorectal neoplasm. *British Journal of Surgery, 76*(3), 280–283.

16. Koga, Y. (2022). Microbiota in the stomach and application of probiotics to gastroduodenal diseases. *World Journal of Gastroenterology, 28*(47), 6702–6715.

17. Marghalani, A. M., Bin Salman, T. O., Faqeeh, F. J., Asiri, M. K., & Kabel, A. M. (2020). Gastric carcinoma: Insights into risk factors, methods of diagnosis, possible lines of management, and the role of primary care. *Journal of Family Medicine and Primary Care, 9*(6), 2659–2663.

18. Martínez, L. E., O'Brien, V. P., Leverich, C. K., Knoblaugh, S. E., & Salama, N. R. (2019). Nonhelical Helicobacter pylori mutants show altered gland colonization and elicit less gastric pathology than helical bacteria during chronic infection. *Infection and Immunity, 87*(7), e00208–e00219.

19. Matsuo, Y., Kido, Y., & Yamaoka, Y. (2017). *Helicobacter pylori* outer membrane protein-related pathogenesis. *Toxins, 9*(3), 101.

20. National Institute of Diabetes and Digestive and Kidney Diseases (NIDDK). (2015). Acid reflux (GER & GERD) in adults. Retrieved from: https://www.niddk.nih.gov/health-information/digestive-diseases/acid-reflux-ger-gerd-adults (accessed on 16 July 2024).

21. Parker, M. (2010). Book review: Krause's food and nutrition therapy Mahan L.K., Escott-Stump S. Krause's food and nutrition therapy. 12th ed. Philadelphia: Saunders; (2007). *Nutrition in Clinical Practice, 25*(3), 314.

22. Ruggiero, P. (2014). Use of probiotics in the fight against *Helicobacter pylori. World Journal of Gastrointestinal Pathophysiology, 5*(4), 384–391.

23. Rust, M., Schweinitzer, T., & Josenhans, C. (2008). *Helicobacter flagella*, motility and chemotaxis. In Yamaoka, Y. (Ed.), *Helicobacter pylori: Molecular Genetics and Cellular Biology*. Caister Academic Press.

24. Salama, N. R. (2020). Cell morphology as a virulence determinant: Lessons from *Helicobacter pylori. Current Opinion in Microbiology, 54*, 11–17.

25. Sun, Z., & Migaly, J. (2016). Review of hemorrhoid disease: Presentation and management. *Clinical Colon and Rectal Surgery, 29*(1), 22–29.

26. Walsh, C. J., Delaney, S., & Rowlands, A. (2018). Rectal bleeding in general practice: New guidance on commissioning. *British Journal of General Practice, 68*(676), 514–515.

27. Warren, J. R., & Marshall, B. (1983). Unidentified curved bacilli on gastric epithelium in active chronic gastritis. *Lancet, 1*(8336), 1273–1275.

28. Zajac, P., Holbrook, A., Super, M. E., & Vogt, M. (2013). An overview: Current clinical guidelines for the evaluation, diagnosis, treatment, and management of dyspepsia. *Osteopathic Family Physician, 5*(2), 79–85.

Chapter 7

SYMPTOMS OF CANCER

Contents

Introduction

A collection of disorders known as cancers are characterized by aberrant cell growth that has the capacity to invade or spread to other bodily regions. In contrast, benign tumors do not metastasize. A lump, unusual bleeding, protracted cough, unexplained weight loss, and altered bowel movements are among the possible warning signs and symptoms. These symptoms may be indicative of cancer, but there are alternative explanations as well. Humans can suffer from more than 100 different types of cancer.

Of cancer-related deaths, tobacco use accounts for about 22% of deaths. An additional 10% can be attributed to being overweight, having a poor diet, not exercising, or drinking too much alcohol. Additional contributing factors comprise specific infections, radiation exposure, and exposure to environmental contaminants. Approximately 16–18% of cancers worldwide are caused by environmental factors such as infection with particular viruses, bacteria, or parasites. The hepatitis B, hepatitis C, human papillomavirus infection, Epstein-Barr virus, human T-lymphotropic virus 1, Kaposi's sarcoma-associated herpesvirus, and Merkel cell polyomavirus are among these infectious agents. Although HIV does not directly cause cancer, it can lead to immune deficiencies that increase the risk of other infections by several 1,000 times (as in the case of Kaposi's sarcoma). Crucially, vaccination against human papillomavirus and hepatitis B has been demonstrated to almost completely remove the risk of cancers brought on by these viruses in those who have received the shots before infection.

These environmental influences alter a cell's genes, at least in part. Usually, a great deal of genetic alteration is needed prior to cancer development. Hereditary genetic defects account for 5–10% of cancer cases. Certain indications and symptoms, as well as screening tests, can identify cancer. Next, medical imaging is usually used to look into it more, and a biopsy is usually used to confirm it.

Avoiding smoking, keeping a healthy weight, consuming less alcohol, eating lots of fruits, vegetables, and whole grains, getting vaccinated against certain infectious diseases, consuming less processed and red meat, and spending less time in the sun can all lower your chance of developing certain cancers. Screening is a good way to detect cervical and colon cancer early. There is debate regarding the advantages of breast cancer screening. A combination of radiation therapy, surgery, chemotherapy, and targeted therapy is frequently used to treat cancer. An essential component of care is managing pain and symptoms. Palliative care is especially crucial for those with advanced illnesses. The type of cancer and the degree of disease at the beginning of treatment determine the prognosis. In the developed world, the five-year survival rate for children under 15 at diagnosis is typically 80%. In the US, the average five-year survival rate for cancer patients of all ages is 66%.

Lung, prostate, colorectal, and stomach cancers are the most prevalent cancer types in men. The most prevalent forms in females are colorectal, lung, cervical, and breast cancer. Skin cancers other than melanoma would make up about 40% of all new cancer cases annually if they were counted. Acute lymphoblastic leukemia and brain tumors are the most common childhood diseases, with the exception of non-Hodgkin lymphoma in Africa. Approximately 165,000 children under the age of 15 received cancer diagnoses in 2012. The chance of developing cancer rises dramatically with age, and developed nations have higher rates of cancer incidence. Rates are rising as more people in the developing world live longer and adopt new lifestyles.

Orientation and Directional Terms

Term	Definition	Illustration
Biopsy	A biopsy is a procedure to remove a piece of tissue or a sample of cells from your body so that it can be tested in a laboratory.	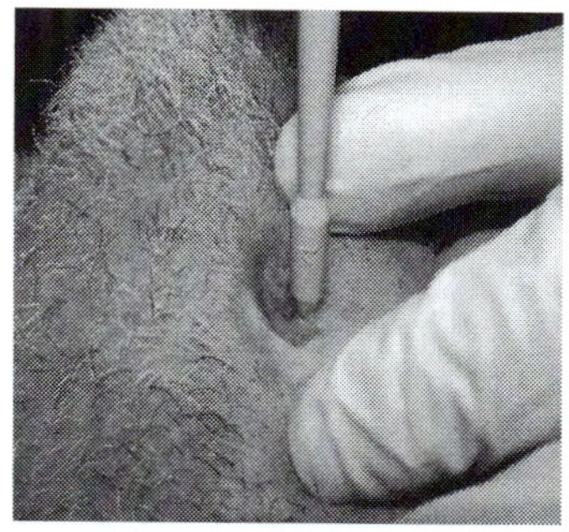
Cancer cells	Cancer cells are cells that divide continually, forming solid tumors or flooding the blood or lymph with abnormal cells	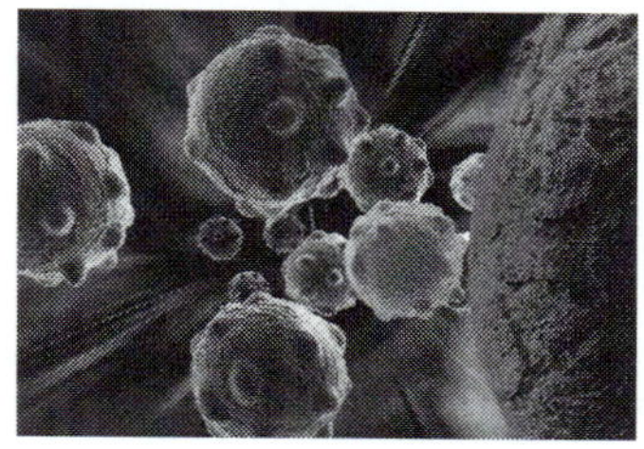
Prostate-specific antigen	Prostate-specific antigen (PSA), also known as gamma-seminoprotein or kallikrein-3 (KLK3), P-30 antigen, is a glycoprotein enzyme encoded in humans by the KLK3 gene. PSA is a member of the kallikrein-related peptidase family and is secreted by the epithelial cells of the prostate gland in men and the paraurethral glands in women.	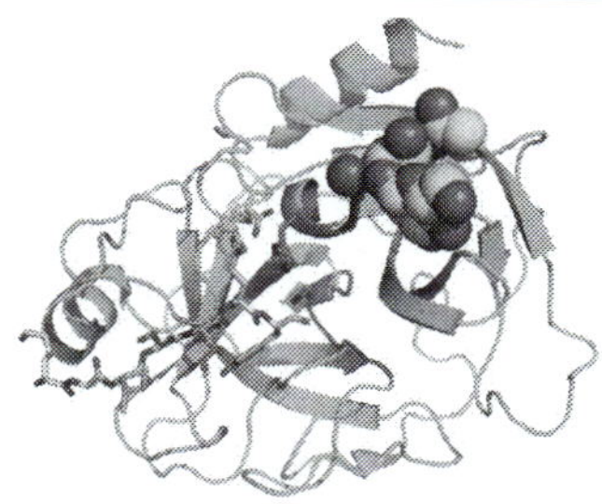
Medical imaging	Medical imaging is the field of medicine in which medical professionals recreate various images of parts of the body for diagnostic or treatment purposes.	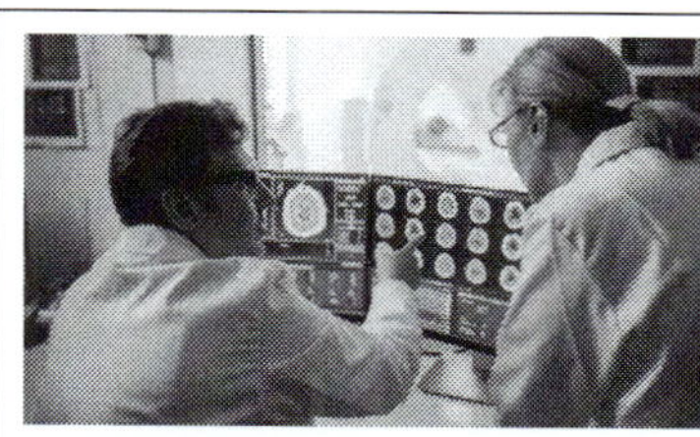
Small cell lung cancer	Small cell lung cancer starts when healthy cells in your lungs mutate or change into cancerous cells. These cells then divide and multiply uncontrollably.	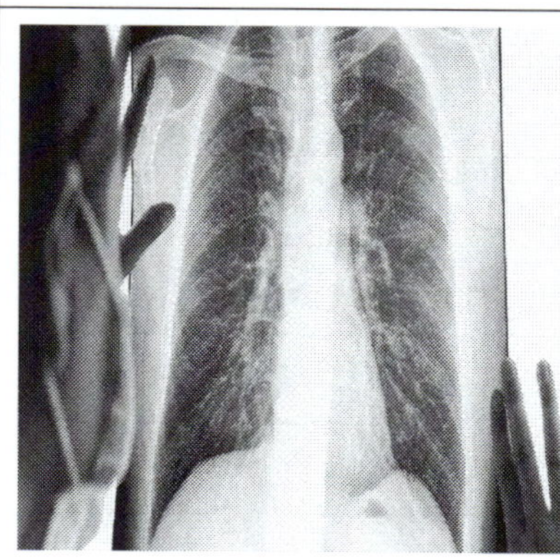

7.1. Lung Cancer

Malignant tumors that originate in the lung are referred to as lung cancer, lung carcinoma, or lung cancer. Genetic damage to the DNA of cells in the airways, frequently brought on by cigarette smoking or hazardous chemical inhalation, is the root cause of lung cancer. Tumor growth results from damaged airway cells' unchecked ability to multiply. Tumors spread throughout the lung and impair lung function if left untreated. Lung tumors eventually spread to other areas of the body through metastasis.

Early-stage lung cancer is typically asymptomatic and only identifiable through imaging tests. Most patients report nonspecific respiratory issues such as coughing, dyspnea, or chest pain as the cancer worsens. Depending on the tumor's size and location, additional symptoms may occur. To find the location and size of any tumors, people suspected of having lung cancer usually go through a battery of imaging tests. A biopsy of the suspected tumor must be performed and examined under a microscope by a pathologist in order to make a definitive diagnosis of lung cancer.

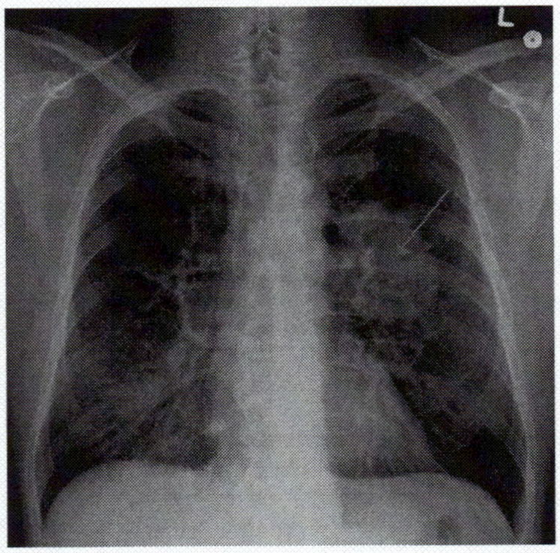

Figure 7.1. *Lung cancer.*

Source: *By James Heilman, MD – Own work, CC BY-SA 3.0, https://commons.wikimedia.org/w/index.php?curid=18076961.*

A pathologist can identify cancerous cells and also categorize a tumor based on the type of cells that made it. About 15% of cases are small-cell lung cancer (SCLC), with adenocarcinomas, squamous-cell carcinomas, and large-cell carcinomas accounting for the remaining 85% of cases, also known as non-small-cell lung cancers, or NSCLC. Following diagnosis, additional imaging and biopsies are performed to establish the stage of the cancer based on its extent of spread (Figure 7.1).

In order to eradicate any remaining cancer cells, radiation therapy and chemotherapy are occasionally administered after surgery to remove the tumor in cases of early-stage lung cancer. Chemotherapy and radiation therapy are used in conjunction with medication treatments that target particular cancer subtypes to treat later-stage cancer. Only about 20% of people survive five years after their diagnosis, even with treatment. Women relative to men, as well as those diagnosed at a younger age and at an earlier stage, have higher survival rates.

Tobacco use is the primary cause of lung cancer in most cases. The remaining ones are brought on by accidental genetic mutations or exposure to dangerous substances like radon gas and asbestos. As a result, initiatives to prevent lung cancer promote quitting smoking and avoiding potentially harmful chemicals. Giving up smoking lowers one's risk of lung cancer and enhances the prognosis of patients who have already been diagnosed with the disease.

Lung cancer is the most common and deadly cancer globally, accounting for 2 million cases and 1 in 8 deaths in 2020. It is uncommon for people under 40 to be diagnosed with lung cancer; the average age of death is 72 years old, and the average diagnosis age is 70. Worldwide variations exist in both incidence and results, contingent upon tobacco use patterns. Lung cancer was an uncommon illness until the 20th century, when cigarettes became popular. As evidence of the connection between smoking and lung cancer grew in the 1950s and 1960s, most major national health organizations issued statements opposing tobacco use.

7.1.1. Signs and Symptoms

Most cases of early lung cancer are symptomless. When symptoms do appear, they are frequently general respiratory issues that vary from person to person, such as coughing, shortness of breath, or chest pain. When someone coughs, they usually report feeling like they are coughing for the first time or that their previous cough is getting stronger or more frequent. One in four people cough up blood, which can vary in size from tiny splotches to large amounts. Shortness of breath affects about half of people with lung cancer, and 25 to 50% report having a dull, enduring chest pain that stays in one spot over time. Some people also have systemic symptoms, such as fever, night sweats, general weakness, appetite loss, and weight loss, in addition to respiratory symptoms.

Some less frequent symptoms point to tumors in specific areas. Thoracic tumors can impair breathing by blocking the trachea or damaging the diaphragm's nerve; they can also make swallowing difficult by compressing the esophagus; they can cause hoarseness by interfering with the larynx's nerves; and they can result in Horner's syndrome by interfering with the sympathetic nervous system. Pancoast tumors, which are tumors at the top of the lung that also cause destruction of the topmost ribs and shoulder pain that travels down the little finger side of the arm, are another common cause of Horner's syndrome. A tumor that has spread throughout the chest may be indicated by swollen lymph nodes above the collarbone. Tumors that invade the area surrounding the heart can result in fluid buildup, arrhythmia (an irregular heartbeat), and heart failure. Tumors that obstruct bloodflow to the heart can cause superior vena cava syndrome, which is characterized by upper body swelling and dyspnea.

Metastases to sites other than the lungs cause symptoms in about one in three patients with lung cancer. Anywhere in the body, lung cancer has the potential to spread, and the symptoms vary according to the site. Headache, nausea, vomiting, seizures, and neurological deficits can all be brought on by brain metastases. Pain, bone fractures, and spinal cord compression can all result from bone metastases. Leukoerythroblastosis, or immature blood cells, can result from metastasis into the bone marrow, which can deplete blood cells. Liver metastases may result in weight loss, fever, right upper quadrant abdominal pain, and enlarged liver.

Hormones that change the body are frequently released by lung tumors, resulting in peculiar symptoms known as paraneoplastic syndromes. Mineral concentrations in the blood can change dramatically when hormones are released inappropriately. The most prevalent is hypercalcemia, or elevated blood calcium, which is brought on by an excess of parathyroid hormone or parathyroid hormone-related protein. Constipation, nausea, vomiting, abdominal pain, increased thirst, frequent urination, and altered mental status are some of the symptoms of hypercalcemia.

In addition, hypokalemia (low potassium) from improper adrenocorticotropic hormone secretion and hyponatremia (low sodium) from excessive antidiuretic hormone or atrial natriuretic peptide synthesis are frequent side effects of lung cancer. Nail clubbing affects about one in three lung cancer patients, and hypertrophic pulmonary osteoarthropathy (which causes nail clubbing, joint pain, and thickening of the skin) affects up to one in ten patients. In patients with lung cancer, a range of autoimmune disorders can manifest as paraneoplastic syndromes. These include autoimmune deterioration of the cerebellum, limbic system, or brainstem; sensory neuropathies; muscle inflammation; and Lambert-Eaton myasthenic syndrome, which results in muscle weakness. Paraneoplastic blood clotting, such as migratory venous thrombophlebitis, heart clots, and disseminated intravascular coagulation (body-wide clots), affects as many as one in twelve lung cancer patients. Skin and kidney paraneoplastic syndromes are uncommon; they can affect up to 1% of patients with lung cancer.

7.1.2. Diagnosis

Imaging tests are performed on a person suspected of having lung cancer in order to assess the presence, extent, and location of tumors. Initially, a chest X-ray is often performed by primary care physicians in order to search for a lung mass. An obvious mass, atelectasis (lung collapse), consolidation (pneumonia), pleural effusion, or widening of the mediastinum (suggestive of spread to lymph nodes there) can all be seen on an X-ray; however, some lung tumors are not visible on one. Many people then have computed tomography (CT) scanning, which can show the locations and sizes of tumors.

It takes a biopsy of the suspected tissue to be histologically analyzed for cancer cells in order to make a conclusive diagnosis of lung cancer. Because lung cancer tumors are located in such a way, biopsies are frequently obtained using minimally invasive methods such as fine needle aspiration, other imaging-guided biopsy through the skin, or a fiberoptic bronchoscope that can retrieve tissue (sometimes guided by endobronchial ultrasound). Those who are unable to have a traditional biopsy procedure performed might instead have a liquid biopsy, which involves taking a sample of bodily fluid that may contain detectable tumor DNA in circulation.

Imaging is another tool used to evaluate the spread of cancer. Finding metastases in the body is frequently accomplished by PET or combined PET-CT scanning. The National Comprehensive Cancer Network advises using magnetic resonance imaging (MRI) or computed tomography (CT) instead of PET scanning to check for brain metastases in patients with non-small cell lung cancer (NSCLC) and large tumors, or tumors that have spread to neighboring lymph nodes, as PET scanning is less sensitive in the brain. A biopsy is frequently performed to confirm the cancerous nature of a suspected metastasis when imaging indicates that the tumor has spread. Most frequently, lung cancer spreads to the liver, brain, bones, and adrenal glands.

When viewed on a chest radiograph or CT scan, lung cancer frequently manifests as a single pulmonary nodule. Up to 30% of people screened in lung cancer screening studies have a lung nodule; most of these turn out to be benign. In addition to lung cancer, numerous other illnesses can also manifest in this way, such as hamartomas and infectious granulomas brought on by histoplasmosis, coccidioidomycosis, or tuberculosis.

7.1.2.1. Classification

Lung cancer is categorized at diagnosis according to the kind of cells that gave rise to the tumor; tumors from distinct cell types grow and react to treatment in different ways. According to the size and appearance of the malignant cells observed under a microscope by a histopathologist, there are two primary forms of lung cancer: non-small-cell lung cancer (NSCLC; 85% of cases) and small cell lung cancer (SCLC; 15% of cases). SCLC tumors are frequently discovered in the main airways, close to the center of the lungs. Their cells have a characteristic nucleus with granular-looking chromatin and no discernible nucleoli. They also appear small with poorly defined boundaries, little cytoplasm, and many mitochondria. Large-cell carcinoma, squamous-cell carcinoma, and adenocarcinoma are the three cancer types that make up NSCLCs. Adenocarcinomas account for approximately 40% of lung cancer cases. Their cells have the ability to produce mucin, resemble glandular cells, and grow in three-dimensional clumps. Squamous-cell carcinomas account for about 30% of all lung cancer cases. They usually happen near wide airways. The tumors are made up of keratin layers sandwiched between sheets of cells. At the core of the tumor, a hollow cavity and related cell death are frequently observed. Large-cell carcinomas, so named because of the large cells with abundant cytoplasm, large nuclei, and prominent nucleoli, make up less than 10% of lung cancer cases. Rarer forms of lung cancer account for about 10% of cases. These comprise uncommon subtypes like sarcomatoid carcinomas and carcinoid tumors, as well as mixtures of the aforementioned subtypes like adenosquamous carcinoma.

Based on the features of the cancer cells' growth, several types of lung cancer are subdivided. Adenocarcinomas can be categorized as solid pattern and micropapillary, acinar and papillary, or lepidic (growing along the surface of intact alveolar walls). Micropapillary and solid pattern adenocarcinomas are the most aggressive, whereas lepidic adenocarcinomas are typically the least aggressive.

To verify the classification of lung cancer, biopsies are frequently stained by immunohistochemistry in addition to being examined for cell morphology. Neuroendocrine cell markers like synaptophysin, chromogranin, and CD56 are present in SCLCs. Apsin-A and TTF-1 are typically expressed by adenocarcinomas, whereas squamous cell carcinomas express p63 and its cancer-specific isoform p40 but do not express either of these two proteins. The distinction between lung cancers is also frequently made using CK7 and CK20. While CK20 is present in many cancers, lung cancer usually lacks it. While CK7 is absent in squamous cell carcinomas, it is present in many lung cancers.

7.1.2.2. Staging

The staging of lung cancer involves determining the extent to which the cancer has spread from its initial site. It is among the variables influencing lung cancer prognosis and treatment.

Generally, SCLC is staged using one of two rather straightforward systems: limited stage or extensive stage. One-third of patients receive a limited stage diagnosis, which means that the cancer is limited to one side of the chest and can be treated with a single radiation field. The cancer has spread to both sides of the chest or to other parts of the body in the case of the other two thirds of patients, who have an "extensive stage" diagnosis.

The Tumor, Node, Metastasis (TNM) staging system developed by the American Joint Committee on Cancer is commonly used to stage NSCLC and, on occasion, SCLC. Stage groups are created by adding the scores for the tumor's size and extent (T), spread to nearby lymph nodes (N), and distant metastases (M).

Relatively small tumors are designated T1, which are subdivided by size: tumors $\leq$ 1 centimeter (cm) across are T1a; 1–2 cm T1b; 2–3 cm T1c. Tumors up to 5 cm across, or those that have spread to the visceral pleura (tissue covering the lung) or main bronchi, are designated T2. T2a designates 3–4 cm tumors; T2b 4–5 cm tumors. T3 tumors are up to 7 cm across, have multiple nodules in the same lobe of the lung, or invade the chest wall, diaphragm (or the nerve that controls it), or area around the heart. Tumors that are larger than 7 cm, have nodules spread in different lobes of a lung, or invade the mediastinum (center of the chest cavity), heart, largest blood vessels that supply the heart, trachea, esophagus, or spine are designated T4. Lymph node staging depends on the extent of local spread: with the cancer metastasized to no lymph nodes (N0), pulmonary or hilar nodes (along the bronchi) on the same side as the tumor (N1), mediastinal or subcarinal lymph nodes (in the middle of the lungs, N2), or lymph nodes on the opposite side of the lung from the tumor (N3). Metastases are staged as no metastases (M0), nearby metastases (M1a; the space around the lung or the heart, or the opposite lung), a single distant metastasis (M1b), or multiple metastases (M1c) (Table 7.1).

Table 7.1. International Staging System for Lung Cancer

Stages	Sizes (in Greatest Dimension)	Invasion
Tx	Tumor cannot be assessed	
T0	No evidence of primary tumor	
Tis	Carcinoma in situ (pre-cancer)	
T1	≤3 cm	Surrounded by lung or visceral pleura. Invades the lobar bronchus but not the main bronchus.
T1a	≤2 cm	
T1b	>2 cm and ≤3 cm	
T2	>3 cm and ≤5 cm	Invades the main bronchus, regardless of distance from the carina but does not invade the carina. Invades the visceral pleura. Invades the hilar region.
T2a	>3 cm and ≤4 cm	
T2b	>4 cm and ≤5 cm	
T3	>5 cm and ≤7 cm	Invades the chest wall, phrenic nerve, and parietal pericardium. Presents satellite nodules in the same lobe.
T4	>7 cm	Invades the diaphragm, mediastinum, heart, great vessels, and trachea. Presents satellite nodules in the different lobes.

Source: *Paing MP, Hamamoto K, Tungjitkusolmun S, & Pintavirooj C, (2019). Automatic detection and staging of lung tumors using locational features and double-staged classifications. Applied Sciences, 9(11), 2329. https://doi.org/10.3390/app9112329.*

7.1.2.3. Screening

Some nations advise using low-dose CT lung scans to screen individuals who have a high risk of developing lung cancer at various intervals. Screening programs have the potential to identify lung tumors in individuals who do not yet exhibit symptoms of lung cancer at an early stage, ideally early enough for the tumors to be effectively treated and reduce mortality. There is proof that routine low-dose CT scans can cut the overall number of lung cancer deaths by up to 20% in individuals who are at high risk of the disease. Notwithstanding evidence of benefit in these populations, there is a chance that a person will receive a "false positive" screening result, which could result in distressing tests, invasive procedures, and unnecessary testing. Radiation-induced cancer is also a possibility, albeit rare. People between the ages of 55 and 80 who have smoked for at least 30 pack years are recommended to undergo annual screening with low-dose CT by the United States Preventive Services Task Force. The European Commission suggests that low-dose CT lung scans be added to cancer screening programs throughout the European Union for individuals who smoke or have smoked in the past. In a similar vein, the Canadian Task Force for Preventative Health advises screening for lung cancer in those who are between the ages of 55 and 74 and who have smoked for more than 30 pack years, whether they are current or former smokers.

7.1.3. Treatment

The exact cell type of the cancer, the extent of its spread, and the patient's health all influence how lung cancer is treated. Radiation therapy, chemotherapy, and surgical tumor removal are common treatments for early-stage cancer. Chemotherapy and radiation therapy are used in conjunction with immune checkpoint inhibitors and more recent targeted molecular therapies for advanced cancer stages. To enhance quality of life, palliative care and lifestyle modifications are incorporated into all lung cancer treatment regimens.

7.1.3.1. Small-Cell Lung Cancer

Treatment for limited-stage SCLC usually consists of chemotherapy plus radiation. The American College of Chest Physicians and the National Comprehensive Cancer Network recommend four to six cycles of a platinum-based chemotherapy, such as carboplatin or cisplatin, in combination with etoposide or irinotecan. This is usually administered in conjunction with the first two chemotherapy cycles and thoracic radiation therapy (45 Gray (Gy) twice daily). Up to 80% of patients who receive first-line therapy experience remission; however, the majority of patients experience a relapse due to chemotherapy-resistant disease. Second-line chemotherapy is administered to patients who relapse. The US FDA has approved topotecan and lurbinectedin for this use. Other occasionally used, similarly effective medications include irinotecan, paclitaxel, docetaxel, vinorelbine, etoposide, and gemcitabine. Preventive cranial irradiation can increase survival in patients with limited-stage disease and lower the risk of brain metastases. Etoposide is first used in combination with either carboplatin or cisplatin to treat extensive-stage SCLC. Radiotherapy is limited to the reduction of tumors that present with extremely severe symptoms. For a small percentage of patients, combining standard chemotherapy with an immune checkpoint inhibitor can increase survival, adding about two months to the average person's life expectancy.

7.1.3.2. Non-small-Cell Lung Cancer

The initial course of treatment for NSCLC in stages I and II typically involves surgically excising the affected lung lobe. Wedge resection or segmentectomy surgery can be used to remove a smaller portion of lung tissue from a patient who is not well enough to undergo complete lobe removal. Patients with tumors positioned in the center of the lung and otherwise in good health may require more intensive surgery called a pneumonectomy, which involves removing the entire lung. A high-volume surgery clinic and skilled thoracic surgeons increase survival rates. Radiation therapy is an option for those who cannot or will not have surgery. The best practice is stereotactic body radiation therapy, which is usually given several times over a two-week period. Chemotherapy may worsen disease outcomes in patients with the earliest stages of the disease and has little effect on those with stage I NSCLC. Chemotherapy for patients with stage II disease is typically started six to twelve weeks following surgery. It consists of up to four cycles of cisplatin (or carboplatin in cases of renal impairment, neuropathy, or hearing loss) coupled with vinorelbine, pemetrexed, gemcitabine, or docetaxel.

The course of treatment for patients with stage III NSCLC varies depending on the illness. For those whose spread has been more restricted, treatment may include radiation therapy and chemotherapy after the tumor and impacted lymph nodes are surgically removed. Individuals with notably large tumors (T4) and those for whom surgery is not feasible receive immunotherapy durvalumab in addition to combination chemotherapy and radiotherapy. While the side effects of combination therapy are more severe, it improves survival when chemotherapy and radiation are administered together rather than separately.

Treatment for individuals with stage IV disease involves a combination of chemotherapy, immunotherapy, radiotherapy, and pain management. Depending on the genetic composition of the malignant cells, targeted therapies may be used to treat a large number of cases of advanced disease. The EGFR inhibitors osimertinib, erlotinib, gefitinib, afatinib, and dacomitinib can be used to treat up to 30% of tumors that have mutations in the EGFR gene that cause an overactive EGFR protein. Of these, osimertinib is known to be superior to erlotinib and gefitinib, and all of them are superior to chemotherapy alone. ALK inhibitors such as crizotinib or its offspring, alectinib, brigatinib, and ceritinib, can be used to treat hyperactive ALK protein, which is present in up to 7% of NSCLC patients. Lorlatinib, a third-generation ALK inhibitor, is an option for treating ALK inhibitor-treated patients who relapse. The MET inhibitors capmatinib or tepotinib can inhibit overactive MET in up to 5% of patients with non-small cell lung cancer. For certain cancers with uncommon mutations, targeted therapies are also an option. Around 2% of NSCLC cancers have hyperactive BRAF, which can be treated with dabrafenib plus the MEK inhibitor trametinib; 1% of NSCLC cancers have activated ROS1, which can be inhibited by crizotinib, lorlatinib, or entrectinib; 1% of NSCLC cancers have overactive NTRK, which can be treated with entrectinib or larotrectinib; and 1% of NSCLC cancers have active RET. Selpercatinib can be used to treat these cancers.

Individuals with non-small cell lung cancer (NSCLC) who are not responsive to existing molecular therapies may be treated with immune checkpoint inhibitors and chemotherapy in combination, which stops cancer cells from deactivating T cells in the immune system. cisplatin plus gemcitabine for squamous cell carcinoma and cisplatin plus pemetrexed for non-squamous cell carcinoma are the recommended chemotherapy drugs, respectively, based on the NSCLC subtype. Immune checkpoint inhibitors work best against tumors that express the PD-L1 protein, though they can also occasionally work against tumors that don't. When treating tumors that express PD-L1, pembrolizumab, atezolizumab, or the combination of nivolumab plus ipilimumab is more effective than chemotherapy alone. The second-line chemotherapy drugs docetaxel and ramucirumab are used to treat patients who relapse on the aforementioned.

7.1.3.3. Palliative Care

Optimizing the quality of life and survival rate of individuals with lung cancer can be achieved by incorporating palliative care, which is a medical approach that focuses on reducing pain and improving symptoms, into treatment from the moment of diagnosis. Breathlessness and pain are two characteristics of lung cancer that are particularly prevalent. Breathlessness can be alleviated with additional oxygen, better ventilation, turning a patient over in bed, and low-dose morphine. Growth of the tumor can narrow or block the airway in 20 to 30% of lung cancer patients, especially in those with late-stage disease, which results in coughing and breathing difficulties. When feasible, obstructing tumors can be surgically removed; however, most of the time, patients with airway obstruction are not healthy enough to undergo surgery. The American College of Chest Physicians advises bronchoscopy, occasionally assisted by thermal or laser ablation, to physically remove the obstructing tissue, try to shrink the tumor with localized radiation (brachytherapy), or open the airway by inserting a stent.

Treatment options for other causes of breathlessness related to lung cancer include direct administration of antibiotics for lung infection, diuretics for pulmonary edema, benzodiazepines for anxiety, and steroids for airway blockage.

Dedicated end-of-life care can help people with advanced disease who are nearing the end of their lives by managing their symptoms and reducing their suffering. Opioid painkillers, which switch from oral to injectable form if the patient loses the ability to swallow, can be used to treat pain and breathing difficulties, which are common in this type of disease. Opioids or cough suppressants can be used to treat common coughing. Some people experience terminal delirium, which is treated with antipsychotic medications, low-dose sedatives, and examining alternative causes of discomfort like low blood sugar, constipation, and sepsis. Terminal delirium manifests as confused behavior, unexplained movements, or a reversal of the sleep-wake cycle. Many people experience terminal secretions in their final days of life, which are collections of fluid in the airways that can make breathing noisy. Although it is not believed to cause respiratory issues, family members and caregivers may become distressed. Anticholinergic drugs can lessen terminal secretions. Cancer-related pain can affect even non-communicative or unconscious patients, which is why painkillers are usually administered until the patient passes away (Kennedy et al., 2018).

7.2. Prostate Cancer

The unchecked growth of cells in the prostate, a gland located beneath the bladder in the male reproductive system, is known as prostate cancer. Early-stage prostate cancer doesn't show any signs. Tests for prostate-specific antigen (PSA) are commonly used in screening procedures to identify abnormal growth of prostate tissue. Prostate cancer is more likely to develop in people with elevated blood PSA levels. Prostate biopsies are necessary for the diagnosis. The pathologist rates the tumors according to their Gleason scores; a higher score indicates a more dangerous tumor if cancer is present. To search for cancer that has spread outside of the prostate, medical imaging is used. A cancer case is categorized into one of four stages based on the Gleason score, PSA levels, and imaging results. A higher stage denotes a more dangerous, more advanced illness.

The majority of prostate tumors stay small and pose no health risks. These are treated with active surveillance, which involves doing routine testing to make sure the tumor has not spread. Radiation therapy can destroy tumors that are more likely to be dangerous, and radical prostatectomy is one surgical method for removing them. Hormone therapy, which lowers levels of androgens (male sex hormones) that prostate cells require to survive, is used to treat patients whose cancer has spread beyond the prostate. Cancer cells may eventually develop resistance to this therapy. Castration-resistant prostate cancer, the most advanced stage of the disease, is treated with docetaxel chemotherapy in addition to ongoing hormone therapy. Certain tumors can metastasize, or spread, to other parts of the body, especially the lymph nodes and bones. Tumors there result in excruciating bone pain, paralysis or weakness in the legs, and finally death (Figure 7.2).

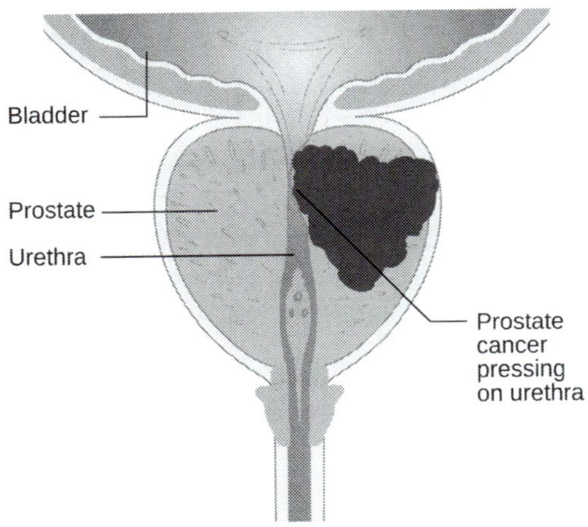

Figure 7.2. *Diagram of a prostate tumor pressing on the urethra (the duct that transports urine from the bladder), which can cause urinary problems.*

Source: *https://upload.wikimedia.org/wikipedia/commons/thumb/5/59/Diagram_showing_prostate_cancer_pressing_on_the_urethra_CRUK_182.svg/800px-Diagram_showing_prostate_cancer_pressing_on_the_urethra_CRUK_182.svg.png.*

The extent of cancer spread at diagnosis determines the prognosis for prostate cancer. 99% of men with prostate-specific tumors survive for more than ten years after being diagnosed. The most dangerous tumors are those that have spread to distant body sites, where the five-year survival rate is only 30–40%.

Prostate cancer is more common in older adults; the average age of diagnosis is 67. Prostate cancer is more common in people with a family history of cancer, especially in those who receive BRCA2 gene variants linked to cancer. Prostate cancer is the second most common cause of cancer and cancer-related death in men, accounting for 1.2 million new cases diagnosed and 350,000 deaths annually. Prostate cancer claims the lives of one in eight men, and one in 40 men pass away from the illness. When men had urinary obstructions surgically treated in the middle of the 19th century, the first reports of prostate tumors were made. Prostate cancer was initially treated primarily with prostatectomy. Radiation therapy and hormone therapy were developed in the middle of the 20th century to enhance the treatment of prostate cancer. Charles B. Gaines received the 1966 Nobel Prize in recognition of his development of hormone therapies for prostate cancer. Huggins and Andrzej W.'s 1977 Prize. Schally.

7.2.1. Signs and Symptoms

Prostate cancer in its early stages often does not show any symptoms. However, as the tumor grows outside of the prostate, it can lead to complications such as erectile dysfunction, blood in urine or semen, and difficulty urinating, including frequent urination and a weak or slow urine stream. Many men over the age of 50 experience urinary issues, often caused by conditions other than prostate cancer such as benign prostatic hyperplasia (enlarged prostate that is not cancerous).

Prostate cancers that have progressed may spread to neighboring lymph nodes and bones, especially those in the head, neck, pelvis, hips, spine, and ribs. They may result in exhaustion, inexplicable weight loss, and bone or back pain that is worse after resting. A bone fracture affects about 25% of people with metastatic prostate cancer. Metastases can harm the surrounding bones. Expanding metastases may also compress the spinal cord, resulting in limb paralysis or weakness in the feet and legs.

7.2.2. Prostate Cancer Screening

Prostate cancer screening is a procedure used to find men who do not exhibit any symptoms or signs of prostate cancer but still have an undetected diagnosis. Early detection of abnormal prostate tissue or cancer may make treatment and recovery easier, but it is not clear if this lowers death rates. When tumors are too small to produce any symptoms, screening tests are used to diagnose the majority of cases of prostate cancer. Prostate-specific antigen (PSA) levels are measured by blood tests, and these are elevated in individuals with enlarged prostates, regardless of the cause—benign prostatic hyperplasia or prostate cancer. One nanogram (ng) of PSA is found in the blood of an average man for every milliliter (mL) of blood tested. It is highly unlikely that someone with below-average PSA levels will get dangerous prostate cancer in the ensuing eight to ten years. Men who have PSA levels above 4 ng/mL are frequently referred for a prostate biopsy because they are at higher risk of developing prostate cancer—roughly 1 in 4 of them will. Men with PSA levels above 10 ng/mL are at even higher risk of developing prostate cancer; more than half of them do so. Since PSA levels can fluctuate for reasons unrelated to prostate cancer, it is frequently advised that men with high PSA levels repeat the blood test four to six weeks later. PSA levels can be raised by benign prostatic hyperplasia, prostate infections, recent ejaculation, and certain urological procedures; they can be lowered by taking 5α-Reductase inhibitors.

To more accurately estimate the risk of developing aggressive prostate cancer, individuals with elevated PSA may be subjected to secondary screening blood tests that measure PSA subtypes as well as other molecules.

Many measure free PSA, which is the percentage of PSA that isn't bound to other blood proteins; this is typically between 10 and 30%. Prostate cancer is more common in men with lower free PSA percentages. Measuring subtypes of free PSA helps several widely used tests, such as the Prostate Health Index (which measures a fragment called –2proPSA) and the 4K score (which measures intact free PSA), identify prostate cancer cases more accurately. Additional testing assesses blood levels of prostate-related proteins like kallikrein-2 (which is also determined by 4K score) or urine levels of mRNA molecules that are frequently found in prostate tumors, such as PCA3 and TMPRSS2 fused to ERG.

Men who are screened for prostate cancer have a lower death rate from the disease, according to several large studies. However, anxiety and unnecessary biopsies and treatments can result from the identification of cancer cases that would not have otherwise affected health. Different guidelines are provided by major national health organizations to weigh the advantages of early detection against the possible risks of treating individuals whose tumors are unlikely to have an impact on their health. According to the majority of medical guidelines, men who are at a high risk of developing prostate cancer because of their age, family history, ethnicity, or past history of high blood PSA levels should be given information about the advantages and disadvantages of PSA testing as well as access to screening tests. According to medical guidelines, men over 70 or those with a life expectancy of less than 10 years are generally advised against screening because the chances of a newly diagnosed prostate cancer affecting their natural lifespan are low. Geographically, men's screening uptake varies: in the US and Western Europe, over 80% of men are screened; in Japan, just 20% of men are screened, and screening is uncommon in areas with a low Human Development Index.

7.2.3. Diagnosis

Men who are suspected of having prostate cancer may have their prostate evaluated with multiple tests. The digital rectal examination is a routine procedure in which a physician feels the prostate nearby by inserting a lubricated finger into the rectum. Tumors feel against the rest of the prostate like hard, asymmetrical lumps. Benign prostatic hyperplasia is another condition that can cause the prostate to harden; approximately 20–25% of people with abnormal results from rectal exams have prostate cancer. According to the guidelines of several urological societies, men with elevated PSA levels should have their prostates evaluated for possible tumors using magnetic resonance imaging (MRI). The results of an MRI can be used to differentiate between people who have and do not have potentially dangerous tumors.

A prostate biopsy is necessary for a conclusive diagnosis of prostate cancer. Typically, transrectal ultrasound imaging, magnetic resonance imaging, or a combination of the two are used to guide the passage of a needle through the rectum or perineum to take a prostate biopsy. To increase the likelihood that any tumors will be discovered, ten to twelve samples are obtained from various prostate regions. A pathologist looks at biopsies under a microscope to identify the kind and quantity of cancerous cells found there. First, a microscope's appearance is used to classify cancers. Adenocarcinomas, which resemble gland tissue, account for more than 95% of prostate cancer cases. The remaining cases are primarily classified as squamous-cell carcinomas, which resemble squamous cells, a type of epithelial cell, and transitional cell carcinomas, which resemble transitional cells.

Tumor samples are then categorized according to the degree of tissue differentiation between the tumor and normal prostate tissue. The greater the degree of differentiation, the higher the likelihood of tumor growth. The pathologist rates various regions of the biopsied tissue using the widely used Gleason grading system, assigning numbers ranging from 3 (most similar to healthy prostate tissue) to 5 (least similar). After that, they add the two numbers that correspond to the biggest regions of the biopsy sample to get a Gleason score. A biopsy with a Gleason score of 6 is the least likely to be cancerous, while a biopsy with a score of 10 is the most likely to be malignant. Gleason scores are commonly grouped into "Gleason grade groups," which predict disease prognosis: a Gleason score of 6 is Gleason grade group 1 (best prognosis). A score of 7 (with Gleason scores 4 + 3, or Gleason scores 3 + 4, with the most prominent listed first) can be grade group 2 or 3; it is grade group 2 if the less severe Gleason score (3) covered more area; grade group 3 if the more severe Gleason score (4) covered more area. A score of 8 is grade group 4. A score of 9 or 10 is grade group 5 (worst prognosis).

A positron emission tomography (PET) imaging technique called PSMA scan, which uses a radioactive label that binds to the prostate protein prostate-specific membrane antigen to identify metastases far from the prostate, is used to determine the extent of cancer spread. Although they can be used as well, CT scans are not as good as MRI at identifying prostate spread. Bone scintigraphy is a test for cancer metastases to the bones.

7.2.4. Management

Prostate cancer treatment varies according to the cancer's stage, likelihood of metastasis, and the health and preferences of the affected individual. Patients with localized diseases that are not likely to spread are frequently more vulnerable to treatment-related side effects than to the disease itself, which is why they are frequently monitored for disease progression. Individuals who are more susceptible to the tumor may be treated with radiation therapy or a prostatectomy, which removes the prostate, occasionally in addition to hormone therapy. Chemotherapy is used to treat patients with metastatic disease, along with radiation therapy or other treatments to relieve the symptoms of metastatic tumors. Every few months, blood PSA levels are checked to determine whether the disease is progressing or relapsing, as well as to evaluate how well the treatments are working.

7.2.4.1. Localized Disease

Men who are diagnosed with low-risk cases of prostate cancer frequently postpone treatment and are subject to active surveillance, which involves periodic testing for tumor growth through digital rectal exams, PSA tests (every six months), MRIs, or repeat biopsies (every one to three years). This program keeps going until increases in tumor size, Gleason grade, or PSA levels point to a higher-risk tumor that might need treatment. At least half of the men never need further direct treatment for their prostate tumors and are kept under active surveillance.

Individuals who choose treatment options such as radiation therapy or prostatectomy experience varying side effects but comparable cancer control rates. There are two ways to deliver radiation: brachytherapy, which involves surgically inserting a radioactive source into the prostate, or intensity-modulated radiation therapy (IMRT), which enables high doses (greater than 80 Gy) to be delivered to the prostate with relatively little radiation to other organs. IMRT is administered over a few sessions, with five days a week of treatments for a few weeks. With the radioactive source permanently implanted into the prostate, where it will eventually exhaust its radioactivity over the course of several months, brachytherapy is usually completed in a single session. Radiation proctitis, or damage to the rectum that can result in bloody stools, diarrhea, fecal incontinence, and pain, can cause erectile dysfunction, infertility, and an increased risk of bladder cancer if it damages adjacent organs with either technique.

With a radical prostatectomy, the prostate's cancerous portion, the seminal vesicles, and the end of the vas deferens—the duct that carries sperm from the testes—are surgically removed. This is usually accomplished in wealthier nations through a process known as robot-assisted surgery, in which a surgeon uses tiny, precise movements made possible by robotic instruments inserted through tiny abdominal incisions. Compared to open surgery, this technique has fewer complications, shorter hospital stays, and less blood loss. Prostatectomy can be done laparoscopically (with a camera and hand instruments passed through tiny abdominal incisions) or openly, using an incision below the scrotum (perineal approach) or above the penis (retropubic approach). This procedure is available in locations where robot-assisted surgery is not available. The rates of cancer control achieved by the four approaches are comparable. Urinary incontinence and erectile dysfunction can arise from surgical incisional damage to adjacent tissue. Older people or those with a history of erectile dysfunction are more likely to experience erectile dysfunction. Age-related incontinence is more common in people with shorter urethras. The competence and experience of the particular surgeon performing the procedure are among the most important factors in determining the outcome of both the surgical side effects and the course of the cancer.

7.2.4.2. Metastatic Disease

Androgen deprivation therapy, also known as chemical castration, is the standard of care for patients with metastatic disease. It involves taking medications that lower the amounts of androgens, or male sex hormones, which prostate cells need to proliferate. By preventing the production or function of testosterone, the main androgen, many medications are used to reduce androgen levels. GnRH agonists, such as leuprolide, goserelin, or triptorelin, are usually injected once a month, or less frequently as necessary, as the first line of treatment. When treatment is started, GnRH agonists raise testosterone levels momentarily, which can exacerbate the condition in patients who have noticeable metastasis symptoms. These patients are instead given GnRH antagonists, such as degarelix or relugolix, which can also quickly lower testosterone levels. Hot flashes, a decline in bone density and muscle mass, a decrease in sex desire, exhaustion, personality changes, and an elevated risk of depression, diabetes, and cardiovascular disease are just a few of the negative effects of testosterone reduction. In over 95% of cases, hormone therapy stops the growth of the tumor, and in as many as 70% of cases, PSA levels return to normal.

7.2.4.3. Supportive Care

The majority of metastatic prostate cancer patients (about 85%) have bone metastases, which are the main cause of the disease's symptoms and demise. Nonsteroidal anti-inflammatory medications are prescribed to people who experience chronic pain. However, "breakthrough pain"—sudden, intense bursts of pain that subside in about 15 minutes—can occur in people with bone metastases before the effects of painkillers take hold. External beam radiation therapy can be used to treat individual pain sites to reduce neighboring tumors. Radium-223 and samarium-153-EDTMP are two radioactive compounds that disproportionately accumulate in bone and can be used to treat more diffuse bone pain by shrinking bone tumors. In a similar vein, as tumors shrink, systemic chemotherapeutics for metastatic prostate cancer can lessen pain. Although they have minimal effect on tumor size, other bone-modifying medications such as denosumab and zoledronic acid can lessen bone pain associated with prostate cancer. Up to 12% of patients with metastatic prostate cancer have spinal cord compression due to metastases, which can result in pain, weakness, numbness, and paralysis. High-dose steroids, radiotherapy, and surgery are all effective treatments for spine inflammation. These methods can also be used to reduce spinal tumor size and relieve pressure on the spinal cord.

Advanced prostate cancer patients experience weakness throughout their body, exhaustion, and sluggishness. This is partially due to gastrointestinal issues, which are frequently accompanied by nausea, constipation, appetite loss, and weight loss. Megestrol acetate or corticosteroids, appetite-increasing medications, antiemetics, or therapies addressing underlying gastrointestinal problems are commonly used to treat these.

Anemia, which is brought on by a mix of the illness itself, inadequate diet, and harm to the bone marrow from cancer therapies or bone metastases, can also result in general weakness. Depending on the underlying cause, anemia can be directly treated with blood transfusions or treated in a variety of ways. Lower limb or vaginal lymphedema is an uncomfortable accumulation of fluid that can be caused by metastases in the lymph nodes or organ damage. These swellings can cause excruciating pain, making it difficult for the affected person to walk normally, urinate, or engage in sexual activity. Treatment options for lymphedema include surgically draining accumulated fluid, applying pressure to promote drainage, and cleaning and tending to nearby damaged skin.

Anxiety and depression are roughly twice as common in prostate cancer patients than in non-patients. Psychoeducation and cognitive behavioral therapy are two psychological interventions that can help lessen anxiety, depression, and overall distress when added to standard prostate cancer treatments.

7.3. Colorectal Cancer

Colorectal cancer (CRC) is the development of cancer from the colon or rectum (parts of the large intestine). It is also referred to as bowel cancer, colon cancer, or rectal cancer. Blood in the stool, altered bowel movements, weight loss, exhaustion, and stomach pain are some possible signs and symptoms. Only a small percentage of colorectal cancer cases are caused by underlying genetic disorders; the majority are caused by lifestyle factors and aging. Dietary habits, obesity, smoking, and inactivity are risk factors. Alcohol use and the consumption of processed and red meat are dietary factors that raise the risk. Inflammatory bowel disorders, such as Crohn's disease and ulcerative colitis, are another risk factor. Familial adenomatous polyposis and hereditary non-polyposis colon cancer are two inherited genetic disorders that can cause colorectal cancer, though they account for less than 5% of cases. It usually begins as a benign tumor that eventually develops into a cancerous one, frequently taking the shape of a polyp.

During a sigmoidoscopy or colonoscopy, a sample of the colon can be used to diagnose colorectal cancer. Medical imaging is then used to ascertain whether the illness has spread. Screening works well to stop and lessen colorectal cancer-related deaths. From the age of 45 to 75, screening is advised using one of several techniques. The suggested starting age was 50, but because colon cancer cases are rising, the recommendation was lowered to 45. Small polyps discovered during a colonoscopy may be removed. To determine whether a large polyp or tumor is malignant, a biopsy may be carried out. During polyp excision, aspirin and other non-steroidal anti-inflammatory medications reduce the possibility of pain. However, because of their adverse effects, it is not advised to use them generally for this purpose (Figure 7.3).

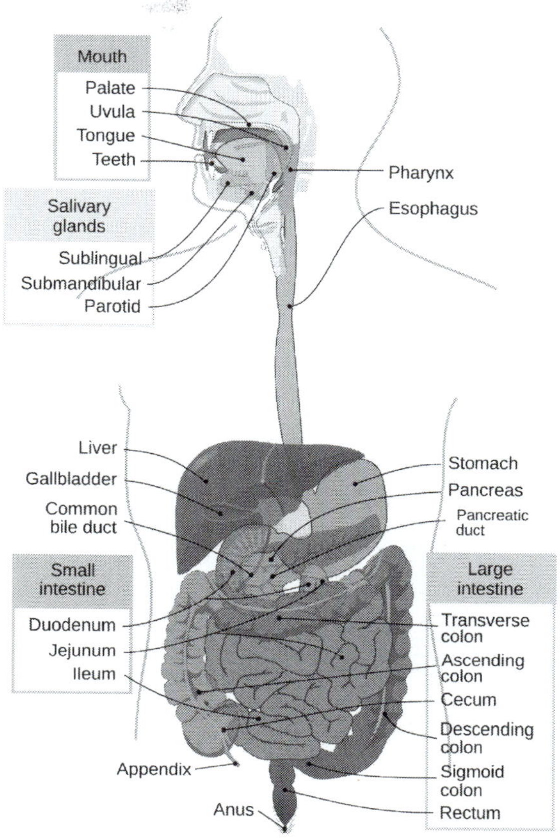

Figure 7.3. *This diagram shows the location of the stomach, small intestine, cecum, ascending colon, transverse colon, descending colon, sigmoid colon, and rectum.*

Source: *By Mariana Ruiz, Jmarchn – Own work, Public Domain, https://commons.wikimedia.org/w/index.php?curid=2898771.*

Treatments for colorectal cancer may involve a mix of chemotherapy, radiation therapy, targeted therapy, and surgery. Surgery may be able to treat cancers that are contained within the colon's wall, but management of cancers that have spread widely is typically limited to symptom relief and quality of life enhancement. In 2014, the five-year survival rate in the US was approximately 65%. The probability of survival varies depending on the patient's general health, the extent of the cancer, and whether or not surgery can remove the entire tumor. Colorectal cancer accounts for approximately 10% of all cancer cases worldwide, making it the third most common type of cancer overall. There were 551,000 disease-related deaths and 1.09 million new cases in 2018. Over 65% of cases are found in developed countries, where it is more prevalent. Compared to men, it is less common in women (Figure 7.4).

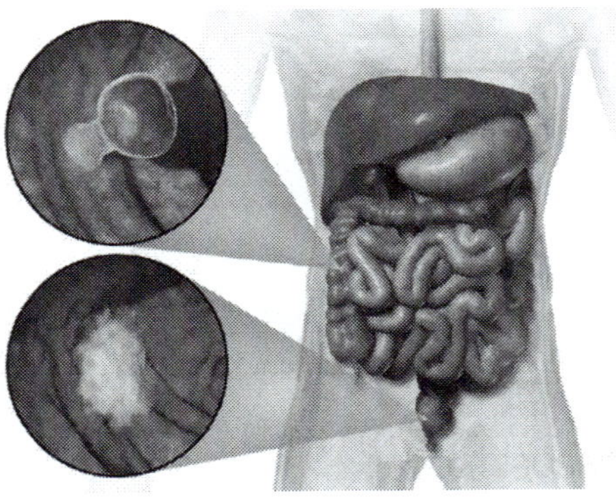

Figure 7.4. *Location and appearance of two example colorectal tumors.*

Source: *https://upload.wikimedia.org/wikipedia/commons/thumb/1/12/Blausen_0246_ColorectalCancer.png/800px-Blausen_0246_ColorectalCancer.png.*

7.3.1. Signs and Symptoms

The location of the tumor in the colon and whether it has metastasized—spread to other parts of the body—determine the signs and symptoms of colorectal cancer. Severe constipation, blood in the stool, a drop in stool caliber (thickness), appetite loss, weight loss, and nausea or vomiting in people over 50 are among the traditional warning indicators. About half of those with colorectal cancer do not experience any symptoms at all.

Anemia and rectal bleeding are considered high-risk symptoms in adults over 50. Generally, weight loss and bowel habit changes should only be taken seriously if they are linked to rectal bleeding.

7.3.2. Cause

A person with little to no genetic risk is involved in 75–95% of cases of colorectal cancer. Older age, male sex, high fat, sugar, and alcohol intake, red meat, processed meats, obesity, smoking, and inactivity are risk factors. Race is also taken into account as a risk factor in the Rectal Cancer Survival Calculator created by the MD Anderson Cancer Center. However, there are concerns about equity regarding whether this could result in unequal clinical decision-making. Roughly 10% of cases have inadequate activity involved. It seems that drinking more than one drink a day increases the risk associated with alcohol. Five glasses of water a day are associated with a lower risk of adenomatous polyps and colorectal cancer. Colon cancer and *Streptococcus gallolyticus* are linked. Since millions of people eat certain strains of the *Streptococcus bovis/Streptococcus equinus* complex every day, they might be safe. Colorectal tumors coexist in 25–80% of patients with *Streptococcus bovis/gallolyticus* bacteremia. In high-risk populations, the seroprevalence of Streptococcus bovis/gallolyticus is thought to be a promising practical marker for the early detection of an underlying bowel lesion. According to certain theories, the bloodstream's antibodies to Streptococcus bovis/gallolyticus antigens or the antigens themselves may serve as indicators of colon cancer development.

7.3.2.1. Inflammatory Bowel Disease

Individuals with inflammatory bowel disease, such as ulcerative colitis and Crohn's disease, have an elevated risk of developing colon cancer. This risk increases over time and with the severity of inflammation. It is recommended for those in high-risk groups to take preventative measures such as aspirin and undergo regular colonoscopies. Endoscopic surveillance can aid in the early diagnosis of colorectal cancer and may decrease the mortality rate associated with colon cancer. Individuals with inflammatory bowel disease make up less than 2% of colon cancer cases annually. The likelihood of developing colorectal cancer after 10, 20, and 30 years for those with Crohn's disease is 2%, 8%, and 18% respectively. For individuals with ulcerative colitis, approximately 16% will develop either a precursor to cancer or colon cancer within 30 years.

7.3.2.2. Genetics

About 20% of cases are in this group, which includes people with a family history involving two or more first-degree relatives (such as a parent or sibling) who have a two- to three-fold increased risk of illness. Higher incidences of colorectal cancer are also linked to some genetic syndromes. The most prevalent of these, accounting for approximately 3% of cases of colorectal cancer, is hereditary nonpolyposis colorectal cancer (HNPCC, also known as Lynch syndrome). Gardner syndrome and familial adenomatous polyposis are two other syndromes that have a strong correlation with colorectal cancer (FAP). Cancer is almost always present in people with these syndromes and accounts for 1% of all cancer cases. Because of the high risk of cancer, a total proctocolectomy may be advised as a preventive measure for individuals with FAP. Because there is a significant risk of rectal cancer if the rectum remains, a colonectomy—the removal of the colon—might not be sufficient as a preventive measure. Serrated polyposis syndrome, which is linked to a 25–40% risk of colorectal cancer, is the most prevalent type of polyposis syndrome that affects the colon.

7.3.3. Diagnosis

The diagnosis of colorectal cancer is made by taking samples from parts of the colon that are suspicious of the development of a tumor. Depending on where the lesion is located, this is usually done during a colonoscopy or sigmoidoscopy. Through microscopic analysis of a tissue sample, it is verified.

7.3.3.1. Medical imaging

On a CT scan, colorectal cancer may occasionally be first detected.

A CT scan of the chest, abdomen, and pelvis detects the presence of metastases. In certain situations, additional imaging tests like PET and MRI might be employed. MRI is especially helpful in determining the tumor's local stage and in determining the best surgical course of action.

To determine which patients experience a full response to neoadjuvant chemotherapy and radiation, MRI is also carried out after treatment is finished. Individuals who show full response on both MRI and endoscopy may be spared needless surgical morbidity and complications, as well as surgical resection. Patients who are chosen for non-surgical treatment of rectal cancer should undergo physical exams, routine MRI scans, and endoscopy procedures in order to identify any tumor regrowth, which can happen in a small percentage of these patients. Periodic follow-up can identify local recurrences when they are still small and treatable with salvage surgery. Furthermore, following chemoradiotherapy, MRI tumor regression grades that are correlated with the long-term survival outcomes of the patients can be assigned.

7.3.3.2. Histopathology

The tumor's histopathologic features are determined through the examination of tissue samples obtained during a biopsy or surgery. A pathology report provides details on the microscopic characteristics of the tumor, including the structure of the tumor cells, how the tumor infiltrates surrounding healthy tissue, and whether the tumor has been fully excised. Adenocarcinoma is the most prevalent form of colon cancer, accounting for 95-98% of cases, with less common types such as lymphoma, adenosquamous, and squamous cell carcinoma also present. Certain subtypes may exhibit more aggressive behavior, requiring the use of immunohistochemistry for accurate diagnosis.

7.3.3.3. Staging

Based on both radiological and pathological findings, the cancer is staged. Tumor staging is based on the TNM system, which takes into account the extent to which the primary tumor has spread as well as the existence of metastases in lymph nodes and farther-off organs, similar to most other types of cancer. In 2018, the eighth edition of the AJCC was released.

7.4. Stomach Cancer

Gastric cancer, also known as stomach cancer, originates from the stomach lining. Most cases are gastric carcinomas, which have various subtypes such as gastric adenocarcinomas. Other types of tumors like lymphomas and mesenchymal tumors can also form in the stomach. Early symptoms include heartburn, upper abdominal pain, nausea, and loss of appetite. Later symptoms may include weight loss, yellowing of the skin and eyes, vomiting, difficulty swallowing, and blood in the stool. If left untreated, the cancer can metastasize to the liver, lungs, bones, abdominal lining, and lymph nodes.

More than 60% of cases have *Helicobacter pylori* infection, which is the most frequent cause. Some varieties of *H. pylori* pose a higher risk than other strains. Other risk factors include obesity, pickled vegetables in the diet, and smoking. 10% of cases are familial, and one to 3% are caused by inherited genetic syndromes like hereditary diffuse gastric cancer. Stomach cancer typically progresses over years in phases. Endoscopy biopsy is typically used to make the diagnosis. Medical imaging is then performed to see if the illness has spread to other body parts. South Korea and Japan, two nations with high incidence of the illness, screen for stomach cancer.

Both quitting smoking and eating a Mediterranean diet reduce the risk of stomach cancer. Preliminary data suggests that managing *H. pylori* lowers the chance in the future. Gastric cancer is curable if caught early enough. A mix of radiation therapy, chemotherapy, surgery, and targeted therapy may be used as treatments. It is also possible to use cancer immunotherapy for specific subtypes of gastric cancer. Palliative care may be recommended if treatment is delayed. Removal of H can cure some types of lymphoma. pylori. Results are frequently dismal, with a five-year survival rate for advanced cases in the West of less than 10%. This is mainly because the majority of patients have advanced disease when they first show symptoms. Five-year survival rates are 31.5% in the US, over 65% in South Korea, and over 70% in Japan—partially because of screening initiatives (Figure 7.5).

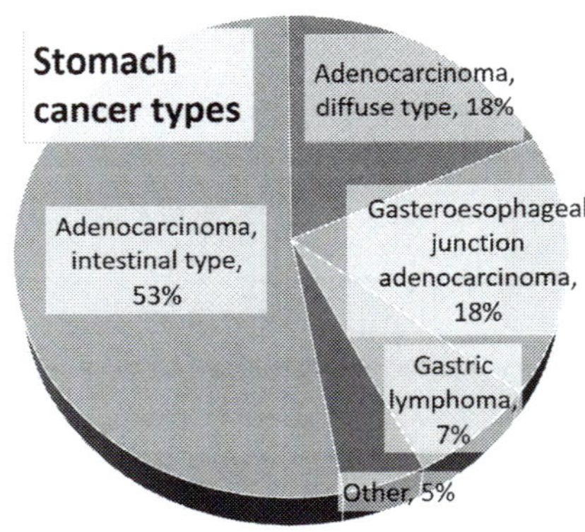

Figure 7.5. *Stages of stomach cancer.*

Source: By Mikael Häggström, M.D. Author info- Reusing images- Conflicts of interest: NoneMikael Häggström, M.D. – Own work, CC0, https://commons.wikimedia.org/w/index.php?curid=101534959.

Stomach cancer accounts for 7% of cases and 9% of deaths worldwide, making it the fifth most common type of cancer and the third greatest cause of cancer-related deaths.

It happened for the first time in 1.033 million people in 2018 and resulted in 783,000 fatalities. It was a major cause of cancer-related deaths in the West prior to the 1930s, but rates among younger generations in the West have significantly decreased, while rates among East Asians remain high. The consumption of salted and pickled foods is thought to have decreased in the West as a result of the invention of refrigeration as a food preservation technique. The most common regions for stomach cancer cases are East Asia and Eastern Europe. In men, it happens twice as frequently as in women.

7.4.1. Signs and Symptoms

In its early stages, stomach cancer is frequently either asymptomatic, meaning it shows no symptoms at all, or it may only cause nonspecific symptoms that can also be found in other disorders that are related to or unrelated to the cancer. One of the primary causes of the cancer's generally bad prognosis is that by the time symptoms are noticed, the disease has frequently progressed to an advanced stage and may have metastasized, or spread to other, possibly distant, parts of the body. The signs and symptoms of stomach cancer include vomiting, diarrhea, constipation, and unexplained nausea. Patients may also have inexplicable weight loss.

Early cancers may present with symptoms such as indigestion or heartburn. However, less than 2% of people referred for endoscopy due to indigestion are found to have cancer. Additional symptoms may include abdominal discomfort and loss of appetite.

Gastric cancers that have grown and infiltrated healthy tissue can result in weakness, exhaustion, post-meal stomach bloating, upper abdominal pain, nausea, and sporadic vomiting. Increased enlargement may result in weight loss, hemorrhaging, vomiting blood, or having blood in the stool, which can occasionally result in anemia and show up as black discoloration (melena). Dysphagia may indicate the presence of a tumor in the heart or the spread of a stomach tumor into the esophagus.

These may be signs of other conditions like tropical sprue, stomach viruses, or gastric ulcers.

7.4.2. Management

Stomach cancer is incurable only if detected early enough (before it has begun to spread). Unfortunately, the disease is typically advanced when stomach cancer is diagnosed because it rarely exhibits symptoms in its early stages.

Radiation therapy, chemotherapy, and surgery are possible treatments for stomach cancer. Clinical trials are investigating novel therapeutic modalities like gene therapy and immunotherapy as well as enhanced applications of existing techniques.

7.4.2.1. Surgery

The only effective treatment for stomach cancer is still surgery. Among the various surgical methods, endoscopic mucosal resection (EMR) is a treatment for early-stage gastric cancer (tumor involving only the mucosa) that was developed in Japan and is offered in select US facilities. In EMR, an electrical wire loop passed through the endoscope is used to remove the tumor along with the mucosa, or inner lining of the stomach, from the stomach wall. The procedure is significantly less invasive than removing the stomach, which is an advantage. A similar method that was developed in Japan and is used to resect a sizable portion of mucosa in a single piece is called endoscopic submucosal dissection. The patient would require a formal stomach resection if the pathologic examination of the removed specimen reveals deep tumor invasion or incomplete resection. The benefits and risks of laparoscopic gastrectomy cannot be ruled out, according to a 2016 Cochrane review, which also found low-quality evidence that there was no difference in short-term mortality between laparoscopic and open gastrectomy (removal of the stomach). Up to 70% of patients who have a total gastrectomy experience post-operative complications like reflux esophagitis and dumping syndrome. Construction of a "pouch," which serves as a "stomach substitute," reduced the incidence of dumping syndrome and reflux esophagitis by 73% and 63% respectively, and led to improvements in quality-of-life, nutritional outcomes, and body mass index.

Patients presenting with metastatic disease may undergo palliative surgery, which, although controversial, has shown mostly positive results in terms of improved survival rates. However, there are concerns over potential complications and delays in chemotherapy.

7.4.2.2. Chemotherapy

There is no clear standard of care for the use of chemotherapy in the treatment of stomach cancer. Regretfully, stomach cancer has not shown a strong sensitivity to these medications. When chemotherapy has been applied, it has typically worked to palliatively shrink the tumor, reduce symptoms, and lengthen the patient's survival. The following medications have been used to treat stomach cancer: mitomycin C, doxorubicin (Adriamycin), BCNU (carmustine), methyl-CCNU (semustine), and more recently, cisplatin and taxotere. Often, these medications are used in different combinations. It is unclear which of these medications, when taken alone or in combination, offers the most advantages. Clinical researchers are investigating the advantages of administering chemotherapy as adjuvant therapy to eradicate cancer cells that remain after surgery or before surgery to shrink the tumor.

7.4.2.3. Targeted Therapy

Treatment with trastuzumab, an inhibitor of the human epidermal growth factor receptor 2 (HER2), has recently been shown to improve overall survival in patients with inoperable gastric carcinoma that is metastatic or locally advanced and over-expressing the HER2/neu gene. Specifically, 13–22% of patients with gastric cancer have overexpressed HER2. It should be noted that HER2 overexpression in gastric neoplasia is heterogeneous and only accounts for a small percentage of tumor cells (more than 5% of tumor cells in less than 10% of gastric cancers overexpress HER2). Because of this, it is necessary to evaluate multiple bioptic samples for HER2 testing, especially in small samples like biopsies where heterogeneous expression is present.

7.5. Breast Cancer

A cancer that originates in the breast tissue is called breast cancer. A lump in the breast, a change in the shape of the breast, skin dimpling, milk rejection, fluid coming from the nipple, a newly inverted nipple, or a red or scaly patch of skin can all be indicators of breast cancer. Shortness of breath, enlarged lymph nodes, yellow skin, and bone pain are possible symptoms in patients whose disease has spread far.

Risk factors for breast cancer include obesity, lack of physical exercise, alcohol consumption, hormone replacement therapy during menopause, ionizing radiation, early age at first menstruation, late childbirth, older age, prior breast cancer history, and family history. 5 to 10% of cases are due to inherited genetic predispositions, including BRCA mutations. Breast cancer typically forms in milk duct and lobule cells. Ductal carcinomas originate from ducts, while lobular carcinomas originate from lobules. There are over 18 sub-types of breast cancer, with some developing from pre-invasive lesions like ductal carcinoma in situ. A biopsy confirms the diagnosis, and further tests determine the extent of the cancer and most effective treatments (Figure 7.6).

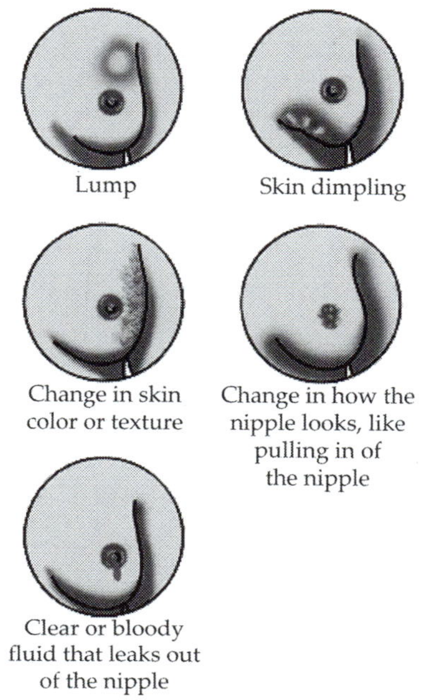

Figure 7.6. *An illustration of breast cancer.*

Source: *By Morning2k – http://www.4woman.gov/faq/cancer-illustrations-with-t.gif, Public Domain, https://commons.wikimedia.org/w/index.php?curid=37747125.*

It is debatable how much is gained from breast cancer screening relative to the risks. The question of whether mammography screening is beneficial or harmful was not resolved by a 2013 Cochrane review, since many women who test positive for the disease turn out not to have it. According to a 2009 review conducted for the US Preventive Services Task Force, screening should be done every two years for women 50 to 74 years old, as there is evidence of benefit in those between the ages of 40 and 70. For people who are highly susceptible to breast cancer, the drugs raloxifene or tamoxifen may be used as a preventative measure. For certain high-risk women, surgical excision of both breasts is an additional preventive measure. Following a cancer diagnosis, a variety of therapies may be administered, such as hormone therapy, targeted therapy, radiation therapy, chemotherapy, and surgery. Surgery comes in many forms, ranging from breast conservation to mastectomy. Breast reconstruction can be done either during or after surgery. Treatments for cancer patients whose disease has spread to other body parts primarily focus on enhancing comfort and quality of life.

7.5.1. Signs and Symptoms

When a breast cancer screening test finds a tumor, the majority of patients with the disease are asymptomatic when they are first diagnosed. The most typical symptom for those who do experience symptoms is a new breast lump. The majority of breast lumps are not cancerous; however, hard, painless lumps with uneven edges have a higher risk of being malignant. Additional signs and symptoms include breast pain or swelling, nipple pain or inversion, and dimpling, thickening, redness, or dryness of the breast skin. Some people may have swollen lymph nodes under their arms or along their collarbone, or they may experience an unusual discharge from their breasts.

Certain rarer types of breast cancer have specific symptoms. Inflammatory breast cancer, which affects up to 5% of all cases of breast cancer, results from cancer cells obstructing a breast's lymph vessels, which causes the breast to swell and turn red over the course of three to six months. Paget's disease of the breast, which causes red, scaly irritation on the areola and nipple similar to eczema, affects up to 3% of breast cancer patients.

Beyond the breast, advanced tumors have the ability to spread (metastasize), most frequently to the bones, liver, lungs, and brain. Swelling, increasing bone pain, and weakening of the bones that results in fractures are all possible effects of bone metastases. Liver metastases can result in skin issues such as rash, itching, or yellowing of the skin (jaundice), as well as nausea, vomiting, and abdominal pain. Chest pain, dyspnea, and persistent coughing are symptoms of lung metastases. Brain metastases can lead to chronic headaches, seizures, nausea, vomiting, and abnormalities in speech, vision, memory, and behavior patterns.

7.5.2. Screening

In an effort to identify breast tumors early, when treatments are more effective, breast cancer screening refers to the process of testing otherwise healthy women for the disease. Low-dose X-ray imaging of the breast, or mammography, is the most popular screening procedure for breast cancer. Every breast is imaged after being compressed between two plates. Tumors can cause tiny dense particles known as microcalcifications, change the shape of the surrounding tissue, or give the breast an abnormally dense appearance. A higher number indicates a higher risk of a cancerous tumor. Radiologists typically report mammogram results on a standardized scale; the six-point Breast Imaging-Reporting and Data System (BI-RADS) is the most widely used worldwide.

Breast density can also be seen on a mammogram; dense breast tissue can hide tumors and appear opaque. Breast density is divided into four groups by BI-RADS. About 90% of breast tumors in the least dense breasts (referred to as fatty breasts) can be found by mammography; however, only 60% of breast tumors in the densest breasts (referred to as extremely dense) can be found. As an alternative, women with particularly dense breasts can undergo screening using tomosynthesis, MRI, or ultrasound, all of which are more sensitive in identifying breast tumors.

At least 20% fewer deaths from breast cancer are caused by routine screening mammography. Most medical guidelines advise women in their 50s to 70s to get screening mammograms every year. Women between the ages of 40 and 49 who undergo screening also have lower breast cancer mortality rates, and some guidelines suggest yearly screening in this age group as well. The majority of guidelines advise combining mammography with MRI screening for women who are highly susceptible to breast cancer in order to improve the likelihood of finding potentially harmful tumors. Breast self-examination, or regularly feeling one's own breasts for lumps or other abnormalities, does not lower one's risk of dying from breast cancer. Clinical breast exams are common; however, it is unknown if they lower the risk of dying from breast cancer. Clinical breast exams involve a medical professional feeling the breasts for abnormalities. In most developed countries, routine breast cancer screening is standard practice; however, in the world's poorest nations, it is still uncommon.

7.5.3. Diagnosis

In order to confirm the presence and location of a suspected tumor, patients who have undergone physical examination or a "diagnostic" mammography should first undergo additional imaging, usually an ultrasound and another diagnostic mammography. The suspected tumor is then biopsied. The most common method for doing a breast biopsy is core needle biopsy, which involves taking tissue samples from the desired area using a hollow needle. When a suspected tumor seems to be filled with fluid, fine-needle aspiration is frequently used to obtain a sample. 10 to 20% of breast biopsies reveal the presence of cancer. Instead, fibrocystic breast changes—a term that includes the benign growth of small pockets of fluid, cell growth, or fibrous tissue—are the cause of the majority of biopsied breast masses.

7.5.4. Management

The health of the affected individual, the molecular features of the cancer case, and the extent of tumor spread at the time of diagnosis all influence how breast cancer is managed.

7.5.4.1. Local Tumors

Surgery is frequently used to remove the tumor along with some surrounding breast tissue in patients whose tumors have not spread outside of the breast. Usually, a lumpectomy (removal of only the tumor) or partial mastectomy (removal of a larger portion of the breast) is the surgical technique used to preserve the greatest amount of healthy breast tissue. Individuals who are unable to receive radiation therapy, have large or multiple tumors, or have a high genetic risk of developing cancers in the future may choose to have the affected breast or breasts completely removed (full mastectomy). Women frequently undergo a sentinel lymph node biopsy, which involves removing the closest lymph node, to lessen the chance that their cancer will spread. A few hours after the dye is injected close to the tumor site, the lymph node it collects in is removed.

Many people receive radiation therapy following surgery in order to lower their risk of cancer returning. Radiation is administered to the entire breast to those who had lumpectomies. Radiation therapy is administered to the chest wall and mastectomy scar in patients who have undergone a mastectomy and are at heightened risk of tumor spread, defined as tumors larger than five centimeters in diameter or cancerous cells in adjacent lymph nodes. Other lymph nodes in the vicinity that have been exposed to cancerous cells will also receive radiation treatment. Usually, radiation is administered five days a week for a maximum of seven weeks. The most common method of delivering radiation therapy for breast cancer is external beam radiotherapy, in which radiation beams are focused onto the desired body parts using a device. Alternatively, some people have brachytherapy, in which a device implanted at the surgical site of the tumor removal contains radioactive material. After adding new radioactive material twice a day for five days, the apparatus is taken out. A person's breast tumor is usually removed with surgery and radiation. In less than 5% of cases, the breast tumor returns after treatment. The breast can be surgically rebuilt following radiation therapy and surgery. This can involve implanting a breast implant or transferring extra tissue from another area of the body.

Chemotherapy lowers the risk of cancer returning within ten years by approximately one-third. However, 1-2% of chemotherapy patients have long-term or potentially fatal side effects. Patients who have a higher risk of cancer recurrence are usually offered chemotherapy in an effort to balance the benefits and risks. The question of who should receive chemotherapy is debatable, and there is no set risk threshold for its administration. Usually administered in two- to three-week cycles, chemotherapy medications are taken in between rest intervals to allow the body to adjust to the side effects of the treatment. There are four to six cycles provided overall. Numerous classes of chemotherapeutic agents, such as taxanes (docetaxel and paclitaxel), DNA alkylating drugs (cyclophosphamide), anthracyclines (doxorubicin and epirubicin), antimetabolites (fluorouracil, capecitabine, and methotrexate), and platinum-based chemotherapies (cisplatin and carboplatin), are effective in treating breast cancer. Chemotherapies from various classes are usually administered in combination, with specific chemotherapy medications chosen in accordance with the patient's condition and the side effects of each chemotherapy drug. Up to 1% of patients treated with cyclophosphamide and anthrocyclines develop leukemia. Congestive heart failure is another side effect that anthrocyclines induce in about 1% of treatments. Peripheral neuropathy caused by taxanes can be permanent in up to 5% of patients. Neoadjuvant therapy, which involves administering the same chemotherapy agents prior to surgery, can reduce tumor size and facilitate their safe removal.

The HER2-targeted antibody trastuzumab, when combined with chemotherapy, lowers the risk of cancer recurrence and death by at least 33% for patients whose tumors are HER2-positive. For a full year, trastuzumab is administered either weekly or every three weeks. Treatment efficacy is marginally increased by the addition of pertuzumab, a second HER2-targeted antibody. Given that anthrocyclines can also harm the heart, trastuzumab is usually not administered in conjunction with it due to the rare possibility that it may impair heart function.

Endocrine therapy, which lowers the levels of estrogens and progesterones that hormone receptor-positive breast cancers need to survive, is beneficial for patients whose tumors are ER-positive or PR-positive after their chemotherapy course. Over the following ten years, tamoxifen treatment lowers the risk of breast cancer death by approximately 40% by blocking the ER in the breast and some other tissues. Although it has more severe side effects, chemically inhibiting the production of estrogen with GnRH-targeted medications (goserelin, leuprolide, or triptorelin) and aromatase inhibitors (anastrozole, letrozole, or exemestane) slightly increases survival. Hot flashes, painful vagina, and pain in the muscles and joints are some of the side effects of estrogen depletion. After surgery and chemotherapy, endocrine therapy is usually advised for a minimum of five years, and it can occasionally be continued for ten years or more.

7.5.4.2. Metastatic Disease

Approximately one in five individuals receiving treatment for localized breast cancer experience tumor metastases, with the most common locations being the adjacent bones (67% of cases), liver (41%), lungs (37%), brain (13%), and peritoneum (10%). Individuals with metastatic illness may be eligible for additional chemotherapy; capecitabine, an anthracycline, or a taxane are usually given first. One chemotherapy drug is started, and then another, until the cancer is under control. Apart from chemotherapeutic medications, gemcitabine, vinorelbine, etoposide, and epothilones can also be useful in treating localized cancer. Regular infusion of denosumab and bisphosphonates, which strengthen bones, is beneficial for individuals with bone metastases. Doing so every three months lowers the risk of bone pain, fractures, and hypercalcemia.

Extra endocrine therapy helps up to 70% of patients with ER-positive metastatic breast cancer. Treatment choices include those for locally advanced cancer, in addition to fulvestrant and toremifene, which are frequently combined with CDK4/6 inhibitors (palbociclib, ribociclib, or abemaciclib). Most patients will benefit from switching to a second endocrine therapy if the first one doesn't work. Additionally, some benefit from a third sequential therapy. Everolimus, an mTOR inhibitor, can be added to further impede the growth of the tumors.

7.5.4.3. Supportive Care

With the right supportive care, the side effects of many breast cancer treatments can be reduced. Almost all chemotherapy patients experience hair loss, nausea, and vomiting. Antiemetic medications can help with nausea and vomiting, and wearing a cold cap while receiving chemotherapy can help with hair loss. Many people report having cognitive problems while receiving chemotherapy. These typically go away a few months after chemotherapy treatment is over. Hot flashes, joint and muscle pain, and dryness or discomfort in the vagina can all be common side effects of endocrine therapy and make it difficult to have sex.

Antidepressants help about half of women with their hot flashes; physical therapy and nonsteroidal anti-inflammatory drugs can treat pain; personal lubricants and counseling can help with sexual issues.

Psychological interventions, like cognitive behavioral therapy, can improve quality of life and have a positive impact on outcomes like mood disturbance, anxiety, depression, and cognitive impairment in women with non-metastatic breast cancer. Following adjuvant therapy, physical activity interventions, yoga, and meditation may also benefit health-related quality of life, cognitive decline, anxiety, fitness, and physical activity in women with breast cancer (Elliss-Brookes et al., 2012).

7.6. Cervical Cancer

Any cancer that develops in the cervix or any of its wall layers is referred to as cervical cancer. The cause is the aberrant proliferation of cells that can infiltrate or disperse throughout the body. Usually, there are no symptoms in the early stages. Subsequent symptoms could be pain during sex, pelvic pain, or irregular vaginal bleeding. Even though bleeding after sex might not be dangerous, it could also be a sign of cervical cancer.

More than 90% of cases are caused by human papillomavirus (HPV) infection; most people with HPV infections, however, do not go on to develop cervical cancer. Approximately 50% of high grade cervical pre-cancers are caused by HPV strains 16 and 18. Although they are not as significant, other risk factors include using birth control pills, smoking, having multiple sexual partners, having a weakened immune system, and beginning sex at a young age. Cervical cancer risk is also influenced by genetic factors. Over the course of 10 to 20 years, precancerous alterations known as cervical intraepithelial neoplasia usually lead to cervical cancer. Squamous cell carcinomas account for about 90% of cases of cervical cancer, adenocarcinomas account for 10%, and other types account for a tiny percentage. Cervical screening is usually used for diagnosis, and then a biopsy is performed. The next step is to undergo medical imaging to see if the cancer has spread.

Up to 90% of cervical cancer cases may be avoided with HPV vaccinations, which offer protection against two to seven high-risk strains of this virus family. Guidelines advise continuing to get regular Pap tests because there is still a chance of cancer. Using condoms and having few or no sexual partners are two more preventative measures. When precancerous changes are identified through cervical cancer screening, either with acetic acid or the Pap test, cancer can be prevented from developing. Radiation therapy, chemotherapy, and surgery may be used in combination for treatment. In the United States, the five-year survival rate is 68%. However, the timing of the cancer's detection has a significant impact on the results.

Cervical cancer ranks fourth globally in terms of both cancer type and cancer-related death rates among women. 266,000 people died from cervical cancer in 2012, out of an estimated 528,000 cases. This represents roughly 8% of all cancer cases and deaths. 90% of deaths and 70% of cervical cancer cases happen in developing nations. With an incidence rate of 47.3 per 100,000 women, it is one of the most common causes of cancer-related deaths in low-income countries. Cervical cancer rates have dropped significantly in developed nations thanks to the widespread implementation of cervical screening programs. Expected scenarios for the global (and particularly in low-income countries) reduction of cervical cancer-related mortality have been reviewed, based on the assumption that the WHO-defined triple-intervention strategies will be used to achieve the recommended prevention targets. The most well-known immortalized cell line in medical research, HeLa, was created from Henrietta Lacks' cervical cancer cells.

7.6.1. Signs and Symptoms

Cervical cancer may show no symptoms at all in its early stages. The presence of malignancy may be indicated by vaginal bleeding, contact bleeding (the most common type being bleeding after sexual activity), or, in rare cases, a vaginal mass. Additionally, vaginal discharge and mild pain during sex are signs of cervical cancer. Metastases may be found in the abdomen, lungs, or other locations in cases of advanced disease.

7.6.2. Causes

Signs of late-stage cervical cancer can include reduced appetite, weight loss, exhaustion, pelvic discomfort, back pain, leg pain, swollen legs, heavy vaginal bleeding, bone fractures, and in rare cases, urinary or fecal incontinence. Bleeding following douching or a pelvic examination is a frequent indication of cervical cancer.

7.6.2.1. Human Papillomavirus

75% of cervical cancer cases worldwide are caused by HPV types 16 and 18, and the remaining 10% are caused by types 31 and 45.

Regardless of gender, women who have multiple sexual partners or whose partners have multiple sexual partners are more likely to develop cervical cancer.

Out of the more than 200 known types of HPV, 12 are considered high-risk (16, 18, 31, 33, 35, 39, 45, 51, 52, 56, 58, and 59), three are considered probable high-risk (26, 53, and 66), and the remaining 12 are considered low-risk (6, 11, 40, 42, 43, 44, 54, 61, 70, 72, 81, and CP6108).

Different strains of HPV can also cause genital warts, a benign tumor of epithelial cells. These serotypes, however, are typically unrelated to cervical cancer. It is not uncommon to have more than one strain present at once, including strains that can cause warts and cervical cancer. Cervical cancer is generally thought to occur only in cases of HPV infection.

7.6.2.2. Smoking

There is an increased risk of cervical cancer with both active and passive cigarette smoking. Current and former smokers have an approximately two to three times higher incidence of invasive cancer among women infected with HPV. Though not as much, passive smoking is also linked to higher risk.

Another factor associated with the development of cervical cancer is smoking. Smoking can raise a woman's risk of cervical cancer in a number of ways, including direct and indirect induction. A smoker's increased risk of developing cervical intraepithelial neoplasia (CIN3), which can develop into cervical cancer, is one direct method of acquiring this disease. CIN3 lesions can be thought of as having a direct connection to cervical cancer because most cases of cancer that result from them do so with the help of the HPV virus, though this is not always the case. The risk of developing CIN3 lesions appears to be higher in individuals who smoke heavily and for an extended period of time than in those who smoke less or never. While there is a connection between smoking and cervical cancer, the primary cause of this kind of cancer is HPV, which is aided by smoking. It also contributes to the development of HPV, and if a woman already has HPV, her risk of developing cervical cancer is increased.

7.6.2.3. Oral Contraceptives

In women who have had HPV, long-term use of oral contraceptives is linked to an increased risk of cervical cancer. The incidence of invasive cancer is approximately three times higher in women who have used oral contraceptives for five to nine years, and the risk is approximately four times higher in those who have used them for ten years or more.

7.6.2.4. Multiple Pregnancies

Cervical cancer risk is higher in those who have had numerous pregnancies. Women with HPV infection who have had seven or more full-term pregnancies are at a four-fold increased risk of developing cancer in comparison to women who have never become pregnant, and at a two- to three-fold increased risk in comparison to women who have only had one or two full-term pregnancies.

7.6.3. Treatment

The availability of surgeons proficient in radical pelvic surgery and the advent of fertility-sparing therapy in developed countries are the main reasons for the variations in cervical cancer treatment across the globe. Treatment options for cervical cancer in less advanced stages usually allow the patient to retain their fertility if they so choose.

Radiation therapy may be used at any stage of the disease when surgical options are not available due to the radiosensitivity of cervical cancers. It is possible that surgical intervention produces better results than radiological methods. Furthermore, chemotherapy is a more effective treatment for cervical cancer than radiation therapy alone. When compared to radiotherapy alone, chemotherapy may improve overall survival and lower the chance of disease recurrence.

Several surgical techniques can be used to effectively treat precancerous cells (cervical intraepithelial neoplasia), which can progress to cancer and early-stage cervical cancer (IA1). Surgical treatment options include ablation, which removes only the areas of the cervix with abnormal tissues, and excision, which removes a portion of the cervix in the shape of a cone. These significantly lower the chance of cancer starting or spreading, but they also raise the possibility of an early birth in subsequent pregnancies. More cervical tissue removed during surgery reduces the chance of the cancer returning, but it also increases the risk of preterm birth. Because of this risk, selecting the appropriate procedure requires careful consideration of the patient's age, her plans for having children, and the location and size of the cancer cells. Low-certainty evidence suggests that peri-operative care strategies like "fast-track surgery" and "enhanced recovery programs" may reduce surgical stress and enhance post-gynecological cancer surgery recovery.

Another treatment option for microinvasive cancer (stage IA) is a hysterectomy, which involves removing the entire uterus along with a portion of the vagina. The lymph nodes are also removed for stage IA2. Options include local surgical techniques like cone biopsy or loop electrical excision. According to the results of a systematic review, additional data is required to make decisions regarding surgical options for women with stage IA2 cervical cancer.

If a cone biopsy is unable to yield clear margins—a biopsy's results indicating that the tumor is encircled by tissue free of cancer, indicating that the entire tumor has been removed—a trachelectomy remains an additional viable treatment option for women who wish to maintain their fertility. This is a less invasive procedure than a hysterectomy because it aims to surgically remove the cancer while protecting the uterus and ovaries. Though few doctors are proficient in this procedure, it is still not regarded as standard of care for patients with stage I cervical cancer that has not spread. Since the extent of the cancer's spread is unknown, even the most skilled surgeon cannot guarantee that a trachelectomy can be carried out until after a surgical microscopic examination. A hysterectomy might still be required if the surgeon cannot confirm under a microscope that the woman's cervical tissue margins are clear while she is under general anesthesia in the operating room. If the woman gives her consent, this can only be done during the same procedure. The surgeon may also need to remove some lymph nodes from around the uterus for pathologic evaluation because of the potential risk of cancer spreading to the lymph nodes in stage 1B cancers and some stage 1A cancers.

There are differing views on whether vaginal or abdominal radical trachelectomy is preferable. Most women recover from a radical abdominal trachelectomy with lymphadenectomy in about six weeks, and the procedure typically only necessitates a two- to three-day hospital stay. Although complications are rare, women who are able to conceive following surgery may experience late miscarriage and premature labor. After surgery, it is usually advised to wait at least a year before trying to get pregnant. If the cancer has been eradicated by the trachelectomy, recurrence in the residual cervix is unlikely. In addition to minimizing any new exposures to HPV through safe sex practices until one is actively trying to conceive, women are advised to practice vigilant prevention and follow-up care, including Pap screenings/colposcopies and biopsies of the remaining lower uterine segment as needed (every 3.4 months for at least 5 years) to monitor for any recurrence.

Radiation therapy or radical hysterectomy with removal of the lymph nodes are two treatment options for the early stages (IB1 and IIA less than 4 cm). Brachytherapy, or internal radiation, and external beam radiation therapy are the two forms of radiation therapy that are administered. In order to lower the risk of relapse, women undergoing surgery and having high-risk features discovered during pathologic examination may receive radiation therapy in addition to or instead of chemotherapy. According to a Cochrane review, there is moderate-to-high certainty evidence that, when compared to no further treatment, radiation therapy reduces the risk of disease progression in individuals with stage IB cervical cancer. On the other hand, scant data was discovered regarding its impact on overall survival.

Radiation therapy combined with cisplatin-based chemotherapy, hysterectomy (which typically necessitates adjuvant radiation therapy), or cisplatin chemotherapy followed by hysterectomy are the available treatment options for larger early-stage tumors (IB2 and IIA greater than 4 cm). In periodic diseases, cisplatin is considered to be the most active single agent when present. For women with early-stage cervical cancer (IA2–IIA), adding platinum-based chemotherapy to chemoradiation appears to increase survival while lowering the chance of recurrence. In comparison to primary chemoradiotherapy, there is insufficient data regarding the advantages and disadvantages of primary hysterectomy for cervical cancer in stage IB2, according to a Cochrane review. Chemotherapy using cisplatin is used in combination with radiation therapy for advanced-stage tumors (IIB-IVA). The combination of hycamtin and cisplatin, two chemotherapy drugs, was approved by the US Food and Drug Administration on June 15, 2006, for women receiving treatment for late-stage (IVB) cervical cancer. Anemia, thrombocytopenia, and neutropenia are serious side effects of combination therapy.

It is unclear whether anticancer drugs, when used following standard care, improve survival rates in women with locally advanced cervical cancer due to lack of sufficient evidence.

Exenteration is the procedure in which the complete removal of the cancer, without any traces of it found at the margins under a microscope, is necessary for the surgery to be considered curative (Elliss-Brookes et al., 2012).

7.7. Skin Cancer

Cancers that originate in the skin are known as skin cancers. They result from the growth of aberrant cells that can infiltrate or spread to different areas of the body. The most common type of cancer in humans to be diagnosed is skin cancer. Melanoma, squamous-cell skin cancer (SCC), and basal-cell skin cancer (BCC) are the three primary forms of skin cancer. Nonmelanoma skin cancer (NMSC) is the term used to describe the first two types of skin cancer as well as several less common types. Although basal-cell cancer is unlikely to spread to distant locations or cause death, it can cause damage to the surrounding tissue and grows slowly. It frequently manifests as a painless elevated patch of skin that may be shiny and have tiny blood vessels running across it, or it may look like a raised ulcerated area of skin. The spread of squamous-cell skin cancer is higher. It may develop into an ulcer, but it typically manifests as a hard lump with a scaly top. Aggressive melanomas are the most common. A mole that has changed in size, shape, or color, has uneven edges, is multicolored, itchy, or bleeds are among the warning signs.

In more than 90% of cases, sun exposure results in UV radiation exposure. There is an increased risk of all three primary forms of skin cancer with this exposure. A thinner ozone layer has contributed to an increase in exposure. Another typical source of UV radiation is tanning beds. Childhood exposure is especially dangerous for basal-cell carcinomas and melanomas. All exposure matters more for squamous-cell skin cancers, regardless of when it happens. 20 to 30% of melanomas start off as moles. Individuals with paler skin tones and those with compromised immune systems due to medication side effects or HIV/AIDS are more susceptible. Biologic diagnosis is made (Figure 7.7).

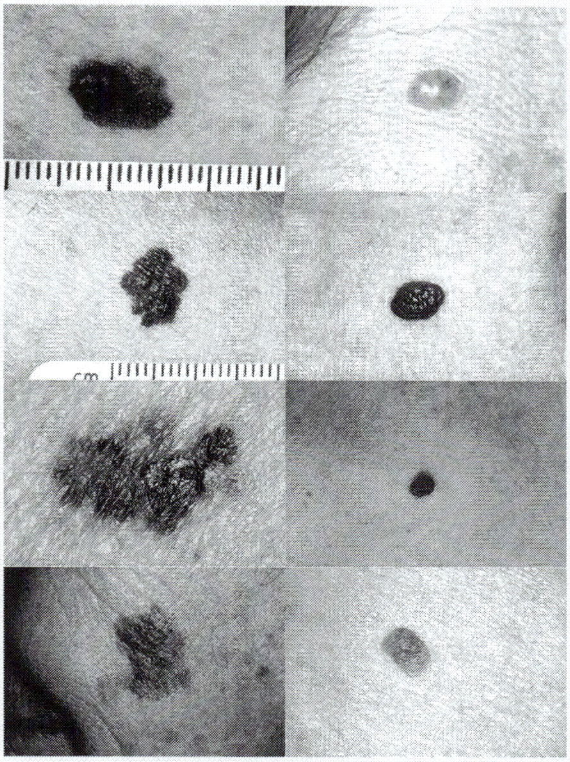

Figure 7.7. *Different types of skin cancer.*

Source: *By Unknown creator; six images merged by User:Stevenfruitsmaak – National Cancer Institute via Skin Cancer Foundation, Public Domain, https://commons.wikimedia.org/w/index.php?curid=5582818.*

Preventing melanoma and squamous-cell skin cancer seems to be achievable through sunscreen use and reducing UV radiation exposure. The relationship between sunscreen use and basal-cell cancer risk is unclear. Skin cancer that is not melanoma is often curable. Surgery is the usual course of treatment, though topical drugs like fluorouracil or radiation therapy are less frequently used. A combination of surgery, chemotherapy, radiation therapy, and targeted therapy may be used to treat melanoma. Palliative care can help patients whose disease has spread to other parts of their body live longer and with a higher quality of life. With over 86% of patients in the UK and over 90% in the US surviving for more than five years, melanoma has one of the highest survival rates among cancers.

At least 40% of cancer cases worldwide are skin cancer, making it the most prevalent type of cancer. Nonmelanoma skin cancer is the most prevalent kind, affecting at least 2-3 million individuals annually. But since accurate statistics are not maintained, this is only an estimate. About 80% of nonmelanoma skin cancers are basal-cell tumors, while 20% are squamous-cell tumors. Skin cancers of the basal and squamous cells seldom cause death. Less than 0.1% of cancer-related deaths in the US were caused by them. Melanoma affected 232,000 individuals worldwide in 2012, and it was the cause of 55,000 deaths. The highest rates of melanoma worldwide are found in white people living in Australia, New Zealand, and South Africa. In the past 20 to 40 years, there has been an increase in the prevalence of the three main types of skin cancer, particularly in areas where White people predominate.

7.7.1. Signs and Symptoms

The symptoms of skin cancer can vary widely. These include non-healing changes in the skin, ulcerations on the skin, discolored skin, and modifications to pre-existing moles, such as enlargement, jagged edges, color changes, changes in feel, or bleeding. A large brownish spot with darker speckles and a painful lesion that burns or itches are common indicators of skin cancer.

- **Basal-Cell Skin Cancer:** When basal-cell skin cancer (BCC) affects sun-exposed areas of the head, neck, torso, or shoulders, it typically manifests as a raised, smooth, pearly bump. There may occasionally be visible tiny blood vessels (known as telangiectasia) inside the tumor. There is often bleeding and crusting in the tumor's core. It is frequently misdiagnosed as an unhealing sore. This type of skin cancer is the least deadly; it can be cured, frequently leaving little to no scars, with the right care.
- **Squamous-Cell Skin Cancer:** Squamous-cell skin cancer (SCC) presents as a red, scaly, thickened patch on skin exposed to the sun. Some may appear as firm nodules or dome-shaped like keratoacanthomas. Ulceration and bleeding can also occur. If left untreated, SCC can progress into a large mass. It is the second most common type of skin cancer, though not as dangerous as melanoma.
- **Melanoma***:* The majority of melanomas range in color from brown to black. A tiny percentage of melanoma are fleshy, pink, or red in color; these are referred to as amelanotic melanoma and are typically more aggressive. A mole's size, shape, color, or elevation can all change, and these are warning signs of malignant melanoma. The emergence of a new mole during adulthood, as well as discomfort, itching, ulceration, redness surrounding the site, or bleeding at the site, are additional indicators. An often-used mnemonic is "ABCDE," where A is for "asymmetrical," B for "borders" (irregular: "Coast of Maine sign"), C for "color" (variegated), D

for "diameter" (larger than 6 mm – the size of a pencil eraser) and E for "evolving."

- **Other:** Merkel cell carcinomas are typically non-tender, skin-colored, red, purple, or other rapidly growing bumps that are neither painful nor itchy. These could be misdiagnosed as a cyst or as another kind of cancer.

7.7.2. Treatment

The type of cancer, its location, the patient's age, and whether it is a primary or recurrent cancer all affect the course of treatment. In young individuals with small-cell basal-cell cancer, the best-in-class treatment (Mohs surgery or CCPDMA) may be recommended. Radiation therapy (which has a slightly lower cure rate) or no treatment at all may be necessary for a difficult-to-excise basal-cell cancer of the nose in an elderly, frail man with numerous complicating medical issues. For large superficial basal-cell carcinoma, topical chemotherapy may be necessary to achieve a good cosmetic outcome; however, for invasive nodular basal-cell carcinoma or invasive squamous-cell carcinoma, it may not be sufficient. Melanoma typically responds poorly to chemotherapy or radiation.

Radiation therapy, topical chemotherapy (5-fluorouracil or imiquimod), and cryotherapy (freezing the cancer off) can all effectively control low-risk diseases; however, their combined overall cure rates may be lower than those of certain types of surgery. Additional treatment options for basal-cell and squamous-cell carcinomas include photodynamic therapy, epidermal radioisotope therapy, topical chemotherapy, electrodesiccation, and curettage.

The goal of Mohs' micrographic surgery (also known as Mohs surgery) is to remove the cancer with the least amount of surrounding tissue possible. The edges are checked right away to determine whether a tumor is present. This offers the chance to achieve the most aesthetically pleasing outcomes with the least amount of tissue removal. Thwis is particularly crucial for regions like the face where there is little room for extra skin. Cure rates are comparable to extensive removal. This technique requires specialized training to execute. An alternative technique called CCPDMA can be carried out by a pathologist who is not experienced with Mohs surgery.

If the disease has progressed (metastasized), additional surgery or chemotherapy might be needed.

The biologic immunotherapy drugs ipilimumab, pembrolizumab, nivolumab, and cemiplimab; BRAF inhibitors, such as dabrafenib and vemurafenib; and the MEK inhibitor trametinib are among the treatments for metastatic melanoma.

The Food and Drug Administration approved the first cancer treatment using tumor-infiltrating lymphocytes (TIL therapy) for melanomas that haven't responded to other treatments in February 2024. Researchers are also conducting advanced clinical trials for a vaccine tailored to a patient's cancer genetic profile.

7.7.2.1. Reconstruction

Currently, the most popular method of treating skin cancer is surgical excision. Recovery of normal function and appearance is the aim of reconstructive surgery. The location and size of the defect determine the reconstruction technique to be used. Face skin cancers are typically more difficult to extricate and reconstruct because the face has many functional and highly visible anatomical features.

Most minor skin defects can be fixed with a straightforward procedure that involves approximating the edges of the skin and sewing them shut. A linear scar will be the outcome of this. The scar won't be noticeable if the repair is done along a wrinkle or natural skin fold. Larger defects might need to be repaired using a microvascular free flap, localized skin flap, pedicled skin flap, or skin graft. Local skin flaps and skin grafts are far more common than the other options on the list.

Skin grafting involves the transplantation of skin from one part of the body to another to cover a defect. The skin graft is stitched onto the edges of the defect and a bolster dressing is applied for seven to ten days to protect and support the healing process. There are two types of skin grafting: split thickness and full thickness. In split-thickness grafting, a thin layer of skin is shaved off from the abdomen or thigh using a shaver. The donor site typically heals within two weeks. In full thickness grafting, a thicker segment of skin is completely removed, requiring the donor site to be sutured closed.

Split thickness grafts are suitable for repairing larger defects, although they may not be as cosmetically appealing as full thickness skin grafts. In contrast, full-thickness skin grafts are more aesthetically pleasing but are only appropriate for small or moderate-sized defects.

Local skin flaps are a technique used to close skin defects by moving tissue from the surrounding area to match the color and quality of the damaged skin. Different types of local flaps can be created to minimize damage to surrounding tissues and improve the overall appearance of the repair. Pedicled skin flaps involve transferring skin with an intact blood supply from a nearby part of the body. For example, a pedicled forehead flap can be used to repair a large skin defect on the nose. Once the flap establishes a new blood supply, the vascular pedicle can be disconnected (Elliss-Brookes et al., 2012).

A Closer Look

Prostate Checks

Prostate problems are common in men, particularly in men over 50 years of age.

- Do you have difficulty in starting to pass urine?
- Do you think it takes you too long to pass urine?
- Do you pass urine in stops and starts?
- Do you dribble urine after you stopped urinating (peeing)?
- Do you have a sensation of not having emptied your bladder completely?
- Do you have to get up more than twice a night to pass urine, but only pass small amounts?

If you are having any of these issues, it is important to schedule an appointment with your healthcare provider. During your visit, your doctor will inquire about your symptoms, conduct a physical exam, and may recommend further testing.

- Digital Rectal Examination (DRE)

During a prostate exam, your doctor will gently feel your prostate by inserting his finger into your rectum while you are lying on your side or bending over. The procedure is quick, lasting only a few minutes, and may cause slight discomfort but is not typically painful.

Blood Test

Tests such as kidney function and prostate-specific antigen (PSA) can be conducted to assess health. PSA, a protein that typically increases in the blood as the prostate grows, can indicate benign prostatic hyperplasia when levels are slightly elevated. Elevated PSA levels may suggest prostate cancer, with higher levels indicating a greater risk.

- ***Urine Flow Test***

You may undergo this procedure at either a medical office or a nearby hospital to evaluate the rate of your urine flow. You will be instructed to urinate into a specialized device known as a urinary flowmeter.

- Ultrasound Scan

How well you can empty your bladder may be determined by an ultrasound scan. Urine remnants are measured by placing a scanner probe on your lower abdomen both before and after you pass urine. This test can only be performed when the bladder is somewhat full, but it is not uncomfortable at all.

- ***Biopsy***

A few microscopic pieces of prostate tissue are removed for analysis in order to determine whether cancer is present. This process is known as a "biopsy." A local anesthetic and antibiotics to lower the risk of infection will be administered to you. A very fine needle inserted through the rectum will remove several (up to twelve) samples of prostate tissue. Next, a microscope is used to examine the tissue to search for cancerous cells. The antibiotics are taken for a few days more.

The biopsy needle is frequently "guided" by ultrasound. A probe the size of a finger is placed in the rectum, or back passage. Through the use of inaudible sound waves, the prostate is imaged on a computer screen by the probe. Even with the local anesthetic, you might still feel a needle prick as each piece of tissue is punctured during the test, which is uncomfortable but not extremely painful.

You might experience blood in your stool, urine, or semen for a few weeks or longer following a prostate biopsy. If an infection develops, you should speak with your doctor because more antibiotics might be required. You might need to visit the hospital if you become uneasy and get a fever. An intravenous antibiotic course might be necessary for you.

- ***MRI Scan***

You might require an MRI if prostate cancer is suspected or confirmed (magnetic resonance imaging). The device, which resembles a slicer going through a loaf of bread, takes multiple photos at various locations throughout the body. This results in precise images of the prostate that, if cancer is present, may demonstrate its extent.

Scans can indicate if secondary tumors have developed in other tissues as well. While some individuals may feel claustrophobic during these tests, they are actually painless (Calanzani et al., 2018).

Prostate cancer biomarkers in the decision- making tool/diagnosis of prostate cancer categorized by molecular markers, approving body, intended use, qualifications, and clinical performance.

Summary

- Cancer is a group of diseases involving abnormal cell growth with the potential to invade or spread to other parts of the body.
- Lung cancer, also known as lung carcinoma, is a malignant tumor that begins in the lung. Lung cancer is caused by genetic damage to the DNA of cells in the airways, often caused by cigarette smoking or inhaling damaging chemicals.
- Treatment for early stage lung cancer includes surgery to remove the tumor, sometimes followed by radiation therapy and chemotherapy to kill any remaining cancer cells.
- Lung tumors often cause the release of body-altering hormones, which cause unusual symptoms, called paraneoplastic syndromes.
- Prostate cancer is the uncontrolled growth of cells in the prostate, a gland in the male reproductive system below the bladder.
- Early prostate cancer usually causes no symptoms. As a tumor grows beyond the prostate, it can damage nearby organs, causing erectile dysfunction, blood in the urine or semen, or trouble urinating – commonly including frequent urination and slow or weak urine stream.
- Prostate cancer screening is the screening process used to detect undiagnosed prostate cancer in men without signs or symptoms.
- The signs and symptoms of colorectal cancer depend on the location of the tumor in the bowel, and whether it has spread elsewhere in the body (metastasis).
- Colorectal cancer diagnosis is performed by sampling of areas of the colon suspicious for possible tumor development, typically during colonoscopy or sigmoidoscopy, depending on the location of the lesion.
- Stomach cancer, also known as gastric cancer, is a cancer that develops from the lining of the stomach. Most cases of stomach cancers are gastric carcinomas, which can be divided into a number of subtypes, including gastric adenocarcinomas.
- Stomach cancer is often either asymptomatic (producing no noticeable symptoms) or it may cause only nonspecific symptoms (which may also be present in other related or unrelated disorders) in its early stages.
- Breast cancer is a cancer that develops from breast tissue. Signs of breast cancer may include a lump in the breast, a change in breast shape, dimpling of the skin, milk rejection, fluid coming from the nipple, a newly inverted nipple, or a red or scaly patch of skin.
- Most people with breast cancer have no symptoms at the time of diagnosis; their tumor is detected by a breast cancer screening test.
- Cervical cancer is a cancer arising from the cervix or in the any layer of the wall of the cervix. It is due to the abnormal growth of cells that can invade or spread to other parts of the body.
- Basal-cell skin cancer (BCC) usually presents as a raised, smooth, pearly bump on the sun-exposed skin of the head, neck, torso or shoulders.

References

1. Abuidris, D. O., Elsheikh, A., Ali, M., et al. (2013). Breast-cancer screening with trained volunteers in a rural area of Sudan: A pilot study. *The Lancet Oncology, 14*(4), 363–370. https://doi.org/10.1016/S1470-2045(13)70004-7.
2. Alexiusdottir, K. K., Möller, P. H., Snaebjornsson, P., et al. (2012). Association of symptoms of colon cancer patients with tumor location and TNM tumor stage. *Scandinavian Journal of Gastroenterology, 47*(7), 795–801. https://doi.org/10.3109/00365521.2012.683254.
3. Bedir, O., Kiziltas, S., Kostek, O., & Ozkanli, S. (2016). The relation of presenting symptoms with staging, grading, and postoperative 3-year mortality in patients with stage I–III nonmetastatic colon cancer. *Turkish Journal of Gastroenterology, 27*(3), 239–245. https://doi.org/10.5152/tjg.2016.16038.
4. Bray, F., Ferlay, J., Soerjomataram, I., Siegel, R. L., Torre, L. A., & Jemal, A. (2018). Global cancer statistics 2018: GLOBOCAN estimates of incidence and mortality worldwide for 36 cancers in 185 countries. *CA: A Cancer Journal for Clinicians, 68*(6), 394–424. https://doi.org/10.3322/caac.21492.
5. Calanzani, N., Nijenhuis, L., Shahaj, O., Weller, D., & Campbell, C. (2018). A systematic review of health system level initiatives promoting the earlier diagnosis of cancer among the adult population in high-income countries. *Journal of Global Oncology, 4*, 38s. https://doi.org/10.1200/JGO.18.00004.
6. Elliss-Brookes, L., McPhail, S., Ives, A., et al. (2012). Routes to diagnosis for cancer—Determining the patient journey using multiple routine data sets. *British Journal of Cancer, 107*(8), 1220–1226. https://doi.org/10.1038/bjc.2012.408.
7. Kennedy, M. P. T., Cheyne, L., Darby, M., et al. (2018). Lung cancer stage-shift following a symptom awareness campaign. *Thorax, 73*(12), 1128–1136. https://doi.org/10.1136/thoraxjnl-2018-211842.
8. Leiva, A., Esteva, M., Llobera, J., et al. (2017). Time to diagnosis and stage of symptomatic colorectal cancer determined by three different sources of information: A population based retrospective study. *Cancer Epidemiology, 47*, 48–55. https://doi.org/10.1016/j.canep.2017.01.007.
9. Lurie, G., Wilkens, L. R., Thompson, P. J., Matsuno, R. K., Carney, M. E., & Goodman, M. T. (2010). Symptom presentation in invasive ovarian carcinoma by tumor histological type and grade in a multiethnic population: A case analysis. *Gynecologic Oncology, 119*(2), 278–284. https://doi.org/10.1016/j.ygyno.2010.07.004.
10. Porta, M., Fabregat, X., Malats, N., et al. (2005). Exocrine pancreatic cancer: Symptoms at presentation and their relation to tumor site and stage. *Clinical & Translational Oncology, 7*(5), 189–197. https://doi.org/10.1007/s12094-005-0047-8.
11. Schliemann, D., Donnelly, M., Dahlui, M., et al. (2018). The 'Be Cancer Alert Campaign': Protocol to evaluate a mass media campaign to raise awareness about breast and colorectal cancer in Malaysia. *BMC Cancer, 18*(1), 881. https://doi.org/10.1186/s12885-018-4775-2.
12. Thompson, M. R., Asiimwe, A., Flashman, K., & Tsavellas, G. (2011). Is earlier referral and investigation of bowel cancer patients presenting with rectal bleeding associated with better survival? *Colorectal Disease, 13*(11), 1242–1248. https://doi.org/10.1111/j.1463-1318.2010.02463.x.

Chapter

8

SYMPTOMS OF DIABETES AND HYPERTENSION

Contents

Introduction

Hypertension, or high blood pressure, can either cause or worsen a number of diabetes-related complications, such as diabetic kidney disease and eye disease. The majority of diabetics eventually develop high blood pressure in addition to other cardiac and circulatory issues. Diabetes causes artery damage and increases the risk of atherosclerosis, or the hardening of the arteries. This may result in hypertension, which, if left untreated, may cause heart problems, kidney failure, and damage to blood vessels.

People with hypertension are more likely to have the following symptoms than those with normal blood pressure readings.

- Coronary artery disease or heart disease
- Strokes
- Peripheral vascular disease, hardening of the arteries in the legs and feet
- Heart failure

Your health is affected even by blood pressure that is "elevated," or between 120/80 and 129/80, which is at the higher end of normal. According to studies, your risk of developing heart disease increases over the course of ten years by two to three times.

Orientation and Directional Terms

Term	Definition	Illustration
Angiotensin-converting enzyme (ACE) inhibitors	ACE inhibitors reduce production of the hormone "angiotensin." This allows the blood vessels to relax and dilate, thereby lowering blood pressure.	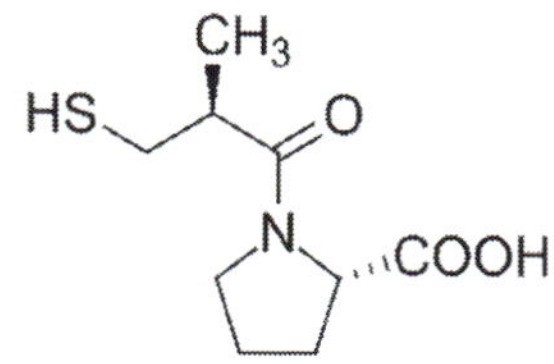
Angiotensin II receptor blockers	These medications block the effects of angiotensin, which is a chemical that causes the arteries to narrow. Without angiotensin, the blood vessels remain open, thereby reducing blood pressure.	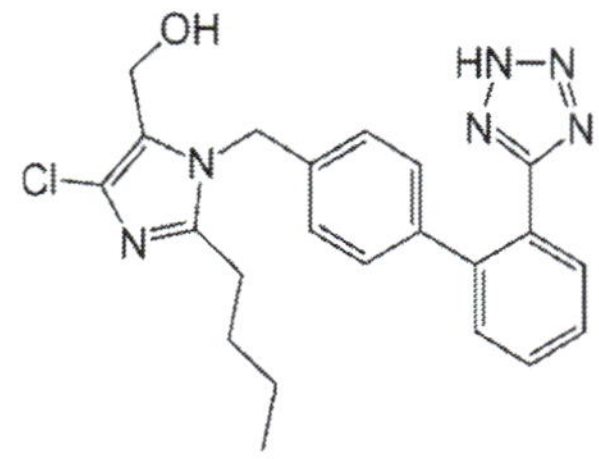
Beta-blockers	These medications cause the following effects on the heart, which help to lower blood pressure: • reducing heart rate • reducing the heart's workload • reducing the heart's output of blood	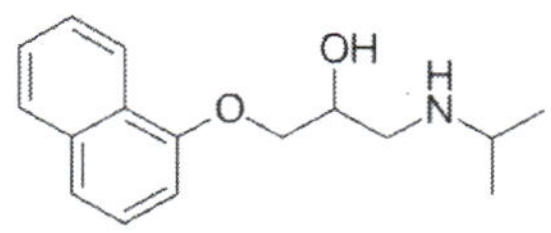
Calcium channel blockers	Calcium causes the smooth muscles of the heart and arteries to contract. Calcium channel blockers prevent this action, resulting in less forceful heart contractions and a relaxation of the blood vessels. Both result in a reduction in blood pressure.	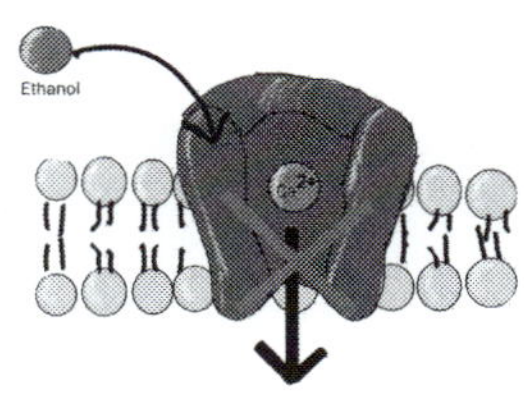
Diuretics	These medications help the body remove excess sodium and water, which reduces blood volume and helps manage blood pressure.	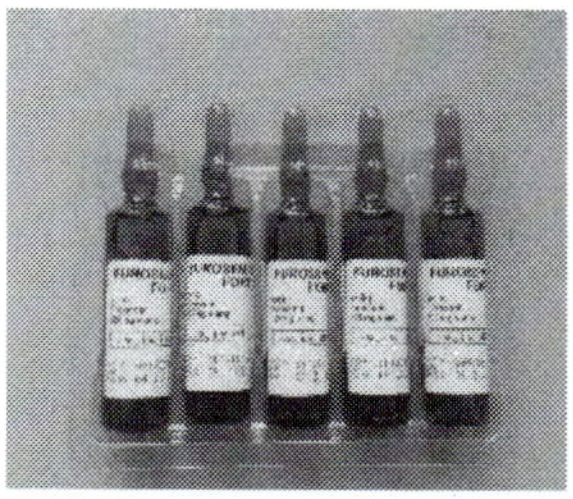
Vasodilators	These are medications that cause the muscular walls of the blood vessels to relax and dilate. This allows blood to flow through more easily, thereby reducing blood pressure.	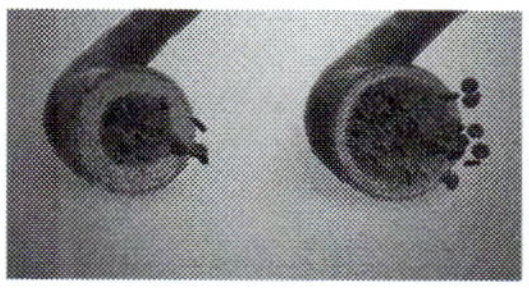

8.1. Diabetes

A collection of prevalent endocrine disorders characterized by persistently elevated blood sugar levels is collectively referred to as diabetes mellitus or just diabetes. Diabetes results from either insufficient insulin production by the pancreas or from the body's cells losing their sensitivity to the hormone's actions. Thirst, polyuria, weight loss, and blurred vision are examples of classic symptoms. The illness can cause problems with the heart, kidneys, eyes, and nerves, among other health issues, if treatment is not received. An estimated 1.5 million deaths annually are attributed to untreated or inadequately treated diabetes.

Although there are other forms of diabetes, type 1 and type 2 are the most common types. Insulin replacement therapy, or insulin injections, is the most popular treatment for type 1, whereas metformin and semaglutide, two anti-diabetic drugs, as well as lifestyle changes, can be used to manage type 2. Some women develop gestational diabetes during pregnancy, but this type usually goes away soon after giving birth.

As of 2021, type 2 diabetes accounted for approximately 90% of all cases of diabetes, with an estimated 537 million people worldwide having the disease, or 10.5% of adults. An estimated 783 million adults, or one in eight, will have diabetes by 2045, a 46% increase from the current estimates. Most notably in low- and middle-income countries, the disease's prevalence is still rising. Diabetes is the seventh leading cause of death worldwide, with rates comparable for men and women. An estimated US$760 billion is spent annually on healthcare related to diabetes worldwide.

8.1.1. Signs and Symptoms

Polyuria, thirst, and weight loss are the traditional signs of untreated diabetes. Several other non-specific symptoms, such as exhaustion, blurred vision, and itching in the genitalia due to a *Candida* infection, may also manifest. It is possible that about half of those who are impacted have no symptoms. Type 2 has a more sneaky onset; patients may go years without experiencing any symptoms. Type 1 manifests suddenly after a pre-clinical phase (Figure 8.1).

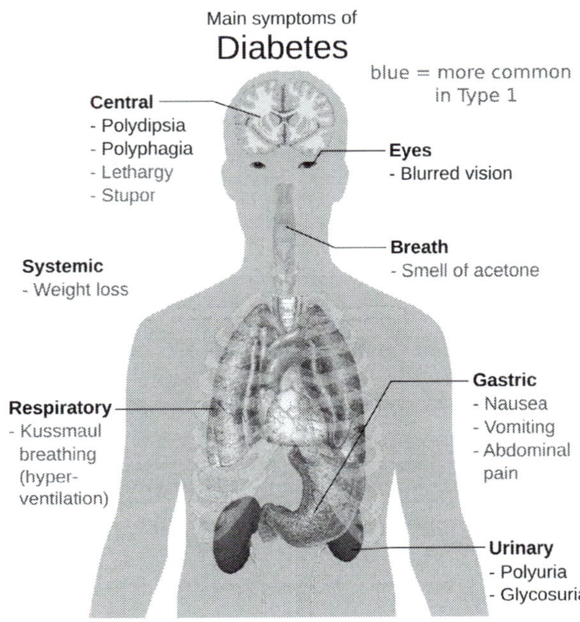

Figure 8.1. *Overview of the most significant symptoms of diabetes.*

Source: By Mikael Häggström, Public Domain, https://commons.wikimedia.org/w/index.php?curid=6055528.

Diabetic ketoacidosis is a medical emergency that primarily affects type 1 diabetes, but it can also affect type 2 if the condition has been present for a long time or if the patient has significant β-cell dysfunction. The overabundance of ketone bodies produced can cause many symptoms, such as acetone breath smell, nausea, vomiting, abdominal pain, deep breathing (also called Kussmaul breathing), and in more extreme situations, unconsciousness. Another emergency condition known as a hyperosmolar hyperglycemic state is characterized by severe hyperglycemia-induced dehydration, which can lead to hypernatremia and potentially a coma.

One known side effect of insulin therapy for diabetes is hypoglycemia. Acute presentations can range from minor symptoms like palpitations, sweating, and trembling to more serious ones like impaired cognition, disorientation, seizures, coma, and in rare cases, death. The glycaemic threshold at which symptoms arise may be lowered by recurrent hypoglycaemic episodes, which means that mild symptoms might not manifest before cognitive decline starts.

8.1.1.1. Long-Term Complications

Diabetes's main long-term effects are related to vascular damage, both macrovascular and microvascular. Diabetes doubles the risk of cardiovascular disease, and coronary artery disease accounts for about 75% of deaths in those with the disease. Peripheral artery disease and stroke are two more macrovascular morbidities. The kidneys, nerves, and eyes are all impacted by microvascular disease. Diabetic retinopathy, or damage to the retina, is the most common cause of blindness in adults who are still in the workforce. Other conditions that can affect the eyes include the onset of glaucoma and cataracts. It is advised that diabetics see an ophthalmologist or optometrist once a year.

More than half of dialysis patients in the US have diabetic nephropathy, which is a major cause of chronic kidney disease. Nerve damage from diabetes can present as diabetic neuropathy, which can cause sensory loss, neuropathic pain, and autonomic dysfunction (diarrhea, erectile dysfunction, and postural hypotension). The most common cause of non-traumatic lower limb amputation is diabetic foot problems, such as ulceration, which can be caused by trauma or loss of pain perception.

It seems likely that there is a causal relationship between type 2 diabetes and gallstones based on a large body of data and multiple cases of gallstone disease. Compared to people without diabetes, those who have diabetes have a higher chance of gallstones. Diabetes and cognitive impairment are related; research indicates that people with diabetes have a higher risk of cognitive decline and experience it at a faster rate than people without the condition. Elderly people with the condition are also more likely to fall, especially if they are receiving insulin.

8.1.2. Causes

The World Health Organization divides diabetes into six categories: hyperglycemia initially discovered during pregnancy, "other specific types," type 1 diabetes, type 2 diabetes, hybrid forms of diabetes (including slowly evolving, immune-mediated diabetes of adults and ketosis-prone type 2 diabetes), and "unclassified diabetes." Contrary to popular belief, diabetes can manifest in a variety of ways in a person.

8.1.2.1. Type 1

Type 1 diabetes is the most common type diagnosed in patients under the age of 20 and accounts for 5 to 10% of cases; however, the term "juvenile-onset diabetes" is no longer used because the disease frequently manifests as an adult. The condition is defined by the death of the pancreatic islets' insulin-producing beta cells, which results in a severe insulin shortage. It is further divided into immune-mediated and idiopathic subtypes (where the cause is unknown). Most cases are immune-mediated, where an autoimmune attack mediated by T cells results in the loss of beta cells and consequently in insulin insufficiency. Patients frequently experience abnormal and erratic blood sugar levels as a result of low insulin and a compromised ability to counteract hypoglycemia. Type 1 diabetes is partially hereditary; the risk of the disease is known to be influenced by some genes, including specific HLA genotypes. Diabetes may develop in genetically predisposed individuals as a result of one or more environmental factors, such as nutrition or viral infections. Although several viruses have been linked, there is currently insufficient proof to back up this theory in human beings.

Any age can develop type 1 diabetes, but most cases are discovered in adulthood. When type 1 diabetes strikes an adult, the diagnosis is known as latent autoimmune diabetes of adults (LADA); it strikes later than in children. Because of this distinction, some people refer to this illness as "type 1.5 diabetes" informally. Based more on age than a cause, adults with LADA are often misdiagnosed as having type 2 diabetes at first. Adults with LADA produce more insulin than those with type 1 diabetes, but not enough to maintain normal blood sugar levels.

8.1.2.2. Type 2

Insulin resistance, which may be coupled with comparatively decreased insulin secretion, is the hallmark of type 2 diabetes. It is thought that the insulin receptor plays a role in the body tissues' impaired ability to respond to insulin. The precise flaws, though, are unknown. Cases of diabetes mellitus resulting from a known defect are categorized differently. 95% of cases of diabetes mellitus are of type 2, which is the most prevalent type. Before fulfilling the requirements for type 2 diabetes, many individuals with the disease show signs of prediabetes, such as impaired glucose tolerance or impaired fasting glucose. Changes in lifestyle or medications that increase insulin sensitivity or decrease the amount of glucose produced by the liver can slow or even reverse the progression of prediabetes to overt type 2 diabetes.

Genes and lifestyle factors are the main causes of type 2 diabetes. Type 2 diabetes is known to be influenced by many lifestyle factors, such as obesity (defined as a body mass index of greater than 30), stress, poor diet, lack of physical activity, and urbanization. 30% of cases in people of Chinese and Japanese descent, 60-80% in people of European and African descent, and 100% in Pima Indians and Pacific Islanders are linked to excess body fat. Individuals without obesity can still have a high waist-to-hip ratio.

Dietary components like drinks with added sugar are linked to a higher risk. The kind of fats in the diet also matters; polyunsaturated and monounsaturated fats lower the risk, while saturated and trans fats raise it. Overindulging in white rice consumption may raise the risk of diabetes, particularly in Chinese and Japanese individuals. For certain people, a sedentary lifestyle may raise their risk of developing diabetes. Unfavorable childhood experiences—abuse, neglect, and problems in the home—raise the risk of type 2 diabetes by 32% in later life. Neglect has the largest impact.

Unhealthy lifestyles (such as poor diet and decreased physical activity) and side effects of antipsychotic medications (particularly metabolic abnormalities, dyslipidemia, and weight gain) are potential risk factors.

8.1.2.3. Gestational Diabetes

In many ways, gestational diabetes is similar to type 2 diabetes; both conditions are characterized by comparatively low insulin responsiveness and secretion. It can get better or go away after delivery and affects 2–10% of pregnancies. It is advised that all expectant mothers undergo testing beginning at approximately 24 to 28 weeks of gestation. Due to the rise in insulin-antagonist hormone levels that takes place during this time, it is most frequently diagnosed in the second or third trimester. However, 5–10% of women with gestational diabetes are found to have another type of diabetes after giving birth, most often type 2. Although it can be completely cured, gestational diabetes needs to be closely monitored by a doctor during the entire pregnancy. Blood glucose monitoring, dietary modifications, and in certain situations, the need for insulin are all possible forms of management.

Untreated gestational diabetes can harm the mother's or fetus's health, even though it may only be temporary. Macrosomia (high birth weight), congenital heart and central nervous system defects, and skeletal muscle malformations are among the risks to the unborn child. Elevated blood insulin levels in a fetus can prevent the production of fetal surfactant and result in respiratory distress syndrome in the infant. Red blood cell degeneration may lead to elevated blood bilirubin levels. Severe cases may result in perinatal death, most often from inadequate placental perfusion brought on by vascular impairment. Reduced placental function may be a sign of labor induction. If there is significant fetal distress or a higher risk of harm from macrosomia, such as shoulder dystocia, a cesarean section may be necessary.

8.1.2.4. Other Types

A rare autosomal dominant inherited form of diabetes known as maturity-onset diabetes of the young (MODY) is caused by one of several single-gene mutations that impair insulin production. It accounts for 1-2% of all cases, which is much less than the three main types. The disease's name alludes to preliminary theories about its nature. There are at least 13 subtypes of MODY because the disease, which is caused by a defective gene, varies in severity and age at presentation based on the particular gene defect. Insulin is frequently not necessary for people with MODY to manage it.

This form of diabetes is extremely rare; it is caused when the body's tissue receptors do not respond to insulin, even in situations where insulin levels are normal. Defects in beta cell function may result from autosomal or mitochondrial genetic mutations. In certain instances, abnormal insulin action could also have a genetic basis. Diabetes can result from any condition that severely damages the pancreas (such as cystic fibrosis and chronic pancreatitis). Diabetes can be brought on by conditions linked to the overproduction of insulin-antagonistic hormones; however, diabetes is usually curable once the excess hormone is eliminated. While some toxins and many medications harm pancreatic beta cells and reduce insulin secretion, other substances—particularly glucocorticoids, which can cause "steroid diabetes"—increase insulin resistance. The World Health Organization (WHO) deprecated the ICD-10 (1992) diagnostic entity, malnutrition-related diabetes mellitus (ICD-10 code E12), upon the introduction of the current taxonomy in 1999. Double diabetes represents yet another possible manifestation of the disease. This occurs when a person with type 1 diabetes develops insulin resistance, which is a sign of type 2 diabetes, or when there is a family history of the disease. It was originally found in 1990 or 1991.

8.1.3. Pathophysiology

With the exception of smooth muscle, where insulin acts through the IGF-1, insulin is the primary hormone that controls the body's ability to absorb glucose from the blood into the majority of cells, including the liver, adipose tissue, and muscle. Thus, the fundamental cause of all types of diabetes mellitus is either an insufficient amount of insulin or an insensitivity of the insulin receptors.

The breakdown of glycogen (glycogenolysis), the liver's stored form of glucose, intestinal absorption of food, and gluconeogenesis—the body's process of producing glucose from non-carbohydrate substrates—are the three main ways that the body gets its glucose. Insulin is essential for controlling the body's glucose levels. Insulin can promote the transport of glucose into muscle and fat cells, prevent the breakdown of glycogen or the process of gluconeogenesis, and promote the storage of glucose as glycogen.

When blood glucose levels rise, usually after eating, beta cells (β-cells) in the pancreatic islets of Langerhans release insulin into the blood. About two thirds of the body's cells use insulin to take up glucose from the blood and use it as fuel, a building block for other molecules, or for storage. Reduced glucose levels cause the breakdown of glycogen to glucose and less insulin release from the beta cells. Insulin functions in the opposite way from glucagon, which is the hormone primarily responsible for this process.

Glucose is not absorbed correctly by the body cells that need it and is not stored correctly in the muscles and liver if there is not enough insulin available, if cells are resistant to the effects of insulin, or if the insulin itself is flawed. Overall, the result is abnormalities in protein synthesis, blood glucose levels that are consistently high, and other metabolic disorders like metabolic acidosis in cases of total insulin insufficiency.

Long-term high blood glucose levels cause the kidneys to reach a reabsorption threshold, which prevents the extra glucose from being absorbed by the body and causes glycosuria, or the passing of excess glucose through urine. This raises the urine's osmotic pressure and prevents the kidneys from reabsorbing water, which increases fluid loss and urine production (polyuria). Dehydration and increased thirst (polydipsia) are caused by the replacement of lost blood volume by osmotically occurring water in body cells and other bodily compartments. Furthermore, a shortage of intracellular glucose increases appetite, which results in overindulgence in food (polyphagia).

8.1.4. Diagnosis

Diagnosing diabetes mellitus involves testing blood glucose levels and looking for any one of the following symptoms:

- Plasma glucose level after fasting ≥ 7 mmol/L (126 mg/dL). Blood is drawn for this test following a period of fasting, i.e., when the patient has had enough time to fast overnight or at least eight hours prior to the test, in the morning before breakfast.
- Two hours following a 75-gram oral glucose load, as measured by an OGTT, plasma glucose levels must be ≥ 11.1 mmol/L (200 mg/dL).
- Signs of elevated blood sugar and plasma glucose levels ≥ 11.1 mmol/L (200 mg/dL), whether during a fast or not.
- Glycated hemoglobin (HbA1C): less than 48 mmol/mol, or less than 6.5% of DCCT.

If there isn't a clear indication of elevated blood sugar, a repeat of any of the aforementioned techniques on a different day should verify a positive outcome. Since formal glucose tolerance testing requires a significant amount of time—two hours—and provides no prognostic advantage over the fasting test, it is preferable to measure a glucose level during fasting. The current definition states that diabetes mellitus can be diagnosed with two fasting glucose readings at or above 7.0 mmol/L (126 mg/dL).

As per the World Health Organization, impaired fasting glucose is defined as having fasting glucose levels between 6.1 and 6.9 mmol/L (110 and 125 mg/dL). Individuals who, two hours after a 75-gram oral glucose load, have plasma glucose levels at or above

7.8 mmol/L (140 mg/dL) but not above 11.1 mmol/L (200 mg/dL) are classified as having impaired glucose tolerance. Of these two prediabetic conditions, the latter is a significant risk factor for both cardiovascular disease and the development of full-blown diabetes mellitus. Since 2003, the American Diabetes Association (ADA) has used a slightly different range of 5.6 to 6.9 mmol/L (100 to 125 mg/dL) for impaired fasting glucose. For assessing the likelihood of cardiovascular disease and death from all causes, glycated hemoglobin performs better than fasting glucose.

8.1.5. Prevention

For type 1 diabetes, there is no known preventive measure. On the other hand, multiple antibodies and islet autoimmunity may be highly predictive of the onset of type 1 diabetes. 85–90% of cases of type 2 diabetes are found worldwide, but they can frequently be avoided or postponed by eating a healthy diet, staying physically active, and maintaining a normal body weight. More than 90 minutes a day of physical activity lowers the risk of diabetes by 28%. Making dietary changes that include eating a diet high in whole grains and fiber as well as selecting healthy fats like the polyunsaturated fats found in fish, nuts, and vegetable oils is known to be beneficial in preventing diabetes. Diabetes can also be avoided by consuming less red meat and other sources of saturated fat, as well as by limiting sugar-filled beverages. Quitting smoking can be a crucial preventive step as well because it is linked to an increased risk of diabetes and its complications.

All over the world, there is a similar correlation between type 2 diabetes and the primary modifiable risk factors (tobacco use, unhealthy diet, excess weight, and physical inactivity). There is mounting evidence that the main factors influencing social, economic, and cultural change—urbanization, population aging, globalization, and the overall environment of health policy—are reflected in the underlying determinants of diabetes.

8.1.6. Comorbidity

Comorbidities in patients with diabetes significantly affect medical costs and related expenses. Research has shown that individuals with diabetes have a higher likelihood of developing atherosclerosis, hypertension, skin, respiratory, and urinary tract infections, as well as chronic kidney disease. These conditions increase the patient's risk of infection and medically necessary complications. Certain infections, like COVID-19, have a higher incidence rate in patients with diabetes mellitus, ranging from 5.3 to 35.5%. The main objective of diabetes management is to maintain adequate glycemic control because it is essential to controlling diabetes and delaying or preventing such complications.

8.1.7. Management

The goal of managing diabetes is to avoid low blood sugar by maintaining blood sugar levels that are relatively normal. Changes in diet, exercise, weight loss, and the use of the proper medications (insulin, oral medications) can usually help achieve this.

Being aware of the condition and actively involved in its treatment is crucial because individuals with well-controlled blood sugar levels experience far fewer and milder complications. A1C levels under 7% are the target for treatment. Additional health issues that could hasten the detrimental effects of diabetes are also taken into consideration. These include obesity with metabolic syndrome, smoking, high blood pressure, and irregular exercise. By lowering the pressure on the foot, specialized footwear is frequently used to lower the risk of diabetic foot ulcers. Every year, diabetic patients should have their feet examined. This examination should include testing for sensation, biomechanics, vascular integrity, and foot structure.

The effectiveness of type 2 diabetes self-management interventions for people with severe mental illness is still understudied, and there is not enough data from research to determine whether these interventions produce outcomes that are comparable to those seen in the general population.

8.1.7.1. Lifestyle

In order to keep their blood glucose levels within reasonable limits over the long term, as well as in the short term, people with diabetes can benefit from dietary modifications, exercise, and education regarding the illness and treatment options. Additionally, lifestyle changes are advised to control blood pressure due to the increased risks of cardiovascular disease.

Losing weight can stop the progression of prediabetes into diabetes type 2, lower the risk of cardiovascular disease, or cause a partial remission of diabetes in those who already have it. For all diabetics, there is no one ideal dietary pattern. While there is no evidence to favor one healthy eating pattern over another, it is common to recommend healthy eating patterns like the DASH diet, the Mediterranean diet, or the low-carb diet. Low or very-low carbohydrate diets are a viable option for people with type 2 diabetes who cannot meet the glycemic targets or where reducing anti-glycemic medications is a priority, according to the American Diabetes Association, which states that "reducing overall carbohydrate intake for individuals with diabetes has demonstrated the most evidence for improving glycemia." Any diet that results in weight loss is beneficial for those with type 2 diabetes who are overweight.

8.1.7.2. Medications

Diabetes medications work by lowering blood glucose levels to treat diabetes mellitus. All diabetes medications, with the exception of insulin and the majority of GLP-1 receptor agonists (liraglutide, exenatide, and others), and pramlintide, are taken orally; for this reason, they are referred to as oral hypoglycemic agents or oral antihyperglycemic agents. There are various classes of hypoglycemic medications, and the choice of the right medication depends on the patient's age, circumstances, type of diabetes, and other medical conditions.

Insulin deficiency is the primary cause of type 1 diabetes. Insulin is therefore the primary treatment for type 1 diabetes and is usually injected subcutaneously. Insulin resistance in cells is the etiology of diabetes mellitus type 2. The most prevalent kind of diabetes is type 2 diabetes mellitus. Treatments include drugs that: (1) raise the pancreatic amount of insulin secreted; (2) raise the target organs' sensitivity to insulin; (3) slow down the rate at which the gastrointestinal tract absorbs glucose; and (4) increase the amount of glucose lost through urination.

In type 2 diabetes, a number of medication classes are recommended for use, frequently in combination. Multiple insulin isoforms or different classes of oral antihyperglycemic medications can be combined therapeutically. The FDA had approved 23 distinct antihyperglycemic medication combinations as of 2020. In 2019, the first triple combination of oral anti-diabetics—dapagliflozin, saxagliptin, and metformin—was approved. In 2020, metformin, linagliptin, and empagliflozin were approved in a triple combination.

8.1.7.2.1. Glucose Control

The majority of drugs used to treat diabetes work in different ways to lower blood sugar levels.

There is general agreement that individuals with diabetes who maintain strict glucose control—keeping blood glucose levels within normal ranges—have fewer complications, including kidney or eye issues. The question of whether this is suitable and economical for older adults, when the risk of hypoglycemia may be higher, is up for debate.

Anti-diabetic drugs are classified into several classes. Insulin is necessary to treat type 1 diabetes; ideally, a "basal bolus" regimen involving long-acting insulin for the basal rate and short-acting insulin with meals most closely resembles normal insulin release. The most common treatment for type 2 diabetes is oral medication (e.g., metformin), though some eventually need to be treated injectably with GLP-1 agonists or insulin.

Given the strong evidence supporting its ability to reduce mortality, metformin is typically advised as the initial line of treatment for type 2 diabetes. It functions by raising the quantity of glucose stored in peripheral tissue and lowering the amount of glucose produced by the liver. In type 2 diabetes, a number of additional drug classes—primarily oral medications—may also lower blood sugar. Sulfonylureas, acarbose, agents that inhibit the enzyme dipeptidyl peptidase-4 (DPP-4) that inactivates incretins like GLP-1 and GIP (sitagliptin), agents that increase the body's sensitivity to insulin (thiazolidinedione), and agents that increase the excretion of glucose in the urine (SGLT2 inhibitors) are some examples of these. When type 2 diabetes is treated, oral medications are usually continued while a long-acting formulation of insulin is added initially.

Insulin is another treatment option for some severe cases of type 2 diabetes. Insulin is gradually increased until glucose targets are met.

8.1.7.2.2. Blood Pressure Lowering

Numerous international guidelines suggest that individuals with diabetes should aim for blood pressure treatment targets lower than 140/90 mmHg because cardiovascular disease is a serious complication of diabetes. On the other hand, there isn't much data to support the lower targets. A follow-up systematic review in 2019 found no evidence of additional benefit from lowering blood pressure to between 130 and 140 mmHg, although there was an increased risk of adverse events. A 2016 systematic review found potential harm to treating to targets lower than 140 mmHg.

According to 2015 American Diabetes Association guidelines, individuals with diabetes and albuminuria should be treated with renin-angiotensin system inhibitors to lower their risk of dying, having cardiovascular events, or progressing to end-stage renal disease. Angiotensin converting enzyme inhibitors (ACEIs) have been shown to be more effective in preventing cardiovascular disease than other renin-angiotensin system inhibitors, such as aliskiren or angiotensin receptor blockers (ARBs). Despite this, a more recent review discovered that ACEIs and ARBs had comparable effects on important renal and cardiovascular outcomes. There is no proof that taking ACEIs and ARBs together offers any extra advantages.

8.1.7.2.3. Aspirin

There is debate surrounding the use of aspirin in diabetics to prevent cardiovascular disease. While routine aspirin use has not been found to improve outcomes in cases of uncomplicated diabetes, it is recommended by some for those who are at high risk of cardiovascular disease. In 2015, the American Diabetes Association recommended that adults with diabetes who are at intermediate risk of cardiovascular disease (10-year cardiovascular disease risk, 5–10%)

use low-dose aspirin. These recommendations are based on expert consensus or clinical experience. People with type 1 or type 2 diabetes who do not yet have a confirmed cardiovascular disease are advised not to take aspirin, according to national guidelines for England and Wales published by the National Institute for Health and Care Excellence (NICE).

8.1.7.3. Surgery

For people with type 2 diabetes and obesity, weight loss surgery is frequently a useful intervention. Following surgery, many are able to maintain normal blood sugar levels with little to no medication, and the risk of long-term death is reduced. However, the surgery carries a less than 1% short-term mortality risk. Currently unknown are the body mass index cutoffs that determine when surgery is warranted. It is advised that individuals who are unable to control their blood sugar levels and weight take this option into consideration. People with type 1 diabetes who experience severe complications from their disease, such as end-stage kidney disease necessitating kidney transplantation, may occasionally be candidates for a pancreas transplant.

8.1.7.4. Self-Management and Support

Care may be provided primarily outside of hospitals in nations with general practitioner systems, like the United Kingdom. Hospital-based specialized care is only utilized in the event of complications, challenging blood sugar control, or research projects. In other cases, a team approach is used to share care between general practitioners and specialists. Research indicates that social prescribing improved type 2 diabetics' blood sugar control just a little bit. Support for home telehealth can be a useful management strategy.

Computer-based self-management interventions that gather customized data to support self-management are part of the technology-enabled educational programs for adults with type 2 diabetes. Effects on blood pressure, cholesterol, weight, depression, eating habits, physical activity, and health-related quality of life, as well as other biological, cognitive, or emotional outcomes, have not been sufficiently demonstrated.

8.1.8. Toxicity and Adverse Effect Management

Hypoglycemia is one of the most frequent side effects of insulin. The most frequent adverse effect of many T2DM drugs is gastrointestinal distress. Metformin should be used cautiously in patients with renal disease and stopped if the estimated glomerular filtration rate (e-GFR) is less than 30 mL/min, as it can cause lactic acidosis. Sulfonylureas may increase the risk of cardiovascular death in diabetic patients and cause hypoglycemia. Thiazolidinediones' negative side effects—namely, increased fluid retention, worsening heart failure, and fractures—have caused them to lose favor in clinical practice. Compared to other medications like metformin, DPP-4 may cause less nausea and diarrhea but may raise the risk of upper respiratory tract infections. Because SGLT-2 inhibitors increase the excretion of glucose in the urine, they may increase the risk of urinary tract infections. SGLT2 inhibitors and GLP-1 Receptor agonists are now thought to be the second line of treatment for patients with ASCVD after metformin.

8.1.9. Prognosis

In the US, diabetes mellitus ranked as the seventh most common cause of death in 2015. The degree of glucose management has a major impact on the prognosis of diabetes mellitus. The risk of problems from diabetes mellitus is greatly increased by chronic hyperglycemia. According to the United Kingdom Prospective Diabetes Study and the Diabetes Control and Complications Trial, people with T1DM and T2DM, respectively, had higher rates of microvascular complications associated with persistent hyperglycemia. Patients with a good prognosis who can return to normal glucose levels during the transition from pre-diabetes to frank diabetes had the potential to slow the course of the disease.

8.1.10. Complications

Whatever the particular form of diabetes, complications include neuropathic, macrovascular, and microvascular problems. Nephropathy, retinopathy, neuropathy, and ASCVD events are examples of microvascular and macrovascular complications that vary depending on the severity and length of poorly controlled diabetes. These complications are particularly common if the condition is co-occurring with other comorbidities such as dyslipidemia and hypertension. Cardiovascular disease is one of the most disastrous effects of diabetes mellitus (ASCVD). A myocardial infarction or stroke will claim the lives of about two thirds of people with diabetes. More than 100 mg/dL of fasting glucose increases the risk of ASCVD in people with type 2 diabetes; however, cardiovascular risk can appear before frank hyperglycemia. In adults in the US between the ages of 20 and 74, diabetes mellitus is another common cause of blindness. Between 12,000 and 24,000 new cases of blindness are caused by diabetic retinopathy each year; laser surgery and glucose management are the usual treatments.

Another important factor contributing to morbidity and death is renal disease. It is the primary cause of end-stage renal disease (ESRD) in the US, and many ESRD patients will require a kidney transplant or start dialysis. Microalbuminuria, or persistent albuminuria in the range of 30 to 300 mg/day, appears to be a reliable early indicator of the onset of diabetic neuropathy. The development of macroalbuminuria (more than 300 mg/24 hr) accelerates the transition to end-stage renal disease. The most popular and preferred method for detecting microalbuminuria is the random spot urine specimen, which is quick, simple, and predictable when measuring the albumin-to-creatinine ratio. The diagnosis of microalbuminuria is supported by two out of three tests conducted over a six-month period that consistently show a level greater than 30 mcg/mg creatinine.

Due mostly to the vasculopathy and neuropathy linked to DM, DM is also the most common cause of limb amputations in the US. Regular foot exams are necessary for many patients who develop neuropathy in order to prevent infection from unseen wounds.

The most important risk factor for the development of diabetic retinopathy is the length of diabetes. It usually appears in type 1 diabetics five years after the disease first manifests. Therefore, it is advised that these patients begin yearly retinal exams approximately five years following diagnosis. Many individuals with type 2 diabetes may already have retinal abnormalities at the time of diagnosis. Nonproliferative retinal disease will affect roughly 10% of patients after ten years, 40% after fifteen years, and 60% after 20 years. It is advised that the annual retinal screening be initiated in these patients at the time of diagnosis. Numerous studies have demonstrated that the development and course of diabetic retinopathy were positively impacted by appropriate glycemic control. Macular edema is furthermore associated with uncontrolled blood pressure. Thus, lowering blood pressure in diabetic patients has an impact on the likelihood that their retinopathy will progress. When macular edema occurs, injections of antibodies against vascular endothelial growth factor (anti-VEGF) agents are typically used as the first line of treatment. Pan-retinal photocoagulation is used in non-proliferative diabetic retinopathy cases. Anti-VEGF medications and pan-retinal photocoagulation are now used in combination to treat diabetic proliferative retinopathy. Patients with diabetes mellitus may experience sudden loss of vision for a variety of reasons, the most common of which is vitreous hemorrhage. Vascular occlusion (central retinal vein or branch vein occlusion involving the macula), retinal detachment, end-stage glaucoma, and ischemic optic neuropathy are less frequent causes that should be taken into account.

Additionally, data indicates that T2DM may also be linked to the development of cancer, particularly bladder cancer, in individuals taking pioglitazone. Metformin users had better cancer-specific survival rates for colorectal, pancreatic, breast, and prostate cancers. On the other hand, it is unknown how metformin affects diabetes patients' cancer. Pregnancy-related diabetes increases the risk of both chronic hypertension and cesarean delivery. Compared to those with T1DM, pregnant patients with T2DM typically have a better prognosis in terms of pregnancy and neonatal complications. Neonatals with diabetes mellitus typically present with macrosomia and hypoglycemia.

Diabetic ketoacidosis (DKA), the most common acute complication of diabetes mellitus, usually manifests in type 1 diabetes. Usually, one of the following causes this condition: insufficient dosage, missed doses, or persistent infection. Tissues in this condition are unable to absorb glucose from the bloodstream due to a lack of insulin. As a substitute energy source, compensation for this leads to the metabolism of lipids into ketones, which results in systemic acidosis, also known as high anion-gap metabolic acidosis. When hyperglycemia and ketosis coexist, it can result in diuresis, acidemia, and vomiting, which can be fatal due to electrolyte imbalances and dehydration. Hyperosmolar hyperglycemic syndrome (HHS) is a critical issue in type 2 diabetes. Excessive thirst, high blood sugar, dry mouth, polyuria, tachypnea, and tachycardia are symptoms that are similar to those of DKA. However, because pancreatic beta cells continue to produce insulin, HHS usually does not manifest with elevated urine ketones, in contrast to DKA. Administering insulin and aggressive intravenous hydration are part of the treatment for DKA or HHS. The treatment of these acute conditions depends heavily on the careful monitoring of electrolytes, especially potassium.

8.1.11. Deterrence and Patient Education

It is important for medical personnel to actively educate patients with diabetes mellitus. Patients who believe that making lifestyle changes for a brief period of time is appropriate are misguided; in order to effectively control their diabetes, lifelong lifestyle changes may be required. Individualized education is more beneficial than group education for patients with poorly controlled diabetes mellitus, according to a randomized, controlled trial. Often, non-clinician healthcare professionals (e.g., nurses, and pharmacists) have more time for individualized instruction and have received substantial training in diabetes education.

8.1.12. Pearls and Other Issues

The development of type 2 diabetes may be significantly influenced by amino acid metabolism. According to studies, people with hyperglycemia have four times as much isoleucine, phenylalanine, and tyrosine. These amino acids were found to be elevated up to 12 years prior to the disease's onset by the researchers. The role of these metabolites in the development, screening, and management of metabolic syndrome (MetS), a cardiometabolic cluster that predisposes patients to type 2 diabetes and cardiovascular disease, has been further clarified by recent studies. Research has indicated that choline, L-carnitine, and trimethylamine-N-oxide are linked to inflammatory pathways and raise the possibility of metabolic dysfunction in individuals who are at risk of developing MetS, meaning they fit the criteria for the condition but do not have cardiovascular disease or type 2 diabetes. Studies have also revealed lower levels of methionine and lysine and higher levels of isoleucine and tyrosine. These metabolites seem to be important contributors to the pro-inflammatory burden of MetS and early indicators of developing MetS.

Insufficient lysine levels have been linked to higher levels of inflammation and increased blood glucose. Therefore, it is believed that a diet rich in lysine may help reduce inflammation. In a recent study, researchers discovered that certain metabolites such as phosphatidylcholine 34:2, GABA, and d-pyroglutamic acid (PGA) were significantly elevated in individuals with early signs of metabolic syndrome and correlated with specific inflammatory markers. These findings highlight the importance of metabolites in the early stages of type 2 diabetes and suggest they may play a role in the inflammation associated with diabetes.

8.1.13. Enhancing Healthcare Team Outcomes

Patients with diabetes are frequently first diagnosed with the disease by primary care physicians. Because diabetes mellitus is a complicated illness, managing it calls for an interdisciplinary team approach. Monitoring the effectiveness of treatments and making sure that patients are properly followed up on can be important tasks for nurse practitioners and physician assistants. In order to help patients learn about appropriate lifestyle modifications and at-home glucose management, nutritionists and diabetes educators can also offer consultations.

The healthcare team may also include nephrologists, podiatrists, neurologists, and ophthalmologists to make sure that patients with DM receive the necessary screenings to avoid life-threatening microvascular complications. Endocrinologists might be consulted if a patient presents with complications or doesn't respond to first treatments. Naturally, pharmacists are essential in assessing appropriate drug delivery and preventing polypharmacy in diabetic patients, who frequently take several medications for the underlying condition and its side effects. They can guarantee appropriate dosage and suggest the most effective regimens to attain glycemic control, as well as inform the patient about the drugs and the course of the disease.

8.2. Hypertension

It is well recognized that having diabetes and hypertension together can compound the negative clinical outcomes associated with both microvascular and macrovascular disease. Therefore, an integrated strategy that combines appropriate glycemic control with optimal blood pressure and lipid control is necessary for effective diabetes management. The pathophysiology of hypertension in diabetes includes immune system abnormalities, detrimental environmental factors, vascular endothelial dysfunction, increased renin-angiotensin-aldosterone system activation, and maladaptive changes in the autonomic nervous system. Numerous excellent randomized controlled trials have demonstrated that lowering high blood pressure in diabetics reduces morbidity. Since most diabetic patients are more likely to develop cardiovascular disease (CVD) than people without the disease, attention must be given to each patient's unique risk factors and co-morbidities with the aim of less than 130/80 mm Hg. The approach to controlling blood pressure in these patients includes good glycemic control, optimizing weight, encouraging exercise, and reducing harmful environmental factors like exposure to air pollution. It is crucial to choose a therapy carefully and to take pertinent side-effect profiles into account. Drug combinations should be selected after careful consideration of the potential for both positive and negative drug interactions. While combined use of these agents is not advised due to poor renal outcomes, angiotensin converting enzyme inhibitors and angiotensin receptor blockers remain preferred agents for the initiation of antihypertensive therapy. When starting therapy for glycemic control, consideration should be given to the antihypertensive, renal, and cardiovascular disease lowering properties of the newer antidiabetic agents, such as SGLT inhibitors and GLP1 receptor agonists.

8.2.1. Symptoms

Rarely does hypertension have symptoms, and the only ways to diagnose it are either through a health screening or by visiting the doctor for a different issue. Some hypertensive individuals report headaches (especially in the morning and in the back of the head), dizziness, lightheadedness, tinnitus (ear buzzing or hissing), blurred vision, or episodes of fainting. Nonetheless, rather than being directly linked to high blood pressure, these symptoms may also be related to related anxiety.

Upon physical examination, ophthalmoscopy-observed alterations in the optic fundus may be linked to hypertension. Grades I through IV indicate the severity of the changes characteristic of hypertensive retinopathy; it may be challenging to distinguish between grades I and II. There is a general correlation between the duration or severity of hypertension and the degree of retinopathy.

8.2.1.1. Secondary Hypertension

Secondary hypertension is defined as hypertension with a known cause that may also present with particular extra symptoms. For instance, Cushing's syndrome commonly results in truncal obesity, glucose intolerance, moon face, a hump of fat behind the neck and shoulders known as a buffalo hump, and purple stretch marks on the abdomen in addition to high blood pressure. Fast heartbeat, bulging eyes, tremor, and increased appetite are all common side effects of hyperthyroidism that lead to weight loss. A localized abdominal bruit to the left or right of the midline (unilateral RAS) or in both locations (bilateral RAS) may be linked to renal artery stenosis (RAS). Aortic coarctation frequently results in absentee or delayed femoral arterial pulses, as well as lower extremity blood pressure that is lower than in the arms. Abrupt episodes of hypertension with headache, palpitations, pale appearance, and profuse sweating are possible symptoms of phenochromotoma.

8.2.1.2. Hypertensive Crisis

A hypertensive crisis is defined as a markedly elevated blood pressure of 180 mmHg or higher at the diastolic or systolic points. Depending on whether end organ damage is present or absent, hypertensive crisis is classified as either a hypertensive emergency or hypertensive urgency. There is no proof of end organ damage from the high blood pressure in hypertensive urgency. In these situations, the BP is gradually lowered over the course of 24 to 48 hours using oral medications.

There is proof that one or more organs have been directly damaged in a hypertensive emergency. The most affected organs include the brain, kidney, heart and lungs, producing symptoms which may include confusion, drowsiness, chest pain and breathlessness. In cases of hypertension emergencies, it is imperative to lower blood pressure more quickly in order to halt the ongoing damage to organs; however, the evidence supporting this approach from randomized controlled trials is lacking.

8.2.1.3. Pregnancy

Approximately 8–10% of pregnancies result in hypertension. Hypertension in pregnancy is diagnosed by taking two readings of blood pressure that are more than 140/90 mmHg, six hours apart. Pre-existing hypertension, gestational hypertension, and pre-eclampsia are three categories for high blood pressure during pregnancy. Premature birth, low birthweight, and stillbirth are among the complications that women with chronic hypertension before becoming pregnant are more likely to experience. Women with high blood pressure who experienced pregnancy complications are three times more likely to develop cardiovascular disease than women with normal blood pressure who did not experience any pregnancy complications. Pre-eclampsia is a dangerous condition that develops in the second half of pregnancy and after delivery. It is characterized by elevated blood pressure and urine that contains protein. Roughly 5% of pregnancies experience it, and it accounts for 16% of maternal deaths worldwide. Additionally, pre-eclampsia doubles the baby's risk of dying shortly after birth. Pre-eclampsia typically shows no symptoms and is identified by routine screening. Pre-eclampsia symptoms include headache, vomiting, pain over the stomach, visual disturbance (often "flashing lights"), and swelling. Periodically, pre-eclampsia can develop into eclampsia, a hypertensive emergency with multiple life-threatening complications, including disseminated intravascular coagulation (a blood clotting disorder), seizures, brain swelling, kidney failure, and pulmonary edema. On the other hand, pregnancy-related new-onset hypertension without protein in the urine is known as gestational hypertension.

8.2.1.4. Children

In neonates and early infants, hypertension may be linked to symptoms such as breathing difficulties, irritability, lack of energy, seizures, and failure to thrive. Hypertension in older infants and children can result in headache, blurred vision, nosebleeds, fatigue, and facial paralysis, along with inexplicable irritability and failure to thrive.

8.2.2. Causes

8.2.2.1. Primary Hypertension

A complex interplay between genetics and environmental factors leads to hypertension. Both common genetic variants with minor effects on blood pressure and rare genetic variants with significant effects on blood pressure have been found. Furthermore, 35 genetic loci associated with blood pressure have been found through genome-wide association studies (GWAS); 12 of these newly discovered genetic loci have an impact on blood pressure. Every newly discovered genetic locus has a sentinel SNP that indicates a correlation with DNA methylation at several neighboring CpG sites. These sentinel SNPs are found in genes associated with renal and vascular smooth muscle function. DNA methylation may play a role in connecting common genetic variation to a variety of phenotypes, despite the fact that the mechanisms behind these connections remain unclear. Single variant test performed in this study for the 35 sentinel SNP (known and new) showed that genetic variants singly or in aggregate contribute to risk of clinical phenotypes related to high blood pressure.

Coronary artery ectasia: The hallmark of coronary artery ectasia (CAE) is an enlargement of the coronary artery that is at least 1.5 times larger than other non-ectasia portions of the vessel. When comparing subjects with hypertension (HTN) to those without, the pooled unadjusted OR of CAE was estimated to be 1.44.

When a western diet and lifestyle are combined, blood pressure increases with age, and there is a considerable chance of developing hypertension later in life. Numerous elements of the surroundings affect blood pressure. In people who are sensitive to salt, consuming a lot of salt causes blood pressure to rise; in certain cases, central obesity and inactivity may be contributing factors. It is unclear what part certain other factors, like caffeine intake and vitamin D deficiency, might play. Hypertension is also a result of insulin resistance, which is linked to syndrome X, also known as the metabolic syndrome, and is prevalent in obesity.

Low birth weight, maternal smoking, and not breastfeeding are examples of early life events that may be risk factors for adult essential hypertension, though it is still unclear how these exposures are linked to adult hypertension. Untreated individuals with hypertension have been found to have higher blood uric acid levels than people with normal blood pressure; however, it is unclear if this is a direct result of their hypertension or if it is a secondary effect of their impaired kidney function. Wintertime average blood pressure may be higher than summertime average. Elevated blood pressure is also linked to periodontal disease.

8.2.2.2. Secondary Hypertension

0Secondary hypertension develops from a known source. The most frequent secondary cause of hypertension is kidney disease. Endocrine disorders such as Cushing's syndrome, hyperthyroidism, hypothyroidism, acromegaly, hyperaldosteronism or Conn's syndrome, renal artery stenosis (from fibromuscular dysplasia or atherosclerosis), hyperparathyroidism, and pheochromocytoma can also result in hypertension. Additional factors contributing to secondary hypertension comprise obesity, sleep apnea, pregnancy, aortic coarctation, excessive alcohol consumption, excessive liquorice consumption, certain prescription medications, herbal remedies, and stimulants like cocaine, coffee, and methamphetamine. It has been demonstrated that drinking water contaminated with arsenic is associated with higher blood pressure. Hypertension and depression have also been related. Additionally, loneliness poses a risk. According to study, men's blood pressure rose with any alcohol consumption, but women's risk increased with more than one or two drinks.

8.2.3. Pathophysiology of Hypertension in Diabetes

Increased activation of the renin-angiotensin-aldosterone system (RAAS), complex interactions between the autonomic nervous system, a maladaptive immune system, and unfavorable environmental factors are all contributing factors to the pathophysiology of hypertension in diabetes. The following factors have been the focus of therapeutic interventions because they are important players in the pathophysiology of hypertension.

8.2.3.1. Sedentary Lifestyle, Excessive Caloric Intake and Insulin Resistance

An increased risk of exacerbating insulin resistance has been linked to adiposity, which can be caused by a sedentary lifestyle and an excessive calorie intake. Insulin resistance has been connected, in turn, to elevated vascular oxidative stress, inflammation, and endothelial dysfunction, which is marked by reduced vascular nitric oxide bioactivity. These factors all contribute to vascular stiffness, which raises blood pressure over time and encourages CVD.

8.2.3.2. Elevated Intravascular Volume

The total sodium content of the body has a strong influence on intravascular volume. The primary extracellular cation in humans is sodium, which has osmotic activity that influences effective arterial blood volume. A positive sodium balance may arise from an imbalance between sodium loss and intake. As a result, the intravascular sodium concentration rises, which increases intravascular volume by encouraging an influx of water along the osmotic gradient. According to the Frank Starling Law, an increase in intravascular volume subsequently causes an increase in venous return to the heart, which increases cardiac output and ultimately raises arterial pressure. Additionally, there is mounting evidence that, in states of obesity and insulin resistance, like those experienced by the majority of T2DM patients, increased activation of sodium inward transport in endothelial cells leads to elevated blood pressure and increased vascular stiffness.

Increasing glomerular filtration and compensatory urinary salt excretion usually lower elevated blood pressure (BP) caused by intravascular volume expansion. Pressure natriuresis is the term used to describe this phenomenon of increased excretion of salt in a state of elevated blood pressure. Unfortunately, secondary changes within the kidney microvasculature and maladaptive changes within the glomerular apparatus itself, which lower glomerular filtration and stimulate sodium reabsorption, mean that this mechanism alone is unable to correct persistently elevated blood pressure. Overt chronic kidney disease (CKD) and end stage renal disease (ESRD), which are both characterized by simultaneous volume overload and persistent hypertension, are the conditions in which these alterations are most noticeable. Restoring normal vascular volume is necessary to control hypertension in CKD/ESRD patients, which can be done with diuretics or dialysis.

8.2.3.3. Premature Vascular Aging

Changes in vessel elasticity can impact blood flow through arteries. Even small reductions in lumen diameter can greatly increase resistance to blood flow. Patients with hypertension often experience negative changes in the structure and function of small arteries and arterioles, leading to vascular remodeling, inflammation, fibrosis, and stiffness. These changes may be due to high blood pressure in individuals with diabetes. Patients with diabetes may show signs of accelerated vascular aging, including impaired relaxation, increased muscle contraction and resistance, and vascular stiffness. These vascular changes can both cause hypertension and worsen its effects on vessel health.

8.2.3.4. Autonomic Nervous System Dysregulation

Autonomic nervous system function plays a significant role in BP regulation. Blood pressure is regulated by both the parasympathetic and sympathetic nervous systems. Increased peripheral vascular resistance, heart rate, ventricle contraction force, and fluid retention are all caused by increased sympathetic activity. The sum of these physiological processes leads to an increase in blood pressure. A decrease in parasympathetic outflow also raises heart rate and causes a relative increase in sympathetic hyperactivity, both of which raise blood pressure. Insulin resistance, sleep apnea, and central obesity are associated with dysregulation of these pathways. Resistant hypertension, an activated RAAS, and elevated sympathetic activity are frequently present in conjunction with hypertension linked to these disorders. Moreover, insulin resistance and the risk of type 2 diabetes are also encouraged by sympathetic nervous system activation. T2DM-related autonomic dysfunction may also exacerbate hypertension by contributing to these alterations. Improvements in insulin sensitivity, better glycemic control, and lower blood pressure are linked to renal denervation, which interrupts the central sympathetic outflow, indicating the importance of these pathways in the etiology of hypertension and diabetes.

8.2.3.5. Renin Angiotensin Aldosterone System (RAAS)

The RAAS pathway is essential for preserving normal blood pressure. The pathophysiology of hypertension is closely associated with RAAS activation due to the elevated levels of plasma aldosterone, which have effects on the kidneys and cardiovascular system. Strong vasoconstrictor angiotensin II directly raises the tone of smooth muscle in the blood vessels. Angiotensin II also increases aldosterone secretion, which encourages the retention of water and salt and raises blood pressure by expanding the volume. Even when there is no increase in angiotensin levels, obesity is linked to higher plasma aldosterone levels. This increase is believed to be partially caused by the expanded adipose tissue's secretion of aldosterone-releasing factors. Since angiotensin converting enzyme (ACE) inhibitors, angiotensin II receptor blockers (ARBs), and increasingly mineralocorticoid receptor antagonists are the mainstays of blood pressure management in people with diabetes, an understanding of the physiology of RAAS is crucial.

Therenal juxtaglomerular cells secrete the proteolytic enzyme renin. Circulating angiotensinogen is broken down by renin into angiotensin I. Angiotensin I is subsequently changed into angiotensin II by ACE in the lung capillaries. Renin production and release are closely regulated by a number of interrelated factors, including sodium chloride concentration in the distal tubule of the nephron, renal perfusion pressure, and sympathetic nervous system stimulation of renin-secreting cells.

When there is hypovolemia-induced renal hypoperfusion, RAAS is physiologically activated. Angiotensin II production rises as a result of a series of events triggered by the juxtaglomerular apparatus's release of renin. Following direct vasoconstriction, angiotensin II increases blood pressure by stimulating aldosterone secretion, which causes salt and water retention and restores intravascular volume.

Obesity and insulin resistance are linked to the overactivation of the RAAS and sympathetic nervous system. An increase in body fat has been connected to higher levels of plasma aldosterone, indicating that the RAAS may be overly active in obese individuals. Both angiotensin II and aldosterone can hinder insulin signaling in traditional insulin-sensitive tissues, leading to issues like impaired vascular relaxation and hypertension. Additionally, these hormones can induce insulin resistance through mechanisms like serine kinase activation and reduced engagement of key signaling pathways, ultimately contributing to vascular dysfunction and increased risk of cardiovascular disease in individuals with obesity and insulin resistance.

8.2.3.6. Renal Dysfunction

In diabetics, there seems to be a reciprocal relationship between hypertension and renal dysfunction. In the context of diabetes, hypertension is acknowledged as a risk factor for chronic kidney disease; however, it is crucial to remember that diabetic nephropathy also plays a role in the development of hypertension. The strongest indication of this reciprocal relationship is seen in type 1 diabetics who do not already have hypertension. Microalbuminuria predates hypertension in this population, according to longitudinal studies, and the prevalence of hypertension increases gradually with worsening kidney disease, reaching nearly 90% in type 1 diabetics with end-stage renal disease. Theorized mechanisms include peripheral vasoconstriction due to endothelial dysfunction, volume expansion secondary to increased renal sodium reabsorption, dysregulated activation of the RAAS, upregulation of endothelin1, and downregulation of nitric oxide.

8.2.3.7. Role of Innate and Adaptive Immunity

Angiotensin II and aldosterone-induced hypertension and vascular disease are associated with increasing evidence of the involvement of both innate immunity and acquired immunity.

8.2.3.8. Environmental and Socioeconomic Factors

Between White and Black Americans, there are notable differences in hypertension. Despite greater awareness and treatment of hypertension among Black Americans compared to White Americans, this disparity is still growing. With disproportionately high rates of morbidity and mortality among communities of color, the recent Covid-19 pandemic has exacerbated this disparity. Some have hypothesized that the social, economic, and environmental injustices that contribute to diabetes, obesity, and hypertension are also responsible for the discrepancy in Covid outcomes.

People living in these communities frequently cannot afford or do not have access to foods that are typically promoted as parts of the DASH diet and are thought to be healthy. Rather, they start consuming low-cost, high-salted, high-calorie foods, which inevitably results in obesity and hypertension. In addition, a lack of secure outdoor areas deters physical activity, and targeted advertising promotes unhealthy choices like smoking. A study of Black and White Americans residing in long-term integrated neighborhoods provides additional evidence for these effects. Although the odds ratio for hypertension was higher in Blacks in the sample population, it was found to have decreased by about 30% when compared to NHANES data in the Exploring Health Disparities in Integrated Communities-South Western Baltimore (EHDIC-SWB) study. The authors came to the conclusion that racial disparities in the prevalence of diabetes and hypertension were significantly explained by social and environmental exposure.

8.2.4. Blood Pressure Measurement and Monitoring

Precise blood pressure measurement is essential for diagnosing and successfully treating hypertension. The majority of the time, blood pressure is measured in a doctor's office using either the oscillometric approach used in automated devices or the auscultatory method of listening to Korotkoff sounds. Because oscillometric devices are more convenient to use and reduce inter-observer variability in manual measurements, the auscultatory method has mostly been replaced by them. But it is crucial to keep in mind that, if certain safety measures are ignored, even automated measurements may turn out to be inaccurate. After the patient has rested for three to five minutes, measurements should be taken while they are seated, ideally with an empty bladder. No exertion, exercise, eating, smoking, or stressful situations for at least half an hour prior to taking a blood pressure reading. In a span of two weeks, three readings will be optimal. To guarantee accurate readings, the device should be calibrated on a regular basis. An incorrect cuff size is a common cause of reading errors. It is advised that the cuff bladder's width be roughly half of the arm circumference and that its length match the patient's arm circumference as measured at the midpoint of the olecranon and acromion processes. Because obesity is becoming more common, using cuffs that are too small can lead to an overestimation of blood pressure. Even with all these safety measures, there can still be a lot of variation in one reading from another, which is why the American Heart Association (AHA) advises getting at least two readings every clinic visit.

A fully automated non-invasive procedure called ambulatory blood pressure monitoring (ABPM) involves placing a blood pressure cuff on the non-dominant arm and taking readings every 15 to 30 minutes for a full day. ABPM has a better prognostic value for target organ damage and cardiovascular outcomes than in-office blood pressure monitoring. The main benefit of ABPM over office monitoring, which depends on individual measurements, is its comprehensiveness. Different blood pressure patterns that cannot be identified with office measurements alone, such as sustained, white-coat, masked, and nocturnal hypertension, as well as non-dipping or reverse-dipping patterns, can be detected with this format. These patterns need to be treated very differently because they are linked to different cardiovascular outcomes. When ABPM readings are consistently normal but office measurements are in the hypertensive range, the condition is known as "white-coat hypertension." This phenomenon is linked to low cardiovascular risk and is not a sign that antihypertensive medication is necessary. It is ascribed to the influence of an observer during the measurement. However, it should be noted that people with white coats are more likely to experience persistent hypertension and should thus undergo routine monitoring. Conversely, "masked hypertension" describes a state in which ABPM readings fall into the hypertensive range, despite office measurements being normal. This phenomenon is linked to elevated cardiovascular risk, similar to what is observed in cases of long-term hypertension. Crucially, masked hypertension is more prevalent in patients with diabetes and obesity. Aggressive antihypertensive therapy is thought to benefit these patients, but no randomized controlled trials have been conducted to support this theory.

Normal blood pressure readings follow a physiologic circadian rhythm, with a drop of over 10% during the night compared to daytime readings. Patients with a non-dipping pattern are those whose blood pressure decreases by less than 10%. This non-dipping pattern has been linked to cardiovascular autonomic neuropathy and is more common in diabetics. Its role in the development of diabetic complications is less clear. Due to its effects on renal hemodynamics, blood flow distribution, and circulating plasma volume, hyperglycemia itself can affect the typical nocturnal dip.

8.2.5. Blood Pressure Targets in Patients with Diabetes

It is impossible to overstate the significance of strict blood pressure management in preventing diabetes-related morbidity. There is growing evidence to support this for both microvascular and macrovascular complications. According to the United Kingdom Prospective Diabetes Study (UKPDS), lowering blood pressure (target blood pressure <150/85 mm Hg) was associated with 44, 32, and 34% lower risks of stroke, diabetes-related deaths, and retinopathy, respectively. Systolic blood pressure reduction was found to have a linear relationship with unfavorable outcomes at as low as 120 mm Hg.

A decrease in diastolic blood pressure was associated with a decrease in CVD, according to the Hypertension On Target (HOT) trial. Interestingly, though, this benefit was limited to patients with diabetes, indicating that a different, possibly more aggressive blood pressure target should be set for this population subgroup.

The initial research study that focused on controlling blood pressure in individuals with diabetes was the Action in Diabetes and Vascular Disease: Preterax and Diamicron MR Controlled Evaluation (ADVANCE) trial. With aggressive reductions in both systolic and diastolic blood pressure, the results demonstrated a significant decrease in microvascular events, cardiovascular deaths, and all-cause mortality (mean achieved blood pressure of 134/74 mm Hg versus 140/76 mm Hg). These were impressive results.

For patients with diabetes, major medical societies such as the American Diabetes Association (ADA) recommend a target blood pressure of less than 130/80 mm Hg. The Normotensive Appropriate Blood Pressure Control in Diabetes (ABCD) trial was the first to look for support for this recommendation. The intensive treatment group's mean blood pressure of 128/75 mm Hg was below the 130 mm Hg systolic target, despite no specific blood pressure target being pursued. Comparing the creatinine clearance (primary outcome) and cardiovascular events over a five-year follow-up period to the placebo group revealed no discernible differences (mean blood pressure 137/81). There were notable improvements in the acute treatment group's albuminuria, stroke risk, and retinopathy progression.

In the ACCORD blood pressure trial, the idea of a systolic blood pressure target of less than 130 mm Hg was contested. In this extensive randomized control trial, a systolic target of less than 120 mm Hg (intensive therapy) was contrasted with a systolic target of less than 140 mm Hg (standard therapy). In terms of the combined CVD outcomes (heart attack, stroke, and cardiovascular death), no discernible difference was found between the two groups with over 4500 patients and a mean follow-up of 4.7 years. Notably, a 40% decrease in the risk of stroke was observed, which is comparable to the outcomes of the ABCD trial. Factors that complicate this study prevent recommendations from being made based on its findings.

The Systolic Blood Pressure Intervention Trial (SPRINT) was the most recent large-scale randomized control trial that looked at a lower systolic blood pressure goal. In this study, the benefits of treatment were compared between groups receiving intensive treatment (whose systolic blood pressure target was less than 120 mm Hg) and standard treatment (whose target was less than 140 mm Hg). At one year, the standard treatment group's mean systolic blood pressure was 136.2 mm Hg, while the intensive treatment group's was 121.4 mm Hg. The intensive treatment group exhibited significantly lower rates of cardiovascular events, both fatal and nonfatal, as well as death from all causes, according to the results. With a hazard ratio of 1.88 ($P<0.001$), serious adverse events that were either definitely or possibly related to the intervention occurred statistically more frequently in the group receiving intensive treatment. 9361 participants with a median follow-up of 3.26 years were included in this study; however, patients with diabetes were not included. Because of its study design, the SPRINT trial cannot be directly applied to the diabetic population, but it does support a lower goal.

According to some experts, the ACCORD trial lacked sufficient power to demonstrate a statistically significant difference for the primary endpoint. The SPRINT primary endpoint was examined in a recent pooled analysis that combined data from the SPRINT and ACCORD trials. Unlike the ACCORD trial, the primary endpoint in this study included not only myocardial infarction, stroke, and CVD death, but also unstable angina and acute decompensated heart failure. The intensive treatment group significantly outperformed the control group in both patients with and without diabetes, according to the final analysis. This implies that there might not be a unique advantage to aggressively lowering blood pressure (i.e., to less than 130/80 mm Hg) in patients with T2DM.

It should be mentioned that blood pressure was measured in the SPRINT and ACCORD trials under very controlled circumstances, which should have resulted in lower readings than in traditional clinic settings. This finding begs the question of whether similar cardiovascular benefits could be obtained in real-world situations by using more lenient targets.

Finally, it should be noted that numerous excellent randomized controlled trials have demonstrated that treating elevated blood pressure in diabetics can reduce their chronic illness. Individuals with type 2 diabetes seem to be especially vulnerable to the harmful effects of high blood pressure on the development and course of cardiovascular disease. Lower treatment targets should be considered when treating hypertension in patients with diabetes, taking into account the patient's preferences, co-morbidities, and individual risk factors. For a young person who would likely benefit from a reduction in stroke risk and a slower progression of retinopathy, a lower blood pressure target, for example, might be more appropriate without causing unwanted side effects like hypotension, syncope, and hyperkalemia—symptoms that are more frequently experienced by the elderly and those with multiple co-morbidities.

8.2.6. Treatment of Hypertension

Diabetes patients can develop resistant hypertension, making treatment of their hypertension difficult. Furthermore, a higher incidence of renal and cardiac comorbidities in diabetics can reduce their tolerance to aggressive antihypertensive therapy. Therefore, a comprehensive treatment plan must address every facet of the intricate metabolic disorders observed in this particular population.

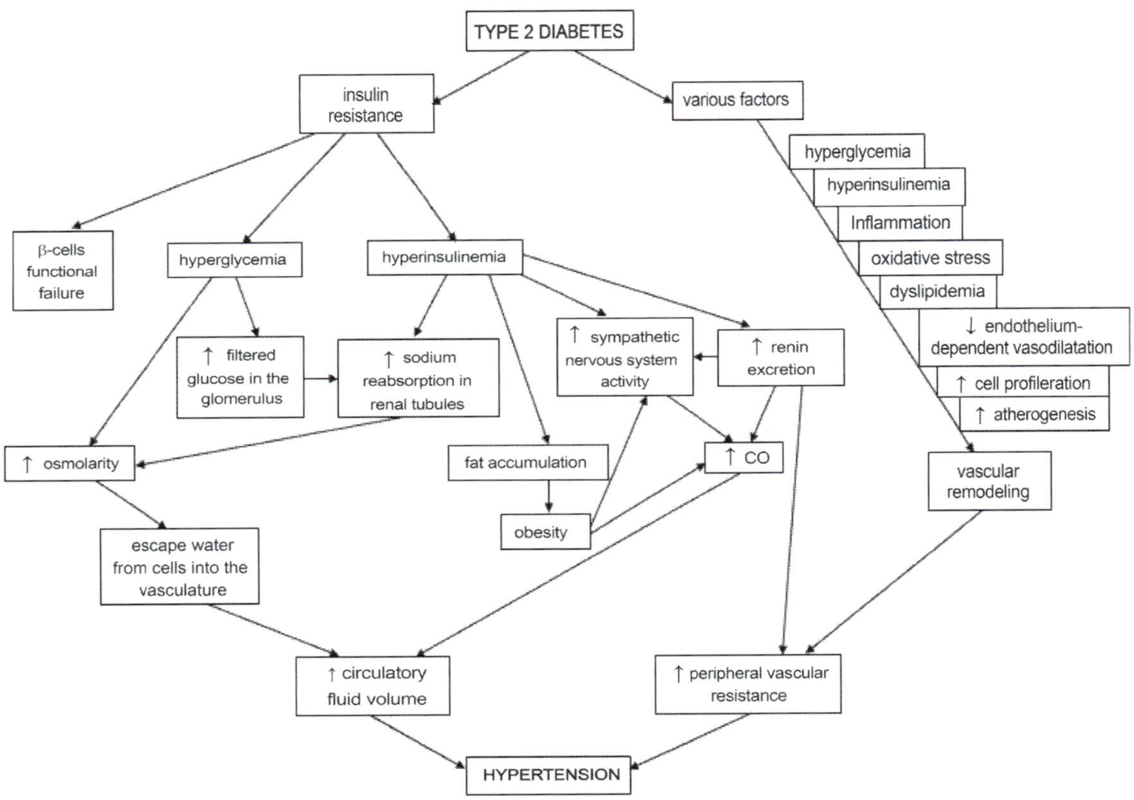

Figure 8.2. *Approach to hypertension in the diabetic patient.*

Source: Przezak A, Bielka W, & Pawlik A. (2022). Hypertension and type 2 diabetes—The novel treatment possibilities. International Journal of Molecular Sciences, 23(12), 6500. https://doi.org/10.3390/ijms23126500.

The treatment of hypertension in relation to type 2 diabetes will be the main topic of this section. We will analyze the benefits and drawbacks of various treatment approaches, breaking them down by drug class. It is imperative to stress the significance of taking accurate blood pressure readings and applying the right techniques, particularly in light of the patient's lifetime consequences. As soon as a patient with diabetes has been diagnosed with hypertension, prompt and intensive treatment must be started. It is also important to remember that, with a few exceptions, the level of blood pressure reduction attained matters more than the specific antihypertensive drug used.

Table 8.1 provides a summary of the different classes of antihypertensive medications that are frequently used. In Figure 8.1, the general connection between hypertension in a diabetic patient is described.

Table 8.1. Antihypertensive Drugs: Age and Dosing Recommendations, Contraindications, and Adverse Drug Reactions

Drug	**Age**	**Initial Dose (mg/kg per Dose)**	**Maximal Dose (mg/kg per Dose)**	**Dosing Interval**	**Contraindications and Adverse Drug Reactions**
ACE inhibitors					**Contraindications:** pregnancy, angioedema. **Common ADR:** cough, headache, dizziness, asthenia. **Severe ADR:** hyperkaliemia, acute kidney injury, angioedema, fetal toxicity
Benazepril	≥6 y	0.2 (up to 10 mg/d)	0.6 (up to 40 mg/d)	1/day	
Captopril	Infants	0.05	6	1–4/day	
	Children	0.5	6	3/day	
Enalapril	≥1 mo	0.08 (up to 10 mg/d)	0.6 (up to 40 mg/d)	1–2/day	
Fosinopril	≥6 y	0.1 (up to 5 mg/d)	40 mg/d	1/day	
	≥50 kg				
	≥50 kg	5 mg/d	40 mg per d		
Lisinopril	≥6 y	0.07 (up to 10 mg/d)	0.6 (up to 40 mg/d)	1/day	
Ramipril	-	1.6 mg/m²/d	6 mg/m²/d	1/day	
Quinapril	-	5 mg/d	80 mg/d	1/day	

ARB					**Contraindications:** pregnancy. **Common ADR:** headache, dizziness. **Severe ADR:** hyperkaliemia, acute kidney injury, fetal toxicity
Candesartan	1–5 y	0.02 (up to 4 mg/d)	0.4 (up to 16 mg/d)	1–2/day	
	≥6 y				
	≥50 kg	4 mg/d	16 mg/d		
	≥50 kg	8 mg/d	32 mg/d		
Irbesartan	6–12 y	75 mg/d	150 mg/d	1/day	
	≥13 y	150 mg/d	300 mg/d		
Losartan	≥6 y	0.7 (up to 50 mg/d)	1.4 (up to 50 mg/d)	1/day	
Olmesartan	≥6 y			1/day	
	≥35 kg	10 mg	20 mg		
	≥35 kg	20 mg	40 mg		
Valsartan	≥6 y	1.3 (up to 40 mg/d)	2.7 (up to 160 mg/d)	1/day	
Thiazide diuretics					**Contraindications:** anuria. **Common ADR:** hypokalemia, dizziness. **Severe ADR:** dysrhythmias, cholestatic jaundice, new-onset DM, pancreatitis.
Chlorthalidone	Child	0.3	2 (up to 50 mg/d)	1/day	
Chlorothiazide	Child	10	20 (up to 375 mg/d)	1–2/day	
Hydrochlorothiazide	Child	1	2 (up to 37.5 mg/d)	1–2/day	
Calcium Channel Blockers					**Contraindications:** hypersensitivity to CCB. **Common ADR:** flushing, peripheral edema, dizziness. **Severe ADR:** angioedema.
Amlodipine	1–5 y	0.1	0.6 (up to 5 mg/d)	1/day	
	≥6 y	2.5 mg	10 mg		
Felodipine	≥6 y	2.5 mg	10 mg	1/day	

Isradipine	Child	0.05–0.1	0.6 (up to 10 mg/d)	Capsule: 2–3/day Extended-release tablet: 1/day	

Abbreviations: ACE—angiotensin-converting enzyme; ARB—AngII receptor blockers; d—dose; ADR—adverse drug reaction; DM—diabetes mellitus; CCB—calcium channel blockers.

Source: Tagi VM, Mainieri F, Chiarelli F. (2022). Hypertension in Patients with Insulin Resistance: Etiopathogenesis and Management in Children. International Journal of Molecular Sciences.; 23(10), 5814. https://doi.org/10.3390/ijms23105814.

8.2.6.1. Lifestyle Modification

One crucial—and frequently disregarded—aspect of treating diabetes and hypertension is changing one's lifestyle. Some lifestyle modifications that seem to be beneficial to health are:

- Reducing salt intake to less than 1.5 g/day
- Increasing consumption of fruits and vegetables (8–10 servings per day)
- Increasing consumption of low- fat dairy products (2–3 servings per day)
- Elevating the intensity of your activity or performing frequent aerobic physical activity (e.g., 30 minutes a day of vigorous walking).
- Losing excess weight
- Limiting alcohol intake to under 2 drinks (30ml of ethanol) for men and 1 drink (15ml of ethanol) for women per day.

Patients with BP <140/90 may benefit solely from lifestyle modification; however, patients with systolic blood pressure (SBP) ≥ 140 and/or diastolic blood pressure (DBP) ≥ 90 mm Hg should ideally receive pharmacotherapy in addition. Most people agree that changing one's lifestyle can effectively lower blood pressure by 5 to 10 mm Hg with only modest antihypertensive effects. However, the added advantages of decreased obesity, increased cardiovascular fitness, and the potential for future medication dosage reductions make these interventions a crucial component of these patients' care.

8.2.6.2. Angiotensin Converting Enzyme Inhibitors

By inhibiting the angiotensin converting enzyme, ACE inhibitors stop angiotensin 1 from becoming angiotensin II. This and other processes result in a reduction in peripheral resistance and blood pressure. By specifically widening the efferent renal arterioles, ACE inhibitors reduce intraglomerular pressure. Patients with diabetic kidney disease benefit from this hemodynamic effect, which is reno-protective. When ACE inhibitor therapy first starts, there may be a sudden increase in serum creatinine. Serum creatinine elevated up to 30% above baseline is normal and does not indicate that therapy should be stopped, but it does highlight the importance of close observation. Since ACE inhibitors have been shown to improve cardiac and renal function, doctors almost always prescribe them as the first line of treatment for patients who have both hypertension and diabetes. It is important to remember that ACE inhibitors' main benefit over other classes of antihypertensive medications is their demonstrated capacity to impede the development of proteinuria.

ACE inhibitors are generally well-tolerated and have a favorable side effect profile. Unlike other antihypertensive medications, the use of these agents is not linked to unfavorable changes in uric acid, glucose, or lipid profiles. As previously mentioned, creatinine elevation is commonly seen and, unless it is severe, should not necessitate stopping therapy. However, another common side effect that can justify stopping treatment is a persistent, dry cough. When taking these medications, patients with hyporeninemic hypoaldosteronism/type 4 renal tubular acidosis, diabetic nephropathy, and long-term diabetes may experience hyperkalemia. ACE inhibitor use is also linked to angioedema, a severe hypersensitivity reaction that is more frequently seen in African American patients. In these patients, the medication should be permanently stopped. Furthermore, because they disrupt the development of the fetal kidney, ACE inhibitors have the potential to be teratogenic, so women who are pregnant or lactating should use caution when taking them.

ACE inhibitors have become the gold standard by which newer classes of antihypertensive drugs are evaluated, particularly in patients with diabetes and diabetic kidney disease, because of their potential advantages and advantageous risk-benefit profile.

8.2.6.3. Angiotensin Receptor Blockers (ARBs)

Angiotensin II is displaced from its receptor by ARBs, which has beneficial effects akin to those of ACE inhibitors. The primary benefit of using ARBs instead of ACE inhibitors is the decreased risk of angioedema and cough. The ARB telmisartan and the ACE inhibitor Ramipril, as well as the combination of these medications, were compared in the ONTARGET trial. This trial demonstrated that telmisartan was generally non-inferior to ramipril in terms of blood pressure control as measured by outcomes like heart failure hospitalization, myocardial infarction, stroke, and cardiovascular deaths. Furthermore, there were significantly fewer cases of cough and angioedema in the telmisartan arm. Additionally, data from the ONTARGET trial demonstrated that while ramipril and telmisartan provided similar renal protection, the combined use of these two medications resulted in worse renal outcomes.

Therefore, it is not advised to use ACE inhibitors and ARBs together at this time. Similar to ACE inhibitors, hyperkalemia is still a possible side effect. Combining these drugs with others that encourage potassium loss through the urine, such as thiazide or loop diuretics, can reduce the risk of hyperkalemia. ARBs used to be significantly more expensive than ACE inhibitors, but this issue has been resolved with the introduction of generic ARBs. These days, ARBs are a common option for treating hypertension, preventing renal problems in diabetic patients, and providing the best care for patients who experience coughing while taking ACE inhibitors.

8.2.6.4. Diuretics

By increasing renal sodium excretion and subsequently decreasing plasma volume, diuretics temporarily lower blood pressure. These modifications in volume status eventually return to normal, but because peripheral vascular resistance is reduced, the antihypertensive effect lasts. Individuals with mild to moderate hypertension and an eGFR greater than 50 can effectively control their blood pressure with hydrochlorothiazide (HCTZ) and related sulfonamide compounds (chlorthalidone). Loop diuretics or a combination of loop diuretics and thiazides is more effective in patients with an eGFR < 30.

Diuretics were found to be just as effective as ACE inhibitors or calcium channel blockers (CCBs) in lowering blood pressure and lowering cardiovascular mortality in patients with diabetes, according to data from the Swedish Trial in Old Patients with Hypertension-2 (STOP Hypertension-2). Hyperglycemia, hyperuricemia, and hypokalemia are examples of metabolic disturbances linked to the use of diuretics. As previously mentioned, taking a diuretic along with an ACE inhibitor, ARB, potassium-sparing diuretic, or aldosterone antagonist can help reduce the risk of hypokalemia that comes with using diuretics. Individuals with type 2 diabetes mellitus who also have concurrent hypertension show worse nighttime blood pressure dipping than those without the disease. For treating hypertension in this patient subgroup, chlorthalidone may be a better option due to its higher potency and longer duration of action.

Calcium Channel Blockers (CCBs)

Dihydropyridines (DHPs) (amlodipine, felodipine, isradipine, nicardipine, nifedipine) and non-DHPs (NDHPs) (verapamil, diltiazem) are the two subclasses of CCBs. Through peripheral vasodilatation, DHPs produce their antihypertensive effect without appreciably altering cardiac conduction or contractility. Although NDHPs also have a slight antihypertensive effect, their main purpose is to treat arrhythmias because they interfere with cardiac automaticity and conduction.

The Avoiding Cardiovascular Events through Combination Therapy in Patients Living with Systolic Hypertension (ACCOMPLISH) trial provides the best support for the use of CCBs over other classes of antihypertensive medications. Benazepril plus hydrochlorothiazide versus benazepril plus amlodipine was the comparison drug in this trial, which was intended for participants with hypertension and a high risk of cardiovascular events. The results showed that the ACE/Diuretic combination arm had more cardiovascular events than the CCB/ACE combination arm. The ALLHAT trial's findings, which showed that thiazide diuretics were not superior to ACE inhibitors, CCBs, or alpha-blockers for blood pressure control or improving cardiovascular or renal outcomes, are not consistent with these findings. In spite of these contradictory findings, the evidence that is currently available places calcium channel blockers in the same category as ACE/ARBs and thiazides when it comes to treating hypertension in individuals who are at high risk of cardiovascular events. The majority of patients tolerate CCBs well. Peripheral edema, flushing, and headache are typical side effects.

8.2.6.5. Adrenergic Receptor Antagonist

Three subclasses of adrenergic receptor antagonists have been identified: alpha-blockers, beta-blockers, and combined alpha- and beta-blockers. When compared to pure beta blockers, alpha-beta blockers such as carvedilol and labetalol result in more significant drops in blood pressure.

Because beta-blockers reduce mortality in patients with heart failure and myocardial infarction, they have become more and more popular. Although there is insufficient evidence, beta-blockers are also commonly used for primary prevention of myocardial infarction. The use of beta-blockers has been linked to glycemic control deterioration, sexual dysfunction, bronchospasm precipitation, and worsening peripheral arterial disease. The reduced perception of hypoglycemia symptoms in diabetic patients is especially concerning.

Additionally, beta-blockers have been shown to affect lipid metabolism and insulin resistance, two aspects that are particularly important for people with diabetes. These side effects, however, differ between medications and are more common with older non-vasodilatory beta-blockers like propranolol, metoprolol, and atenolol. For example, in patients with type 2 diabetes, a randomized control trial comparing metoprolol and carvedilol showed that, at doses titrated to achieve comparable blood pressure control, metoprolol was associated with worsened glycemic control compared to carvedilol. Additionally, the same study showed that carvedilol improved lipid profile by reducing non-HDL cholesterol, triglycerides, and total cholesterol. On the other hand, using metoprolol was linked to a higher requirement for statin-based lipid-lowering therapy. Likewise, it has been demonstrated that the highly selective beta-1-blockers labetalol and nebivolol, which have nitric oxide-dependent vasodilatory qualities, enhance insulin resistance. One possible mechanism is unopposed activation of the alpha-adrenergic system. Additionally, nebivolol improves endothelial function by promoting endothelial cell growth and reducing cellular stiffness.

8.2.6.6. Mineralocorticoid Receptor Antagonists

Steroidal mineralocorticoid receptor antagonists, spironolactone and eplerenone, as well as new non-steroidal antagonist finerenone, have shown great effectiveness in individuals with resistant hypertension, a condition that is more prevalent in those with obesity and diabetes. These medications have also been found to decrease mortality in heart failure patients by counteracting the harmful effects of aldosterone on heart function. When added to patients already receiving ACE inhibitors or ARB, finerenone has been shown to decrease urinary albumin excretion compared to a placebo. The FIDELIO-DKD trial further demonstrated that finerenone not only improves cardiovascular outcomes but also slows the progression of kidney disease.

Since steroidal MR antagonists are frequently combined with ACE inhibitors or ARBs, it is especially important to keep an eye out for the common side effect of hyperkalemia. With the more recent non-steroidal MR antagonists, this is not as much of an issue. Menstrual irregularities and gynecomastia are two more possible side effects of spironolactone. Eplerenone is an aldosterone antagonist that is more selective and infrequently exhibits anti-androgenic properties. Many of these worries should be dispelled by the more recent non-steroidal MR antagonists, which are expected to be used more frequently to treat hypertension in diabetic patients.

8.2.6.7. Direct Renin Inhibitors

The FDA approved Aliskiren, the first-in-class direct renin inhibitor, in 2007. Although it offers end-organ protection and is a potent antihypertensive, its precise role in the hypertension treatment regimen is still unknown. When combined with ARB, aliskiren improves left ventricular hypertrophy and exhibits synergism. Its side effect profile is comparable to that of ARBs, and potassium level monitoring is advised. A randomized control trial called the Aliskiren Trial in Type 2 Diabetes Using Cardiovascular and Renal Disease Endpoints (ALTITUDE) assessed the effectiveness of Aliskiren when combined with either ARBs or ACE inhibitors for patients with T2DM. Safety concerns and an increase in cardiovascular events led to its premature termination. Furthermore, the combination resulted in increased hypotension and hyperkalemia. These side effects might have been caused by the use of combination therapy similar to what was used in the ONTARGET trial. As of right now, patients with type 2 diabetes should not take Aliskiren in addition to ACE inhibitors or ARBs to treat their hypertension. ACE inhibitors and ARBs intolerance can be treated with aliskiren due to its antiproteinuric effect.

8.2.7. Diabetes Medications with Antihypertensive Effects

Some anti-diabetic drugs have mildly antihypertensive effects. These should be remembered, particularly in patients taking antihypertensive medications concurrently. If vigilance is not used, these patients may develop hypotensive symptoms. However, a number of these medications protect the cardiovascular system, probably due in part to their ability to lower blood pressure, which makes them desirable for people with elevated cardiovascular risk. Thiazolidinediones, dipeptidyl diphosphatase (DPP-4) inhibitors, glucagon-like peptide 1 (GLP-1) receptor agonists, and sodium glucose cotransporter 2 (SGLT 2) inhibitors are anti-diabetic drugs that possess these characteristics. GLP-1 receptor agonists seem to have the biggest impact on blood pressure of all of these classes.

Blood pressure was observed to decrease in a meta-analysis of 16 randomized control trials that contrasted the GLP-1 agonists exenatide and liraglutide with placebo and other antihyperglycemic medications. In comparison to a placebo, exenatide reduced systolic blood pressure by about 6 mm Hg. Comparing liraglutide to a placebo, a mean drop in systolic blood pressure of roughly 5 mm Hg was observed. Regardless of baseline readings, a randomized control trial examining the hemodynamic effects of dulaglutide also revealed a decrease in systolic blood pressure. Less than 5 mm Hg of systolic blood pressure reduction has been observed with the other classes of anti-hyperglycemic drugs. The effects of the SGLT2 inhibitors on blood pressure were investigated early on because of their ability to lower volume and sodium levels. Canagliflozin and dapagliflozin demonstrated slight BP reductions in phase 2 and 3 trials, both by less than 4 mm Hg. This result was validated by a recent meta-analysis, which found that all other major SGLT2 inhibitors currently available on the market reduced blood pressure on average by 3.6/1.7 mm Hg when compared to a placebo. This decrease is similar to what is observed when hydrochlorothiazide is taken at a low dose. Although the precise mechanism of BP reduction is not fully understood, weight loss, natriuresis, and osmotic diuresis are thought to be involved. Significantly, it has been demonstrated that these drugs can lower the risk of cardiovascular disease and renal disease in diabetic patients.

8.2.8. Impact of Comorbidities on Choice of Antihypertensive Regimen

A considerable fraction of people with diabetes experience microvascular and macrovascular complications at some point in their lives, despite improvements in diagnosis and treatment. In fact, a lot of patients have advanced problems when they are diagnosed. These comorbidities have potential benefits and drawbacks that should be taken into account when selecting an antihypertensive regimen. Since ACE inhibitors and ARBs are most effective in treating proteinuria and chronic kidney disease, they are typically prescribed to patients with these conditions. Conversely, beta-blockers have not been shown to improve mortality when used in the absence of established coronary artery disease or heart failure with reduced ejection fraction (HFrEF). However, they have been shown to be beneficial in these conditions. As a result, their use ought to be limited to suitable environments. Because they can cause reflex vasoconstriction in patients with peripheral arterial disease, beta-blockers should be avoided in these cases. Because beta-blockers can conceal hypoglycemia symptoms and thereby increase hypoglycemia unawareness, they should also be avoided in patients with a history of brittle diabetes and frequent hypoglycemia. For diabetics with heart failure, mineralocorticoid antagonists should be a part of their antihypertensive regimens because they have demonstrated benefits in HFrEF.

8.2.9. Resistant Hypertension

The term "resistant hypertension" refers to blood pressure that is higher than 140/90 mm Hg even after a treatment plan that includes appropriate lifestyle changes, a diuretic, and two additional antihypertensive medications given at the recommended dosages. It presents an unique therapy dilemma for endocrinologists. Remember that a number of other disorders must be ruled out in order to diagnose resistant hypertension. It is imperative to rule out medication non-adherence and address obstacles like cost and side effects. ABPM can be used to evaluate white coat hypertension, which can be extremely resistant to treatment or, on the other hand, linked to unbearable side effects at home that cause non-adherence to medication. Ultimately, it is important to search for secondary causes of hypertension. Secondary hypertension can be caused by a wide range of conditions, including illicit drug use, hyperaldosteronism, renal artery stenosis, and obstructive sleep apnea. The different endocrine disorders that present with hypertension, such as Cushing's syndrome, pheochromocytomas and paragangliomas, primary hyperaldosteronism, and hypo- and hyperthyroidism, are of particular interest to the consulting endocrinologist. Since many of these conditions have unique clinical presentations, it is not recommended to pursue a thorough and costly evaluation in the absence of encouraging signs and symptoms. Given its strong correlation with obesity and diabetes, obstructive sleep apnea warrants particular attention and should be taken into account whenever a patient has resistant hypertension. Upon diagnosis, specific therapies can often lead to an immediate improvement in blood pressure in secondary hypertension cases.

The most successful course of treatment is usually pharmacological therapy with the addition of mineralocorticoid receptor antagonists after resistant hypertension has been diagnosed and any secondary causes have been ruled out. When these medications are added to patients' current regimens of ACE inhibitors, ARBs, diuretics, and calcium channel blockers, they are beneficial for treating type 2 diabetes. As previously mentioned, mineralocorticoid receptor antagonists also lessen proteinuria and have additional cardiovascular advantages. On the other hand, hyperkalemia is more likely when a mineralocorticoid receptor antagonist is added to a medication regimen that already contains an ACE inhibitor or an ARB. Thus, serum potassium and creatinine levels for these patients need to be checked on a regular basis.

8.2.10. Special Considerations in Type 1 Diabetes

Patients with type 1 diabetes currently comprise between 5% to 8% of all Americans with diabetes (1). Patients with type 1 diabetes, in contrast to those with type 2 diabetes, usually experience renal disease prior to hypertension. Proteinuria usually develops before hypertension does, according to longitudinal studies of type 1 diabetics. But just like in patients with type 2 diabetes, once hypertension sets in, it quickens the progression of both microvascular and macrovascular disease. Sadly, not much information is available about type 1 diabetes. An ACE inhibitor is substantially more effective than blood pressure control alone in preventing the decline of renal function in insulin-dependent diabetic nephropathy, according to a randomized trial. As a result, recommendations for antihypertensive treatment, such as a preference for ACE inhibitor or ARB therapy, are extrapolated from patients with T2DM.

Furthermore, because beta-blockers tend to encourage hypoglycemia and can conceal hypoglycemic symptoms, it is best to avoid them as tight glycemic control with insulin is the cornerstone of care for these patients.

The role that glycemic control plays in preventing hypertension in individuals with type 1 diabetes may be the most unique feature of this condition. Over the course of a 15-year follow-up period, data from the Diabetes Control and Complications Trial (DCCT) and the Epidemiology of Diabetes Intervention and Complications (EDIC) trials demonstrated that intensive therapy reduced incident hypertension by 24%. It is interesting to note that the subjects' incident hypertension decreased years after they began intensive control, indicating that the relationship between hyperglycemia and hypertension is not direct but rather is mediated by long-term complications from diabetes, like diabetic nephropathy.

8.2.11. COVID-19 and Antihypertensive Therapy in Individuals with Diabetes

People with multiple medical comorbidities have been disproportionately affected by the ongoing novel SARS-CoV-2 coronavirus (COVID-19) pandemic. An extensive observational study conducted in China, for example, revealed that patients with severe infections had up to 23.7% hypertension and 16.2% diabetes, compared to only 13.4% and 5.7%, respectively, of patients with non-severe infections. It is now thought that the increased risk of negative outcomes associated with COVID-19 in patients who have diabetes and hypertension is related to both the immunosuppressive effects of these comorbidities directly and to common socioeconomic themes like limited access to wholesome foods and high-quality healthcare. Subsequent investigations into the pathophysiology of COVID-19 infection in this patient subset raised concerns about the involvement of ACE inhibitors and ARBs. The finding that the novel coronavirus attaches itself to human cells through the angiotensin converting enzyme 2 specifically sparked worries that drugs like ACE inhibitors and ARBs that raise this enzyme's levels could hasten the infection process with the novel coronavirus. Nevertheless, no clinical evidence has been found to support this theory as of yet, and policy statements from the American Society of Hypertension, the American College of Cardiology (ACC), the American Heart Association (AHA), and the Heart Failure Society of America (HFSA) have all been released. These organizations strongly advise patients to stick to their regular antihypertensive treatment plan. It is not advised to stop therapy for COVID-19 infection at this time due to the numerous advantages these classes of medications provide for patients with diabetes or hypertension.

8.2.12. Recent Guidelines

A blood pressure reading of more than 130/80 mm Hg is now considered hypertension, and the pre-hypertension category was removed completely from the high blood pressure clinical practice guidelines published by the ACC/AHA Task Force in 2017. Since this new definition lowers the diagnostic threshold, it immediately reclassifies a significant number of diabetics as hypertensive, which increases the incidence and prevalence of hypertension in the diabetic population. According to these guidelines, patients with diabetes who have a blood pressure reading higher than 130/80 mm Hg should start pharmaceutical therapy because it is believed that they are more likely to develop cardiovascular disease. It is advised to compute the 10-year risk of atherosclerotic cardiovascular disease (ASCVD) in the general population. When blood pressure exceeds 130/80 mm Hg, pharmacotherapy should be started in individuals with an ASCVD risk of more than 10%; the remaining patients can be treated with lifestyle changes alone.

The conventional cut off of 140/90 mm Hg for the diagnosis of hypertension in people with diabetes is still in place in the 2021 position statement on cardiovascular risk management in diabetes published by the American Diabetes Association (ADA). The ASCVD risk calculator is included in the ADA guidelines' treatment algorithm, just like it is in the ACC/AHA guidelines. The target blood pressure is established based on the score, which is not the case with the ADA guidelines. Therefore, those with diabetes who score less than 15% should aim for a blood pressure target of less than 140/90 mm Hg, while those who score more than 15% should, if safely achievable, target a blood pressure goal of less than 130/80 mm Hg. This strategy is based on findings from the SPRINT and other trials, which showed a correlation between the absolute baseline cardiovascular risk and the benefit from lowering blood pressure. The significance of individualized treatment targets and taking patient preferences and provider judgment into account when establishing blood pressure goals is also emphasized by these guidelines.

For patients with stage 2 hypertension—defined as a blood pressure reading higher than 160/100 mm Hg—pharmacologic therapy using two medications from different classes is advised by both the ACC/AHA guidelines and the ADA guidelines. This suggestion is supported by data from numerous trials that demonstrate combination therapy is both safer and more effective than monotherapy at controlling blood pressure. In patients with stage 2 hypertension, combination therapy also minimizes target organ damage by accelerating the achievement of target levels and lowering blood pressure more quickly. In order to maximize patient adherence, the ADA guidelines also support the use of single pill fixed dose combinations. It should be highlighted, though, that single pill combinations are frequently challenging to titrate, which can result in an intolerance to the maximal dosage of one component and suboptimal dosing of the other. This is especially important for beta-blockers, ARBs, and ACE inhibitors, which all have benefits that are dose dependent and should always be increased to the highest dose that can be tolerated.

A Closer Look

Insulin

The pancreas, an organ situated behind the stomach, produces the hormone insulin. Insulin is derived from the Latin word insula, which means island, and refers to specific regions found within the pancreas known as the islets of Langerhans. The islets of Langerhans are composed of various hormone-producing cells, the most prevalent of which are beta cells, which generate insulin.

The pancreas then secretes insulin into the bloodstream, where it is subsequently transported to various bodily regions. Insulin regulates the body's utilization of carbohydrates, which are present in specific food types, among its many other functions. The human body breaks down carbohydrates to create glucose, a form of sugar. Cells use glucose as their primary energy source. Insulin facilitates the uptake of glucose by cells in the muscles, liver, and adipose tissue, enabling them to use it as an energy source for proper bodily function. Cells cannot use glucose as fuel without insulin, and they will begin to malfunction. When blood glucose levels are too low, excess glucose that the cells are not able to use will be transformed and stored as fat. Insulin also inhibits the breakdown of fat and protein, among its other metabolic effects.

The two primary functions of insulin are to permit glucose to enter cells for energy production and to keep blood glucose levels within normal ranges. In healthy individuals, the body's need for metabolism and food intake are balanced by tightly controlling the release of insulin. This is a complicated process, and the pancreas and other gut and hormones also play a role in controlling blood sugar. Blood glucose levels rise when we eat because glucose is absorbed into the bloodstream from our gut. The pancreas releases insulin in response to this increase in blood glucose levels, allowing glucose to enter and be utilized by cells. Insulin release decreases and blood glucose levels return to normal as glucose travels through the cells. Insulin release is also triggered by other hormones produced by the gut in response to food and proteins found in food. Adrenaline and other hormones released during acute stress prevent insulin from being released, raising blood glucose levels to help the body deal with the stressful event.

Glucagon, another hormone the pancreas produces, and insulin function together. Glucagon's function is to raise blood sugar levels if they fall too low, while insulin's function is to lower blood sugar levels if necessary. Through the use of this system, the body maintains control over blood glucose levels, allowing for optimal bodily function. Should someone unintentionally inject more insulin than necessary, e.g., cells will take up too much blood glucose because they use more energy or consume less food than they planned. This results in hypoglycemia, or abnormally low blood glucose levels. The body attempts to restore normalcy by releasing stored glucose from the liver in response to hypoglycemia. A person may experience symptoms of low blood glucose.

When hypoglycemia occurs, the sympathetic nervous system, a specialised group of nerves, triggers the body's initial "fight back" reaction. Palpitations, perspiration, hunger, trembling, anxiety, and pale complexion are symptoms of low blood sugar that typically alert the patient so that it can be treated. However, because the brain almost exclusively uses glucose as an energy source to function correctly, it will also be impacted if the initial blood glucose level is too low or if it is not treated right away and keeps falling. Severe cases may result in coma, disorientation, fits, and dizziness.

Some drugs used for people with type 2 diabetes, including sulphonylureas (e.g., gliclazide) and meglitinides (e.g., repaglinide), can also stimulate insulin production within the body and can also cause hypoglycaemia. The body reacts as it would if an injection of excess insulin had been administered. In addition, there is a rare tumor known as an insulinoma that affects 1-4 people per million. It is a tumor of the pancreatic beta cells. Hypoglycemia symptoms are present in patients with this kind of tumor.

Individuals who have diabetes may experience issues with insulin synthesis, insulin function, or both. Although there are other, less common forms of diabetes, type 1 and type 2 diabetes are the most common types.

Individuals with type 1 diabetes have limited or no production of insulin due to the destruction of beta cells by antibodies. Without enough insulin, the body is unable to transport glucose from the blood into cells, resulting in high blood sugar levels. Excess glucose may spill into urine, leading to increased urination and thirst. Dehydration may occur, potentially causing confusion. Without sufficient glucose for energy, the body relies on alternative sources such as fat and muscle, leading to fatigue and weight loss. Patients risk getting seriously sick if this keeps up. This is a result of the body producing acids as waste products in an attempt to repurpose fat for energy. If medical assistance is not obtained, this may ultimately result in a coma and death. To stay alive, people with type 1 diabetes must inject insulin.

Type 2 diabetes may result from insulin's improper interaction with its receptor. There are two primary causes of type 2 diabetes, and the severity of the condition varies with the severity of the underlying issues. First off, the patient may not be producing enough insulin to meet the body's needs because their beta cells may be having issues producing the hormone. Unlike the "absolute insulin deficiency" associated with type 1 diabetes, this is "relative insulin deficiency." Second, the insensitivity and lack of response to the insulin in the bloodstream occurs in the insulin receptors, which are the parts of the cell where insulin acts. This results in an improper functioning of the available insulin. Insulin resistance is the term for this, and it is highly prevalent in type 2 diabetes and obesity. Overweight individuals appear to have more malfunctioning of these receptors. Some type 2 diabetics may show very little symptoms at first, with the elevated blood glucose only being noticed when a routine blood test is scheduled for another reason; other people may show symptoms akin to those of type 1 diabetics, including thirst, frequent urination, dehydration, hunger, fatigue, and weight loss. Certain patients with type 2 diabetes can manage their symptoms by losing weight and/or making dietary changes; others will require medication, and still others will require insulin injections to lower their blood glucose levels.

Summary

- Diabetes mellitus, often known simply as diabetes, is a group of common endocrine diseases characterized by sustained high blood sugar levels. Diabetes is due to either the pancreas not producing enough insulin, or the cells of the body becoming unresponsive to the hormone's effects.
- The classic symptoms of untreated diabetes are polyuria, thirst, and weight loss. Several other non-specific signs and symptoms may also occur, including fatigue, blurred vision, and genital itchiness due to *Candida* infection.
- Diabetes is classified by the World Health Organization into six categories: type 1 diabetes, type 2 diabetes, hybrid forms of diabetes (including slowly evolving, immune-mediated diabetes of adults and ketosis-prone type 2 diabetes), hyperglycemia first detected during pregnancy, "other specific types," and "unclassified diabetes." Diabetes is a more variable disease than once thought, and individuals may have a combination of forms.
- Insulin is the principal hormone that regulates the uptake of glucose from the blood into most cells of the body, especially liver, adipose tissue and muscle, except smooth muscle, in which insulin acts via the IGF-1. Therefore, deficiency of insulin or the insensitivity of its receptors play a central role in all forms of diabetes mellitus.
- The coexistence of diabetes and hypertension is known to have a multiplicative effect on adverse clinical outcomes with respect to both microvascular and macrovascular disease. Effective management of diabetes should therefore include a multifaceted approach combining optimal control of blood pressure and lipids with appropriate glycemic control.
- Hypertension is rarely accompanied by symptoms, and its identification is usually through health screening, or when seeking healthcare for an unrelated problem. Some people with high blood pressure report headaches (particularly at the back of the head and in the morning), as well as lightheadedness, vertigo, tinnitus (buzzing or hissing in the ears), altered vision or fainting episodes. These symptoms, however, might be related to associated anxiety rather than the high blood pressure itself.
- The pathophysiology of hypertension in diabetes can be traced to maladaptive changes and complex interactions between the autonomic nervous system, a maladaptive immune system, enhanced activation of the renin-angiotensin-aldosterone system (RAAS) as well as adverse environmental factors.
- Accurate measurement of BP is key for both diagnosis and effective management of hypertension. BP measurement is most often conducted in the medical office, where it can be performed either through the auscultatory technique of listening to Korotkoff sounds or the oscillometric technique employed in automated devices.
- Several anti-diabetic medications possess modest antihypertensive properties. These should be kept in mind especially in patients concurrently receiving antihypertensive drugs who may experience hypotensive symptoms if caution is not exercised.

References

1. Atkinson, M. A., McGill, D. E., Dassau, E., & Laffel, L. (2020). Type 1 diabetes mellitus. In *Williams Textbook of Endocrinology* (pp. 1403–1437). Elsevier.
2. Boughton, C. K., & Hovorka, R. (2020). The artificial pancreas. *Current Opinion in Organ Transplantation, 25*(4), 336–342. https://doi.org/10.1097/MOT.0000000000000786.
3. Brownlee, M., Aiello, L. P., Sun, J. K., Cooper, M. E., Feldman, E. L., Plutzky, J., et al. (2020). Complications of diabetes mellitus. In *Williams Textbook of Endocrinology* (pp. 1438–1524). Elsevier. ISBN 978-0-323-55596-8.
4. Butler, A. E., & Misselbrook, D. (2020). Distinguishing between type 1 and type 2 diabetes. *The BMJ, 370*, m2998. https://doi.org/10.1136/bmj.m2998.
5. Cashen, K., & Petersen, T. (2019). Diabetic ketoacidosis. *Pediatrics in Review, 40*(8), 412–420. https://doi.org/10.1542/pir.2018-0231.
6. Dayan, C. M., Korah, M., Tatovic, D., Bundy, B. N., & Herold, K. C. (2019). Changing the landscape for type 1 diabetes: The first step to prevention. *The Lancet, 394*(10205), 1286–1296. https://doi.org/10.1016/S0140-6736(19)32127-0.
7. Dean, P. G., Kukla, A., Stegall, M. D., & Kudva, Y. C. (2017). Pancreas transplantation. *The BMJ, 357*, j1321. https://doi.org/10.1136/bmj.j1321.
8. Delli, A. J., & Lernmark, A. (2016). Type 1 (insulin-dependent) diabetes mellitus: Etiology, pathogenesis, prediction, and prevention. In J. L. Jameson (Ed.), *Endocrinology: Adult and Pediatric* (7th ed., pp. 672–690). Saunders. ISBN 978-0-323-18907-1.
9. DiMeglio, L. A., Evans-Molina, C., & Oram, R. A. (2018). Type 1 diabetes. *The Lancet, 391*(10138), 2449–2462. https://doi.org/10.1016/S0140-6736(18)31320-5.
10. Domenech, M., & Coca, A. (2016). The role of diet in the prevention of cardiovascular disease. In *Hypertension and Cardiovascular Disease* (pp. 171–180). Springer International Publishing. https://doi.org/10.1007/978-3-319-39599-9_12.
11. Forbes, J. M., & Cooper, M. E. (2013). Mechanisms of diabetic complications. *Physiological Reviews, 93*(1), 137–188. https://doi.org/10.1152/physrev.00045.2011.
12. Kahn, C. R., Ferris, H. A., & O'Neill, B. T. (2020). Pathophysiology of type 1 diabetes mellitus. In *Williams Textbook of Endocrinology* (14th ed., pp. 1349–1370). Elsevier.
13. Karslioglu French, E., Donihi, A. C., & Korytkowski, M. T. (2019). Diabetic ketoacidosis and hyperosmolar hyperglycemic syndrome: Review of acute decompensated diabetes in adult patients. *The BMJ, 365*, l1114. https://doi.org/10.1136/bmj.l1114.
14. Katsarou, A., Gudbjörnsdottir, S., Rawshani, A., Dabelea, D., Bonifacio, E., Anderson, B. J., et al. (2017). Type 1 diabetes mellitus. *Nature Reviews Disease Primers, 3*, 17016. https://doi.org/10.1038/nrdp.2017.16.
15. Lent-Schochet, D., Silva, R., McLaughlin, M., Huet, B., & Jialal, I. (2018). Changes to trimethylamine-N-oxide and its precursors in nascent metabolic syndrome. *Hormone Molecular Biology and Clinical Investigation, 35*(2). https://doi.org/10.1515/hmbci-2018-0021.
16. Martínez, E., Portillo, N., Lizarralde, E., Grau, G., Vela, A., Rodríguez, A., & Rica, I. (2018). For debate: Paediatric T1DM: DKA is still a problem. *Pediatric Endocrinology Reviews, 16*(2), 233–239. https://doi.org/10.17458/per.vol16.2018.mk.

17. Moore, T. J. (2003). *The DASH Diet for Hypertension: Lower Your Blood Pressure in 14 Days–Without Drugs*. Pocket Books.

18. Murphy, H. R., Steel, S. A., Roland, J. M., Morris, D., Ball, V., Campbell, P. J., & Temple, R. C., East Anglia Study Group for Improving Pregnancy Outcomes in Women with Diabetes (EASIPOD). (2011). Obstetric and perinatal outcomes in pregnancies complicated by type 1 and type 2 diabetes: Influences of glycemic control, obesity and social disadvantage. *Diabetic Medicine, 28*(9), 1060–1067. https://doi.org/10.1111/j.1464-5491.2011.03284.x.

19. Norris, J. M., Johnson, R. K., & Stene, L. C. (2020). Type 1 diabetes-early life origins and changing epidemiology. *The Lancet Diabetes & Endocrinology, 8*(3), 226–238. https://doi.org/10.1016/S2213-8587(19)30412-7.

20. Ramakrishnan, N., Denna, T., Devaraj, S., Adams-Huet, B., & Jialal, I. (2018). Exploratory lipidomics in patients with nascent metabolic syndrome. *Journal of Diabetes and its Complications, 32*(8), 791–794. https://doi.org/10.1016/j.jdiacomp.2018.03.008.

21. Reddy, P., Leong, J., & Jialal, I. (2018). Amino acid levels in nascent metabolic syndrome: A contributor to the pro-inflammatory burden. *Journal of Diabetes and its Complications, 32*(5), 465–469. https://doi.org/10.1016/j.jdiacomp.2018.01.010.

22. Redondo, M. J., Steck, A. K., & Pugliese, A. (2018). Genetics of type 1 diabetes. *Pediatric Diabetes, 19*(3), 346–353. https://doi.org/10.1111/pedi.12597.

23. Repaske, D. R. (2016). Medication-induced diabetes mellitus. *Pediatric Diabetes, 17*(6), 392–397. https://doi.org/10.1111/pedi.12406.

24. Rickels, M. R., & Robertson, R. P. (2019). Pancreatic islet transplantation in humans: Recent progress and future directions. *Endocrine Reviews, 40*(2), 631–668. https://doi.org/10.1210/er.2018-00154.

25. Rock, C. L. (2004). Diet modifications to control hypertension: The multifactorial approach. In *Metabolic Issues of Clinical Nutrition* (pp. 155–167). KARGER. https://doi.org/10.1159/000080661.

26. Shapiro, A. M., Pokrywczynska, M., & Ricordi, C. (2017). Clinical pancreatic islet transplantation. *Nature Reviews Endocrinology, 13*(5), 268–277. https://doi.org/10.1038/nrendo.2016.178.

27. Shim, K., Gulhar, R., & Jialal, I. (2019). Exploratory metabolomics of nascent metabolic syndrome. *Journal of Diabetes and its Complications, 33*(3), 212–216. https://doi.org/10.1016/j.jdiacomp.2018.12.006.

28. Smith, A., & Harris, C. (2018). Type 1 diabetes: Management strategies. *American Family Physician, 98*(3), 154–156. PMID 30215903. Retrieved from: https://www.aafp.org/afp/2018/0801/p154.html (accessed on 16 July 2024).

29. Sperl-Hillen, J., Beaton, S., Fernandes, O., Von Worley, A., Vazquez-Benitez, G., Parker, E., & Spain, C. V. (2011). Comparative effectiveness of patient education methods for type 2 diabetes: A randomized controlled trial. *Archives of Internal Medicine, 171*(22), 2001–2010. https://doi.org/10.1001/archinternmed.2011.561.

30. Tseng, C. H. (2011). Diabetes and risk of bladder cancer: A study using the national health insurance database in Taiwan. *Diabetology, 54*(8), 2009–2015. https://doi.org/10.1007/s00125-011-2116-5.

31. von Scholten, B. J., Kreiner, F. F., Gough, S. C., & von Herrath, M. (2021). Current and future therapies for type 1 diabetes. *Diabetology, 64*(5), 1037–1048. https://doi.org/10.1007/s00125-021-05398-3.

32. Wang, T. J., Larson, M. G., Vasan, R. S., Cheng, S., Rhee, E. P., McCabe, E., & Gerszten, R. E. (2011). Metabolite profiles and the risk of developing diabetes. *Nature Medicine, 17*(4), 448–453. https://doi.org/10.1038/nm.2307.

33. Wolsdorf, J. I., & Garvey, K. C. (2016). Management of diabetes in children. In *Endocrinology: Adult and Pediatric* (pp. 854–882.e6). Elsevier. https://doi.org/10.1016/B978-0-323-18907-1.00049-4.

34. Yin, M., Zhou, J., Gorak, E. J., & Quddus, F. (2013). Metformin is associated with survival benefit in cancer patients with concurrent type 2 diabetes: A systematic review and meta-analysis. *The Oncologist, 18*(12), 1248–1255. https://doi.org/10.1634/theoncologist.2013-0101.

Chapter 9

SYMPTOMS OF JOINT DISEASE

Contents

Introduction

A broad range of illnesses marked by pain, inflammation, and decreased ability to move one or more body joints. Millions of people worldwide suffer from this illness, which severely reduces their mobility and quality of life. The three most prevalent forms of joint disease are gout, rheumatoid arthritis, and osteoarthritis; each has its own causes, signs, and therapies. The most common type of joint disease, osteoarthritis, usually develops with age or as a result of trauma to the joint or overuse. The tissue that cushions the ends of the bones in a joint, cartilage, gradually breaks down as a result of it, causing pain, stiffness, and a reduction in range of motion. Osteoarthritis can affect the hands and fingers in addition to weight-bearing joints like the spine, hips, and knees.

In contrast, rheumatoid arthritis is an autoimmune disease in which the synovium—the lining of the membranes surrounding the joints—is mistakenly attacked by the body's immune system. If treatment for this persistent inflammation is not received, it frequently results in deformities and disability by causing swelling, pain, and eventually erosion of the joint tissues. Rheumatoid arthritis, in contrast to osteoarthritis, can impact several joints at once and cause systemic symptoms like fever, fatigue, and weight loss. Another type of joint disease called gout is caused by an accumulation of uric acid crystals in the joints, which can cause sudden, intense episodes of pain, swelling, and redness. The big toe is typically affected by gout. Genetics, a diet high in purines (found in foods like red meat and seafood), obesity, and specific medical conditions or medications are some of the factors that can cause gout.

Whatever the exact kind, joint disease can have a major impact on day-to-day functioning by producing pain, stiffness, and difficulty with everyday tasks. Moreover, long-term joint inflammation can cause deformity and damage to the joints, limiting mobility and lowering overall quality of life. In order to determine the degree of inflammation and rule out other potential causes, the diagnosis usually consists of a combination of the patient's medical history, physical examination, imaging studies (such as MRIs or X-rays), and laboratory testing. The goals of joint disease treatment are to enhance joint function, reduce disease progression, and relieve symptoms. A multidisciplinary approach is frequently used to treat this, including medication (such as corticosteroids, disease-modifying antirheumatic drugs, or nonsteroidal anti-inflammatory drugs), physical therapy, dietary and lifestyle changes (like exercising and losing weight), assistive devices (like braces or splints), and occasionally, surgery (like joint replacement or arthroscopic surgery) (Klippel et al., 2013; Firestein et al., 2021).

COrientation and Directional Terms

Term	Definition	Illustration
Rheumatism	Rheumatism or rheumatic disorders are conditions causing chronic, often intermittent pain affecting the joints or connective tissue.	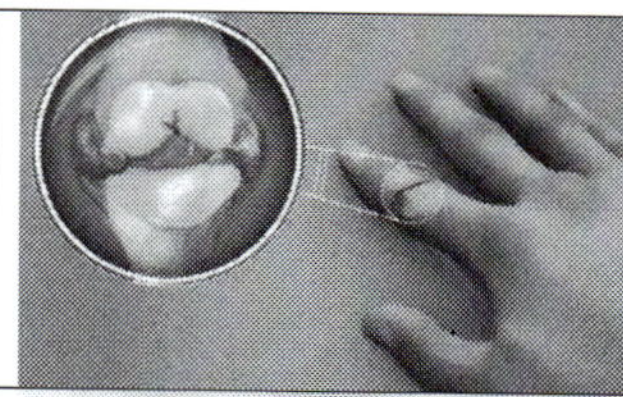
Brucellosis	Brucellosis is an infectious disease caused by bacteria. People can get the disease when they are in contact with infected animals or animal products contaminated with the bacteria.	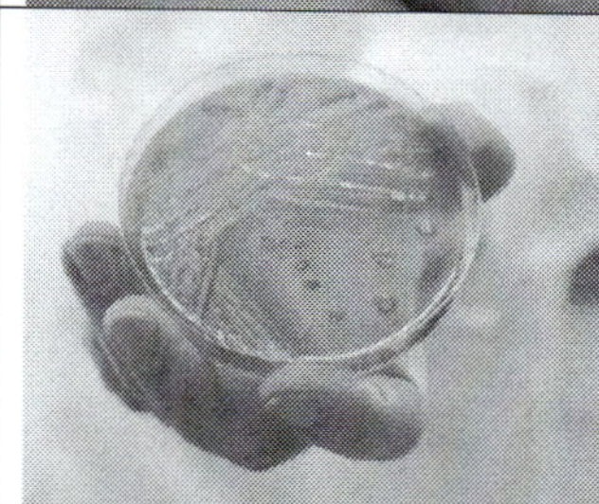
Microorganisms	An organism of microscopic size, which may exist in its single-celled form or as a colony of cells.	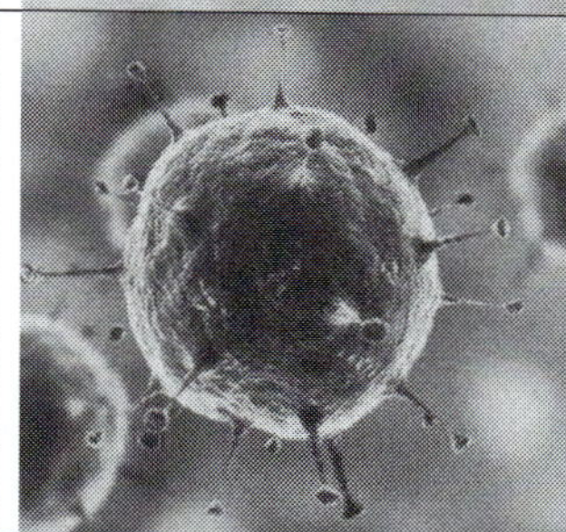
Osteomyelitis	A serious infection of the bone that can be either acute or chronic. It is an inflammatory process involving the bone and its structures caused by pyogenic organisms that spread through the bloodstream, fractures, or surgery.	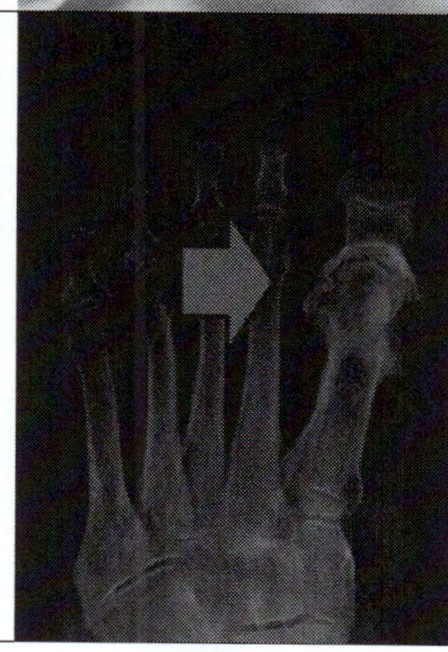
Staphylococci	A genus of Gram-positive bacteria in the family Staphylococcaceae from the order Bacillales. Under the microscope, they appear spherical, and form in grape-like clusters. Staphylococcus species are facultative anaerobic organisms.	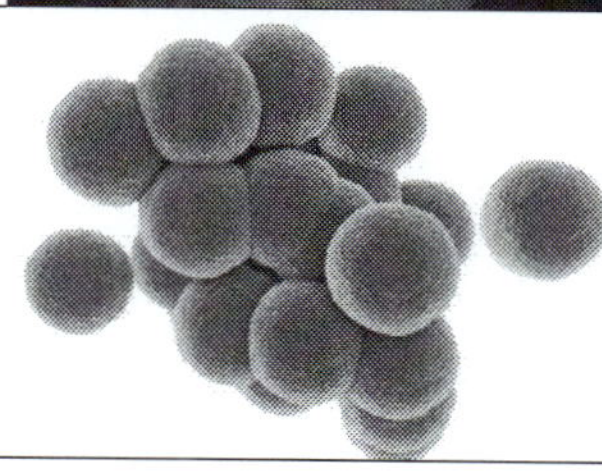

9.1. Understanding the Joint Diseases

Any illness or injury that affects a person's joints is considered a joint disease. The most well-known joint disease is undoubtedly arthritis, but there are numerous others as well. Joint diseases can range widely in duration from extremely brief to extremely long, excruciatingly painful to just bothersome; they can affect a single joint or multiple joints throughout the skeleton. For the purposes of this article, two main categories are distinguished: noninflammatory joint diseases, in which inflammation may be present to some extent (such as following an injury) but is not a primary feature, and inflammatory joint diseases, in which inflammation is the primary set of signs or symptoms.

9.1.1. Inflammatory Joint Diseases: Types of Arthritis

The general word for inflammatory joint disease is arthritis. Whatever the reason, joint inflammation can result in pain, stiffness, swelling, and sometimes even redness around the joint. It is typical for fluid to diffuse into the joint cavity, and analyzing this fluid can be a useful step in identifying the type of disease. It is possible for the inflammation to be so severe and of such a kind that it destroys the underlying bone and joint cartilage, resulting in deformities that cannot be repaired. In these situations, adhesions between the articulating members are common; the fusion that results in loss of motion is known as ankylosis. Synovitis is the term used to describe inflammation that is limited to the synovial membrane, which lines a joint. Simply put, arthritis refers to joint pain; the term itself, as it is commonly used, suggests that there are no other symptoms associated with arthritis. Rheumatism, which is not the same as these, refers to any type of discomfort experienced by the articular apparatus, which includes the joints as well as bursas, ligaments, tendons, and tendon sheaths. It does not always indicate an inflammatory state. Spondylitis is the term for joint and spinal inflammation.

9.1.1.1. Bursitis

Bursitis, also known as bursal synovitis, is the inflammation of a synovial bursa, the lubricating sac that lies over a joint or between tendons and muscles or bones. In cases of gout and rheumatoid arthritis, bursas can occasionally be impacted in addition to joints and tendon sheaths. It is rare but possible for infectious agents carried by the bloodstream or introduced through punctured wounds to cause bursitis. When brucellosis (undulant fever) strikes, the prepatellar bursa, which is situated on the underside of the kneecap, is particularly vulnerable to involvement. Local mechanical irritation appears to be the cause of bursitis in most cases. The irritation, which typically affects the shoulder, knee, or hip region, is caused by one's job. Calcium salts may or may not be deposited as a result of the inflammatory response. In many cases, it is difficult to distinguish bursitis from other painful rheumatic conditions of the soft tissues.

The subdeltoid bursa, which is located above the shoulder joint, is impacted by the most prevalent type of bursitis. In this case, the main abnormality is not bursitis; rather, it is the result of calcification and degeneration of the adjacent rotator tendon. Calcium deposits and inflammation in the tendon are not usually the result of direct injury; in fact, people who work heavy labor are less likely to be affected than those who work less demanding jobs. Only when tendon debris extends into the bursa proper is it affected; this intrusion is the main source of excruciating shoulder pain. The condition is rare in young children and most common in middle age. The condition affects women twice as often as it does men. It could start suddenly and without warning. Raising the arm is difficult and there is a lot of pain and tenderness. Analgesics and resting the arm can help reduce pain; corticosteroids can help reduce inflammation; and carefully progressed exercises can help reduce the chance of chronic shoulder stiffness. Several months might elapse before full recovery occurs. Trochanteric bursitis, a chronic inflammation of the bursa at the side of the hip joint, progresses in a similar way (Figure 9.1).

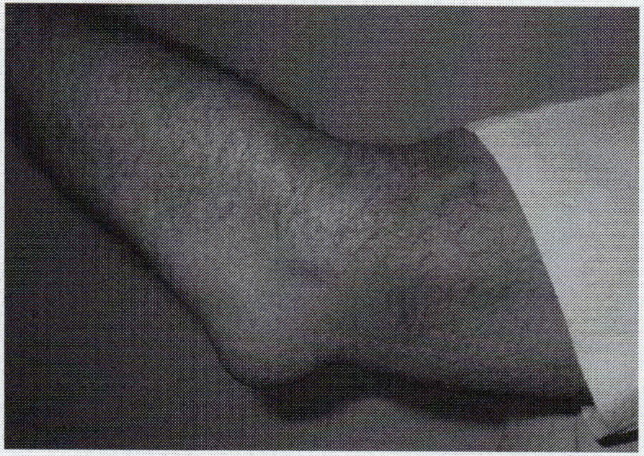

Figure 9.1. *Bursitis of the elbow.*

Source: *By en:User:NJC123 – en:Image:Bursitis_Elbow_WC.JPG, Public Domain, https://commons.wikimedia.org/w/index.php?curid=2814450.*

A classic example of the more obviously traumatizing types of bursitis is "beat knee," a bursitis that appears below the kneecap as a result of intense or protracted pressure on the knee. Bloody fluid causes the bursa to swell and, if left behind, could permanently thicken the bursa walls. Treatment for subdeltoid bursitis is essentially the same and entails preventing further irritation to the extent that it is feasible. An injury to the skin above causes a good percentage of these lesions to become infected.

9.1.1.2. Infectious Arthritis

Numerous microorganisms, including fungi, viruses, and bacteria, as well as occasionally animal parasites, can cause infections in joints. Three pathways exist for infection: direct contact, bloodstream penetration, and spread from nearby bone infections (osteomyelitis). Although it can also happen during joint surgery, puncturing wounds are typically the source of direct contamination. Synovial blood vessels are a potential entry point for blood-borne infections into the joints. However, osteomyelitis foci typically appear first in the long bones close to the joint or near the end of the shaft. The infection then spreads to the joint through pathological or natural fractures in the cortex, or outer layer, of the bone. Characteristically, hematogenous (blood-borne) infectious arthritis usually affects large joints (hip and knee) rather than small ones, affecting one joint (monarthritis) or a small number of joints (oligoarthritis) as opposed to many joints (polyarthritis). Similar to infections elsewhere in the body, joint infections frequently result in fever and other systemic signs of inflammation.

The rapid formation of pus in infections caused by bacteria like pneumococci, hemolytic streptococci, and staphylococci can cause damage to joint cartilage. Joint tuberculosis can lead to open channels to the skin and significant bone loss in the surrounding area. Pott disease, another name for tuberculous spondylitis, is the most prevalent type of this infection. It mostly affects young children. Antibiotics like streptomycin and anti-tuberculous drugs like rifampin and isoniazid are used in treatment. An organism native to the arid regions of the United States southwest, *Coccidioides immitis*, is the cause of a common fungal infection in the country. Similar to tuberculosis, joint involvement typically occurs after lung to bone seeding. Similar to tuberculosis, brucellosis has a special affinity for the spine. The most likely brucellar organism to cause disease of the skeleton is Brucella suis. In leprosy (Hansen disease), deformities and harmful alterations in the joints result from either leprosy bacillus infection of the nerves or infection by other bacteria. Rubella, also known as German measles, and serum hepatitis are two of the more common viral infections that can cause discomfort in the joints. Typically, these infections are transient and do not result in permanent damage. Additionally, several tropical types of synovitis are viral. Guinea worms are parasitic nematodes that infect humans in tropical regions. The infection known as draunculiasis, or "Guinea worm disease," can affect the joints.

Gonorrhea is one of the sexually transmitted illnesses that is made more difficult by infectious arthritis. Early penicillin therapy may offer a speedy recovery and shield the joint from the severe damage that might otherwise occur. Reactive arthritis, also known as Reiter disease, typically goes better on its own over a few months and can be brought on by food poisoning or infections with certain STDs. Reactive arthritis is characterized by inflammation of the urethra, the eyes' conjunctiva, and the joints. With the exception of congenital syphilis and the disease's most advanced stages, syphilis does not seem to directly infect the joints. In newborn infants, the latter often results in damaging inflammation of the growing cartilaginous ends of the bones. If left untreated, it causes deformity and growth restriction in the affected area; however, if penicillin is administered early on, recovery may be total. Another kind of congenital syphilitic lesion is the button joint. Although it causes knee swelling, it is a relatively benign condition that affects children between the ages of 6 and 16 and is actually an inflammation of the synovial membrane. Children with congenital syphilis may occasionally develop lesions in their joints that are indicative of tertiary syphilis. Similar skeletal lesions are seen in yaws, a nonvenereal infection caused by an organism closely related to that which causes syphilis. Although almost completely eradicated, the condition still affects people living in tropical regions.

9.1.1.3. Rheumatoid Arthritis and Allied Disorders

There is no known cause for any of the several forms of arthritis that mimic infectious joint disease. The most common of these is rheumatoid arthritis. While this disorder can manifest at any age, the fourth and fifth decades are the most common times for it to do so. Juvenile rheumatoid arthritis is the name given to a type that affects children. The same joints on both sides of the body are usually affected by rheumatoid arthritis. Though the fingers, wrists, and knees are especially vulnerable, almost any movable joint may be affected. When the afflicted individual wakes up, the joints are extremely stiff. Fatigue and anemia suggest that rheumatoid arthritis affects more than just the joints; a more widespread systemic involvement is present. There may occasionally be a slight fever. In places other than the joints, lesions can also occur. The disease is largely responsible for the involvement of bursas, tendons, and tendon sheaths. Nodules in the subcutaneous tissue at the elbow's point or elsewhere affect about one in five affected individuals. Additionally, pericardium—the membrane that surrounds the heart—and small arteries can occasionally exhibit inflammatory alterations.

The illness progresses very differently in each individual and is distinguished by a startling propensity for exacerbation and spontaneous remission. Joint cartilage is destroyed as a result of ongoing joint inflammation. The degree of cartilage damage associated with rheumatoid arthritis greatly influences the degree of articular (joint) disability. Adhesions may form between the articular surfaces if the injury is severe enough to cause large areas of bone to lose their cartilage. These adhesions eventually mature into mature fibrous or bony connective tissue, a condition known as ankylosis that causes a firm union between the bony surfaces, impairs joint motion and may cause complete immobility. In other cases, the joint becomes unstable and partially dislocates due to the loss of bone and cartilage as well as the weakening of tendons, ligaments, and other supporting structures. In a tiny percentage of cases, the illness progresses quickly and is characterized by unrelenting joint degeneration and signs of diffuse vasculitis, or blood vessel inflammation. Over several months, therapeutic exercises, analgesic medications, and rest are beneficial for many affected individuals. Roughly one-third of cases of the illness worsen and result in significant disability. If appropriate physical therapy is not received, the joints may suffer significant deformity and ankyloses.

Immunologic responses are now strongly suggested to be a major contributing factor in the development of rheumatoid arthritis. Rheumatoid factor, an immunoglobulin that functions as an antibody and reacts with another class of immunoglobulin, is present in the blood of about 80–90% of people with rheumatoid arthritis. The plasma cells found in tissue injury sites produce this immunoglobulin. Evidence exists to support the theory that this agent is one or more viruses or viral antigens that have persisted in the tissues of the joints. Nonsteroidal anti-inflammatory drugs (NSAIDs) and corticosteroid medications may help reduce pain and inflammation even though there is no known cure. Corticosteroids have certain drawbacks, including increased vulnerability to infection and peptic ulcers, and their efficacy typically wanes with time. Direct injection of corticosteroids into joint tissues may even exacerbate joint damage in certain individuals. Disease-modifying antirheumatic medications (DMARDs) prevent additional joint damage, which may slow the disease's progression. In order to correct established deformities, surgery is frequently beneficial. Sometimes a moderately dry climate seems to be advantageous, but usually not enough to make a move that would cause significant disruption to the affected person's life worthwhile. Rheumatoid arthritis can occasionally be closely associated with conditions that don't seem to be related. Rheumatoid arthritis coexists with Sjögren syndrome in approximately one-third of cases, and elevated levels of rheumatoid factors are typically found in the blood. Felty syndrome is characterized by rheumatoid arthritis, splenic enlargement, and decreased blood cell counts, especially white blood cells. While the quantity of blood cells returns to normal after the spleen is removed, the arthritis is unaffected.

While they share similarities with rheumatoid arthritis, a number of other forms of polyarthritis are distinguished by the absence of rheumatoid factors in the blood. Psoriatic arthritis, which is linked to the skin condition psoriasis, is distinct from rheumatoid arthritis in that it primarily affects the outer joints of the fingers and toes instead of the inner ones, and it also causes more bone loss. Chronic intestinal conditions such as cirrhosis, Whipple disease, inflammatory bowel disease, ulcerative colitis, and regional enteritis are linked to other kinds of arthritis. Although it primarily affects the spine and sacroiliac joints, ankylosing spondylitis, also known as Marie-Strümpell disease or Bechterew disease, can also affect some peripheral joints, including the hip. Both the edges of the intervertebral disks and the tiny synovial joints in the spine are affected. The spine stiffens as bone fills in the gaps between these structures. Men are affected by ankylosing spondylitis about eight times more frequently than women. Compared to rheumatoid arthritis, the age of onset is lower. The two conditions are largely treated in the same way overall, however phenylbutazone works better for ankylosing spondylitis than for rheumatoid arthritis (Klippel et al., 2013; Firestein et al., 2021).

9.1.1.4. Collagen Diseases

The reason the diseases involving collagen are named so is that anomalies arise in the connective tissue that contains collagen in each case. Joint issues are often associated with these mainly systemic diseases. Systemic lupus erythematosus (SLE) is one of these illnesses that can impact any bodily organ or structure. The fact that 25% of people with SLE have positive rheumatoid factor serological tests, and possibly the same number of patients with rheumatoid arthritis have positive lupus erythematosus tests, suggests a connection with rheumatoid arthritis. Skin tightness and thickening are symptoms of generalized scleroderma, another collagen disease. Other organs, especially the gastrointestinal tract, experience similar alterations. Rheumatoid fever is frequently included in the category of collagen illnesses. As the name implies, there are some similarities to rheumatoid arthritis, but the distinctions are more pronounced. Subcutaneous nodules and arthritis are common in both conditions, and pericardial inflammation is often present. However, rheumatic fever's joint symptoms usually subside quickly, whereas rheumatoid arthritis's are more severe. Regarding cardiac involvement in the two disorders, the opposite is true. Streptococcal infection does not seem to be a significant cause of rheumatoid arthritis, but it does seem to be a well-established cause of rheumatic fever. About 25% of children with low blood levels of gamma globulins experience arthritis that closely resembles rheumatoid arthritis. The body's processes for producing antibodies are impaired in this situation.

9.1.1.5. Miscellaneous Arthritides

It seems that a hypersensitivity reaction is connected to several forms of arthritis. Reddish nodules that form on the front of the legs are the typical sign of the skin condition erythema nodosum. Most of the time, different joints may experience pain, and occasionally swelling may also manifest. The lung's hilus, where the bronchus, blood vessels, and nerves enter the body, has enlarged lymph nodes. Over the course of several weeks or months, the synovitis goes away. Drug hypersensitivity, infections like tuberculosis, coccidioidomycosis, and leprosy, and sarcoidosis—a systemic disease in which nodules form in the lymph nodes and other organs and structures of the body—are linked to numerous cases of erythema nodosum. This type of synovitis affects 10 to 15% of sarcoidosis patients. Unknown in origin, palindromic rheumatism is typified by one- or two-day attacks that have no lasting consequences. However, palindromic rheumatism rarely goes away entirely, and rheumatoid arthritis develops in about one-third of cases. A fairly common condition that affects older adults, polymyalgia rheumatica is characterized by pain and stiffness in the muscles surrounding the hips and shoulders, but there does not appear to be any involvement of the actual joints. There does appear to be some connection to giant cell arteritis, a form of inflammatory arterial disease. Under corticosteroid or nonsteroidal anti-inflammatory drug therapy, polymyalgia rheumatica is typically not associated with significant systemic abnormalities (Klippel et al., 2013; Firestein et al., 2021).

9.1.2. Noninflammatory Joint Diseases: Injury and Degenerative Disorders

9.1.2.1. Traumatic Joint Diseases

Joint blunt trauma can range in severity from minor sprains to obvious fractures and dislocations. A sprain is defined as an injury to a ligament, tendon, or muscle that results from an abrupt twist and brief partial dislocation (subluxation) of a joint. These tissues have some minor hemorrhage and healing usually occurs over a few days. More severe strains have the potential to tear tendons and ligaments. The ligaments and tendons are often torn from their bony attachments instead of being ripped into segments because of their strength. As long as the edges of the tears are not completely severed from one another, fibrous union can repair ligamentous, tendinous, and capsular tears. The most common cause of internal knee deformities is tearing of the semilunar cartilages (menisci). The medial meniscus is typically the one that is injured. These tears, which occur most frequently in athletes, occur when the knee twists while the foot stays planted on the ground. One common symptom is locking of the knee. The semilunar cartilages are not very repairable, so they need to be surgically removed. Other possible outcomes of injuries include hemarthrosis, or bleeding into the joint. To allow the capsular and other tears to heal, the majority of traumatic dislocations are treated with extended immobilization. Surgical repairs are necessary in certain cases. Bone fractures that occur near joints may or may not extend into the joint space. Whether they do or not, arthritic complications are likely to arise unless the normal contour of the joint is restored.

9.1.2.2. Degenerative Joint Disease

All adults have osteoarthritis to some extent by the time they reach middle age, as it is a common disorder. Insofar as its suffix suggests that the ailment is essentially inflammatory, the term "osteoarthritis" is misleading. It is commonly referred to as osteoarthrosis, arthrosis deformans, or degenerative joint disease for this reason. Spondylosis is the term used when there is involvement of the spine. Osteoarthritis does not usually result in deformities that are incapacitating, unlike rheumatoid arthritis, which is a systemic disease. Most of the time, there are no noticeable symptoms associated with the milder anatomical changes. Abrasive wear away of the articular cartilage and reshaping of the adjacent ends of the bones are the characteristics that define the changes. Consequently, masses of newly proliferating bone—known as osteophytes—protrude from the joint margins. Depending on where and how severe the lesions are, osteoarthritis can present with different clinical symptoms. Malum coxae senilis, the most incapacitating form of the disorder, is localized in the hip joint. Similar to osteoarthritis in other joints, hip osteoarthritis can be categorized as primary or secondary. The alterations in secondary osteoarthritis are a result of some prior abnormality in the joint's structure or posture. However, even a thorough examination is unable to find such an abnormality in roughly half of the cases; in these cases, the osteoarthritis is referred to as primary.

Hip dislocation or subluxation, or congenital dysplasia, is likely the most common cause of osteoarthritis. This word describes an improper fit between the acetabulum, the pelvic socket, and the head of the femur, the long bone of the thigh. Evidence suggests that swaddling or carrying infants in headboards—maneuvers that maintain the thighs extended—causes a high number of cases to develop during infancy. The hip joint has often not fully developed before the child can walk, and this extension pushes the head of the femur out of its normal position. Hip osteoarthritis that strikes people in their 30s or 40s, when they are still relatively young, usually progresses over time and necessitates surgery. An osteotomy, which reshapes the upper end of the femur to better distribute the load on the joint, is one of the two rather different surgical strategies used. The other involves removing the diseased tissue and replacing it with an artificial joint. In addition to the quickly progressing varieties, hip osteoarthritis is also commonly seen in the elderly. Since the lesions become more frequent and severe with age, aging also plays a significant role in the development of other types of degenerative joint disease.

These kinds of factors have led to the belief that senescent deterioration of joint tissue and improper mechanical loading are the primary causes of degenerative arthritis. Osteoarthritis is a rare consequence of single injuries unless they cause a permanent deformity in the joint. However, repeated microtrauma, or small injuries, is more likely to occur from activities like heavy pneumatic drill vibrations or specific sports. Certain studies have linked spinal involvement to heavy weight lifting. Osteoarthritis frequently develops in the first metatarsophalangeal (MTP) joint, which is situated between the big toe and the remainder of the foot and naturally bears heavy loads. Osteoarthritis of the first MTP joint is linked to repeated microtrauma and wearing high-heeled shoes regularly. Osteoarthritis can also result from specific hormonal abnormalities and congenital joint deformities. Treatment options include rest and appropriate exercise, preventing injuries, using analgesics, NSAIDs, and corticosteroids to relieve pain, and various forms of physical therapy, in addition to surgery such as that seen in the hip and occasionally the knee. The surgical implantation of a synthetic cartilage implant can help treat painful osteoarthritis of the first MTP joint and preserve big toe mobility.

A common and recognizable softening of the kneecap's articular cartilage in young people, especially young athletes, is called chondromalacia patellae. As the knee is bent and straightened out, it causes "catching" and pain in the patella, or kneecap, area. Pathologically, the alterations are identical to those that take place at the beginning of osteoarthritis. Physical therapy, NSAIDs, and rest are all part of the treatment. Surgery might be necessary in more severe cases of chrondromalacia patellae. One common and somewhat similar disorder is degeneration of the intervertebral disks between the vertebrae of the spine. This frequently affects young and middle-aged adults severely. A slipped disk is the result of the pulpy center of the disk pushing out through rips in the fibrous outer ring. The nucleus pulposus, the displaced center, impinges on the nearby nerve roots when this occurs in the lumbosacral region, resulting in sciatica, or shooting pains in the sciatic nerve's distribution. In addition to spondylosis and intervertebral disk degeneration, structural anomalies in the area may also be linked to pain in the small of the back. The most common of these is spondylolisthesis, a condition in which one lumbosacral vertebral body is anteriorly displaced onto another. Bed rest and mechanical support from an abdominal brace are effective treatments for the episodes. Exercises that strengthen muscles and muscle relaxants may also be beneficial. Back strains can be avoided to stop recurrences. Surgery is only used to remove the protruding tissue when neurological defects and severe pain are unresponsive to less drastic measures.

9.1.3. Congenital and Hereditary Abnormalities

Congenital defects can develop during fetal life or shortly after delivery; they are not always passed down from one generation to the next. The inherited defects can be either structural or manifest later in life as a result of a systemic metabolic defect that is present from conception, while the latter abnormalities are typically structural. The topic of congenital hip dysplasia has already been raised. In this condition and in several other congenital disorders, the joint proper may initially be normal; the distortion of the bone and joint occurs only after other supporting tissues have changed the proper relationships. Many joints are malformed from birth in arthrogryposis multiplex congenita (multiple congenital crooked joints), especially the hip. The deformities are caused by muscle weakness, which can occasionally be brought on by spinal cord injury. A congenital deformity known as clubfoot (talipes equinovarus) causes the foot to twist inward and downward due to excessively short ligaments and tendons. The muscles are not usually at fault. The lateral curvature of the spine, or idiopathic scoliosis, typically manifests in the early stages of adolescence. The tissues have a great deal of latitude that allows for the correction of these deformities as well as the prevention of their progression. Because of this, the mainstay of treatment involves applying splints and other mechanical supports as soon as the condition is identified. When all other options are exhausted, surgery is the next step.

In the lumbosacral spine, structural differences are frequent and frequently innocuous. A congenital condition known as spondylolysis is caused by incompletely ossified interarticular portions of a vertebra's neural arches. This condition predisposes to forward slipping of the vertebra later in life, which in turn causes the congenital form of spondylolisthesis mentioned previously. In contrast, spina bifida occulta is the term used to describe the condition in which there is a failure of bony fusion between the left and right halves of the neural arch. Articular manifestations are present in several metabolic diseases that are influenced by genetics. The most common of these is gout. Sodium acid urate crystals are deposited in and around the joints as chalklike masses. Gouty arthritis flare-ups are excruciatingly painful. The big toe is more likely to become involved; this is referred to as podagra. Ochronotic arthropathy is caused by an additional, less common, inborn metabolic error. It is characterized by hyaline cartilage pigmentation and degeneration as well as improper tyrosine and phenylalanine amino acid breakdown, which results in a significant buildup of homogentisic acid in bodily fluids, including urine. When urine is exposed to air, it can turn black, a condition known as alkaptonuria. Severe degenerative alterations take place in the spine and peripheral joints after many years.

Calcium pyrophosphate crystals are deposited in the joint cartilages of chondrocalcinosis, also known as pseudogout, another metabolic disease. The illness comes in multiple forms. There may be no symptoms at all, or the symptoms may be so bad as to confuse them with rheumatoid arthritis. Certain cases are hereditary. Defects in the metabolism of connective tissue matrices give rise to a group of relatively uncommon hereditary diseases known as mucopolysaccharidoses, which also affect joints. Hurler syndrome, for instance, is characterized by abnormal skeletal growth in addition to heart failure and mental retardation. Most impacted individuals do not make it through adolescence. On the other hand, neither mental impairment nor cardiac insufficiency are linked to Morquio disease, a severe form of dwarfism that is inherited recessively. Spine X-rays show that the vertebral bodies have a recognizable flattened and misshapen appearance. It is common to see severe and premature degenerative changes in the spinal and peripheral joints. Precocious osteoarthritis and spondylosis are the first abnormalities to appear in a vaguely similar, though much milder, group of conditions known as polyepiphyseal dysplasias (abnormal development of some epiphyses—the ends or outlying portions of bones separated from the main body of the bone by cartilage) in childhood. On X-ray examination, preexisting alterations in the skeleton that resemble a milder version of Morquio disease may be found. The most severely impacted joint is the hip. Certain inheritances are recessive, while others involve dominance. The hallmark of Marfan syndrome is abnormalities in the fibrous components of connective tissue matrices. This is a condition that affects many organs, with articular manifestations being less significant. However, the joints are extremely loose, and in roughly half of the affected individuals, painful complications arise (Klippel et al., 2013; Firestein et al., 2021).

9.1.4. Secondary Joint Diseases

9.1.4.1. Hemorrhagic Joint Diseases

Hemarthrosis, or bleeding into the joints, is one of the most serious consequences of hemorrhagic diseases. It is the main disability resulting from hemophilias, aside from potentially fatal bleeding episodes. The majority of people who have these clotting defects are usually impacted in their early years of life. Although relatively minor injuries are typically the cause of bleeding into the joints, there may be multiple residual deformities and loss of movement in the affected part. In the absence of a systemic bleeding tendency, recurrent bleeding into a single joint is indicative of pigmented villonodular synovitis, a tumor characterized by aberrant synovial membrane thickening and coloration. Despite the name, this is not a primary inflammatory disease of the joints. Large joints are impacted, typically in the lower limbs.

9.1.4.2. Aseptic Necrosis

Joint cartilages are not harmed by blood supply problems because they do not contain blood vessels. Nevertheless, aseptic necrosis—tissue death not brought on by infection—of the bone adjacent to the joints is linked to some joint disorders. It is not always clear what exactly caused the blood supply to fail. One apparent reason is fractures. The contributing factors to decompression sickness, also known as caisson disease, are tiny gas bubbles that are created in the bloodstream as a result of an overly rapid decompression. Decompression syndromes mostly affect tunnel workers and divers. Acute cases often result in death and take the shape of "bends." But even in those who have not had the bends, a significant number of workers in these fields eventually develop secondary osteoarthritis and large infarcts (areas of dead tissue) in their bones. Similar alterations in sickle cell anemia are most likely caused by blood clotting associated with the aberrant red blood cell structure. For other forms of adult aseptic necrosis, there isn't a completely convincing theory. The hip is the joint most affected in each case. A similar condition called osteochondritis dissecans occurs when a fragment of bone that underlies the cartilage breaks off and becomes lodged in the joint cavity. Most of the time, the individual who is injured can recall hurting the joint. The most common location is the knee. Typically, the illness strikes in the second and third decades of life. A surgical procedure is required to remove the displaced fragment, which produces a creaking sound when the joint is moved.

Growing children experience two distinct patterns of aseptic necrosis with joint involvement. One kind, called slipped epiphysis, is characterized by an epiphysis that has been partially or completely torn away, usually due to an injury. Particularly vulnerable is the epiphysis at the top of the thigh bone. Similar lesions occur in Osgood-Schlatter disease, but they affect a growth center (anterior tibial tubercle) slightly away from the joint instead of right next to it. The second kind of aseptic necrosis in children does not result from the part being mechanically torn away. The most common location is in the thighbone head; Legg-Calvé-Perthes disease is the term for necrosis at this location. It affects kids between the ages of three and thirteen, with boys experiencing it far more frequently than girls. The most noticeable symptom is persistent pain. Severe lesions left untreated cause the hip joint to develop deformity, stop growing, and develop arthritis.

9.1.4.3. Endocrine Factors

Acromegaly is the only joint lesion that is unmistakably connected to a ductless (endocrine) gland malfunction. An anterior pituitary tumor's excessive growth hormone secretion is the cause of this illness. The hormone promotes the growth of bone, soft tissues, and joint cartilage in the skeleton. This results in the disease's typical enlargement of the fingers. Osteoarthritic degeneration is especially prone to occur in the larger joints. Though it appears not to cause joint disease, cretinism, a condition associated with hypothyroidism, causes dwarfism and abnormally developed bony epiphyses. However, because of how severe diabetes affects the nervous system, it can cause Charcot joint (see below) in people with diabetes mellitus.

9.1.4.4. Neurogenic Arthropathy

When the sensory mechanisms of joints are compromised, a severe degenerative disease associated with nerve lesions called neurogenic arthropathy, or Charcot joint, arises. According to the current theory, these joints experience excessive strain because they are unable to receive the stimuli from internal organs and structures that are required for a normal restriction of motion. Consequently, there is severe structural disintegration and tearing of the supporting tissues. The most common causes of neurogenic arthropathy are diabetes mellitus, leprosy, syringomyelia (a disease in which cavities form in the gray substance of the spinal cord), and tabes dorsalis, a late form of syphilis that affects the posterior columns of the spinal cord. The disease typically affects one joint or a subset of joints, depending on where the nerve defect is located. Considering the severe distortion of the joint, pain is often minimal. The mainstays of the challenging treatment plan are immobilization and weight-bearing restriction.

9.1.4.5. Hypertrophic Osteoarthropathy

The ends of the bones close to the joints enlarge and hurt in about 5 to 10% of people with primary tumors in the chest. The periosteum is where new bone grows, and abnormalities within the joints themselves only rarely occur. It is unclear exactly how the abnormality in the chest causes hypertrophic osteoarthropathy, a disease of the bones and joints characterized by abnormal bone growth, but since the condition is typically promptly relieved by cutting the vagus nerve, there is reason to suspect that the vagus nerve is involved. The tumor's removal also relieves it. This disorder causes the tips of the fingers to take on the shape of a club; this is a painless lesion that can also happen in many other situations.

9.1.4.6. Reflex Sympathetic Dystrophy

Rarely does reflex sympathetic dystrophy—also known as shoulder-hand syndrome because pain in the shoulder is linked to hand pain, edema, and stiffness—occur after an external injury. It frequently has no apparent cause and most often occurs after a heart attack (myocardial infarction) or is linked to a disease in the neck vertebrae. The syndrome typically starts with shoulder pain and stiffness, which is quickly followed by hand pain and swelling along with vascular (blood vessel) changes in the hand's skin. The vascular alterations and swelling go away over several months, but the skin and soft tissues tighten. These alterations can occasionally go away entirely, but other times they leave behind irreversible contractures—i.e., flexion and decreased range of motion as a result of the fingers' tightening. Mineral loss happens in the fingers, wrist, and shoulder bones. The condition is managed with the administration of corticosteroids, therapeutic exercises, and blocking (interruption of functioning) of the sympathetic nerves serving the area.

9.1.4.7. Tumors of Joints

Joint tumors are not common. The benign disease known as synovial chondromatosis causes the soft tissues of the joint to develop numerous cartilaginous nodules. The lesion usually affects young or middle-aged adults and is limited to one joint, usually the knee. The excision of a portion of the synovial membrane is typically the cure, and it may or may not cause pain or swelling. Rarely does the tumor turn malignant. When islands of bone are present in the cartilaginous nodules, the lesion is referred to as synovial osteochondromatosis. Similar to synovial chondromatosis, synovial osteochondromatosis is frequently a primary or spontaneous disorder with no known etiology. However, it frequently develops as a side effect of other synovial diseases, including osteoarthritis and rheumatoid arthritis. Malignant tumors known as synoviomas, also known as synovial sarcomas, are rare tumors that develop in the tissues surrounding joints, such as the bursas, fasciae, intermuscular septa, or divisions, and the capsule. While they can happen to anyone at any age, teenagers and young adults experience them most frequently. Usually, the legs are more affected than the arms. The tumors metastasized both locally to the lungs and nearby lymph nodes. X-ray sensitivity of synoviomas is not very high, and medication therapy has not proven to be successful in treating them. The recommended course of treatment is radical excision, which may involve amputation of the affected portion, if distant spread has not yet taken place at the time the condition is discovered (Klippel et al., 2013; Firestein et al., 2021).

9.2. Problems of Arthritis

Any condition that affects the joints is commonly referred to as arthritis. In most cases, stiffness and joint pain are symptoms. Additional indications could be warmth, redness, swelling, and a restricted range of motion in the afflicted joints. Certain forms of arthritis can also impact other organs. Onset may occur gradually or abruptly. Arthritis comes in more than 100 varieties. Rheumatoid arthritis and osteoarthritis, a degenerative joint disease, are the most prevalent types. Osteoarthritis typically affects the fingers, knees, and hips and develops with age. An autoimmune condition that frequently affects the hands and feet is rheumatoid arthritis. Septic arthritis, fibromyalgia, lupus, and gout are some other types. They are all categories of rheumatoid arthritis. As part of the treatment, the joint may be rested and heated or cooled in turns. Exercise and weight loss may also be beneficial. The type of arthritis may determine the recommended course of treatment. These could include ibuprofen and paracetamol (acetaminophen), two painkillers. There are situations when a joint replacement could be helpful.

Rheumatoid arthritis affects roughly 0.24% of the population, whereas osteoarthritis affects over 3.8% of people. About 1-2% of people in the West will experience gout at some point in their lives. In the United States, over 20% of people suffer from some form of arthritis, compared to approximately 15% in Australia. Overall, as people age, the disease becomes more prevalent. People frequently miss work due to arthritis, which can also lower their quality of life. The word comes from the Greek words arthr-, which means "joint," and -itis, which means "inflammation." One or more joints that are swollen and tender is called arthritis. Joint stiffness and pain are the primary signs of arthritis, and they usually get worse with age. Rheumatoid arthritis and osteoarthritis are the two most prevalent forms of arthritis. The hard, slick tissue called cartilage, which covers the ends of bones where they meet to form joints, deteriorates as a result of osteoarthritis. The disease known as rheumatoid arthritis occurs when the body's immune system targets the joints, starting with the joint lining. Gout can result from uric acid crystals, which occur when there is an excess of uric acid in the blood. Other types of arthritis can be brought on by infections or underlying medical conditions like lupus or psoriasis. The type of arthritis determines the different treatments. Improving quality of life and reducing symptoms are the main objectives of arthritis treatment.

9.2.1. Causes of Arthritis

A range of joint disorders characterized by inflammation, pain, stiffness, and reduced range of motion are collectively referred to as arthritis, a common and frequently incapacitating condition. Arthritis is caused by a variety of factors, many of which are complex interactions between environmental, genetic, and lifestyle factors. Osteoarthritis, or age-related joint wear and tear, is one of the main causes of arthritis. Growing older causes pain and stiffness because the cartilage that cushions the ends of bones gradually deteriorates. In addition, a person's susceptibility to specific kinds of arthritis is mostly determined by their genetic makeup. Certain individuals may be more prone to developing arthritis at a younger age or enduring more severe symptoms due to inherited factors that can affect the structure and integrity of joints. Autoimmune dysfunction, in which the body's immune system unintentionally targets its tissues, including the joints, is another frequent cause of arthritis. The autoimmune disease rheumatoid arthritis is typified by inflammation of the synovium, which is the lining of the joint capsule. If treatment for this chronic inflammation is not received, joint damage and deformity may result. In those who are vulnerable, environmental factors like infections or exposure to specific toxins can cause or worsen autoimmune reactions. Reactive arthritis and other types of inflammatory joint disease can result from infections, including bacterial or viral infections, which can also cause inflammatory arthritis. Furthermore, when uric acid crystals build up in the joints due to metabolic disorders like gout, arthritis can result, causing abrupt, excruciating pain and inflammation. Similar to pseudogout, acute arthritis attacks are brought on by the accumulation of calcium pyrophosphate crystals in the joints.

Lifestyle choices can have a big impact on how arthritis starts and progresses. For instance, obesity increases the amount of stress placed on weight-bearing joints, hastening cartilage deterioration and raising the risk of osteoarthritis. On the other hand, exercise supports general joint health by preserving joint strength and flexibility. On the other hand, overuse or repetitive joint stress, as from specific jobs or sports, can raise the risk of arthritis developing after an injury. In addition, changes in hormones, especially in women, can affect the severity and onset of arthritis. Certain types of arthritis, like lupus or rheumatoid arthritis, may have worsening symptoms due to hormonal changes that occur during pregnancy or menopause. Additionally, joint pain and inflammation may be exacerbated by hormonal imbalances linked to diseases such as hypothyroidism. Arthritis is also influenced by environmental factors such as smoking, pollution, and food habits. For example, smoking has been associated with a higher risk of developing rheumatoid arthritis and may exacerbate symptoms in those who have already been diagnosed with the illness. Some dietary choices, like eating too much red meat, processed foods, or sugary drinks, can increase inflammation in the body and aggravate arthritis symptoms.

9.2.2. Symptoms of Arthritis

Depending on the kind and severity of the disease, arthritis can present with a wide range of symptoms. The most typical symptoms include stiffness, swelling, pain in the joints, and a reduction in range of motion. Depending on what causes the arthritis in the first place, these symptoms can appear suddenly or develop gradually over time. One of the main signs of arthritis is pain, which can range from a little discomfort to excruciating, incapacitating pain. One or more joints may be the source of the pain, which is frequently made worse by pressure or movement in the affected area. While osteoarthritis pain may worsen with activity and improve with rest, inflammatory types of arthritis, like rheumatoid arthritis, typically cause more widespread, continuous pain. Another typical sign of arthritis is joint swelling or inflammation. Rheumatoid arthritis and psoriatic arthritis are examples of inflammatory arthritis conditions that usually cause visible swelling and redness around the affected joints. This is because the immune system of the body attacks the synovium, which is the lining of the joint capsule. Because osteoarthritis damages and irritates the joints, swelling may be less noticeable but can still happen.

One of the most common symptoms of arthritis is stiffness, especially in the morning or after periods of inactivity. Mobility and flexibility may be restricted by joint stiffness, which may become less severe with movement but may linger all day. Some stiffness associated with arthritis can worsen to the point of joint deformity, which can impair quality of life and make daily tasks difficult. Another common symptom of arthritis is decreased range of motion, which is caused by pain, inflammation, and joint damage that limits joint mobility. This movement restriction can interfere with a number of daily activities, including walking, climbing stairs, and grasping objects. During times of active inflammation, fatigue, muscle weakness, and a general sense of malaise can all be additional symptoms of arthritis. Furthermore, some forms of arthritis, like lupus and rheumatoid arthritis, can impact several organs and systems in the body, resulting in a variety of symptoms outside of joint problems. It is crucial to remember that arthritis symptoms can change over time, going through phases of improvement known as remission and periods of worsening known as flare-ups. Implementing suitable treatment strategies to effectively manage symptoms and prevent further joint damage requires early recognition and diagnosis of arthritis. For a precise diagnosis and individualized treatment plan, it is critical to speak with a healthcare provider if you're dealing with chronic joint pain, swelling, or stiffness.

Pain, which can vary in severity, is a common symptom in virtually all types of arthritis. Other symptoms include swelling, joint stiffness, redness, and aching around the joint(s). Arthritic disorders like lupus and rheumatoid arthritis can affect other organs in the body, leading to a variety of symptoms (Figure 9.2). Symptoms may include:

- Inability to use the hand or walk
- Stiffness in one or more joints
- Rash or itch
- Malaise and fatigue
- Weight loss
- Poor sleep
- Muscle aches and pains
- Tenderness
- Difficulty moving the joint

It is common in advanced arthritis for significant secondary changes to occur. For example, arthritic symptoms might make it difficult for a person to move around and/or exercise, which can lead to secondary effects, such as:

- Muscle weakness
- Loss of flexibility
- Decreased aerobic fitness

These changes, in addition to the primary symptoms, can have a huge impact on quality of life.

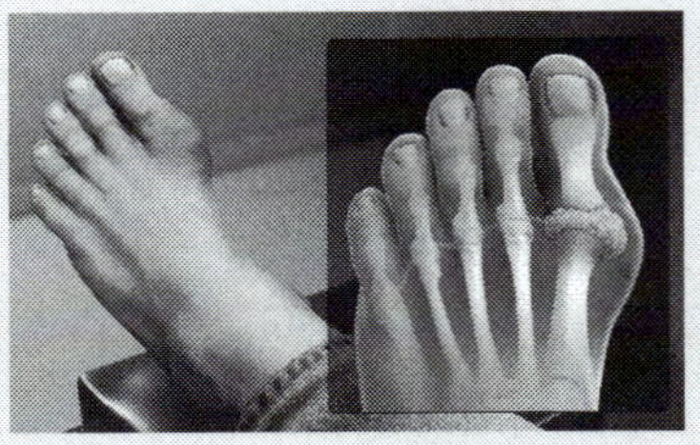

Figure 9.2. *An illustration of a gout-affected foot.*

Source: https://upload.wikimedia.org/wikipedia/commons/thumb/0/0b/Gout_Signs_and_Symptoms.jpg/1280px-Gout_Signs_and_Symptoms.jpg.

9.2.2.1. Disability

In the US, arthritis is the most common cause of disability. Every day, more than 20 million people with arthritis experience significant functional limitations. People with arthritis often have absenteeism and make frequent doctor visits. People with arthritis may find it difficult to engage in physical activity, and some may end up bedridden. An estimated $100 billion is spent on arthritis cases overall, with lost wages accounting for nearly half of that amount. Nearly 1 million hospital admissions and nearly 45 million outpatient visits to medical facilities are caused by arthritis each year. When combined with the aforementioned symptoms, decreased mobility can make it difficult for a person to maintain an active lifestyle, which raises the risk of obesity, high cholesterol, or heart disease. Individuals who have arthritis also have a higher chance of developing depression, which can be brought on by a variety of things, such as anxiety about their symptoms getting worse.

9.2.3. Diagnosis

Depending on the type of suspected arthritis, additional tests like blood and radiological examinations may be used to confirm the diagnosis, which is made by a clinical examination performed by a qualified healthcare provider. Pain is a possible side effect of all arthritis. Depending on the location and type of arthritis, different pain patterns may occur. Rheumatoid arthritis is typically worse first thing in the morning and causes stiffness that lasts longer than 30 minutes. The diagnosis is guided by certain aspects of the disorder's history. The rapidity and timing of the onset, the pattern of joints involved, the symmetry of the symptoms, the stiffness and tenderness in the morning, the gelling or locking with inactivity, the aggravating and relieving factors, and other systemic symptoms are important features. It could involve assessing joints, monitoring motions, looking for rashes or nodules on the skin, and looking for signs of pulmonary inflammation. A physical examination could support the diagnosis or point to a systemic illness. Radiographs are frequently used to monitor development or assist in determining severity. To make the diagnosis, X-rays of the afflicted joints and blood tests are frequently carried out. If a particular type of arthritis is suspected, screening blood tests should be performed. Rheumatoid factor, antinuclear factor (ANF), extractable nuclear antigen, and particular antibodies are a few examples of these (Table 9.1).

Table 9.1. Synovial Fluid Examination

Type	WBC (per mm^3)	% Neutrophils	Viscosity	Appearance
Normal	<200	0	High	Transparent
Osteoarthritis	<5000	<25	High	Clear yellow
Trauma	<10,000	<50	Variable	Bloody
Inflammatory	2,000–50,000	50–80	Low	Cloudy yellow
Septic arthritis	>50,000	>75	Low	Cloudy yellow
Gonorrhea	~10,000	60	Low	Cloudy yellow
Tuberculosis	~20,000	70	Low	Cloudy yellow
Inflammatory: Arthritis, gout, rheumatoid arthritis, rheumatic fever.				

Source: *https://en.wikipedia.org/wiki/Arthritis.*

Patients with rheumatoid arthritis frequently have elevated levels of C-reactive protein (CRP) or erythrocyte sedimentation rate (ESR, sometimes referred to as sed rate), which show that the body is undergoing an inflammatory process.

Two other frequently performed blood tests are rheumatoid factor (RF) and anti-cyclic citrullinated peptide (anti-CCP) antibodies. While negative results help rule out this autoimmune condition, positive results indicate the possibility of rheumatoid arthritis.

Imaging tests used to diagnose and track arthritis include MRIs, ultrasounds, and X-rays. Additional imaging tests for rheumatoid arthritis that could be taken into consideration are bone scanning, dual-energy X-ray absorptiometry (DEXA), computed tomography (CT), and positron emission tomography (PET).

9.2.3.1. Osteoarthritis

The most prevalent type of arthritis is osteoarthritis. It affects not only humans but also other animals, including cats and horses, but most commonly dogs. It can impact the body's larger and smaller joints equally. This covers the hands, wrists, feet, back, hips, and knees in humans.

This includes the stifle (knee), elbow, hip, shoulder, and back in dogs. Osteoarthritis is primarily a condition brought on by normal joint wear and tear, though injuries can also cause the condition to develop.

The disease known as osteoarthritis starts in the cartilage and eventually erodes the two opposing bones into one another. The ailment initially manifests as mild discomfort experienced during exercise, but it can quickly become constant and even happen while at rest (Figure 9.3).

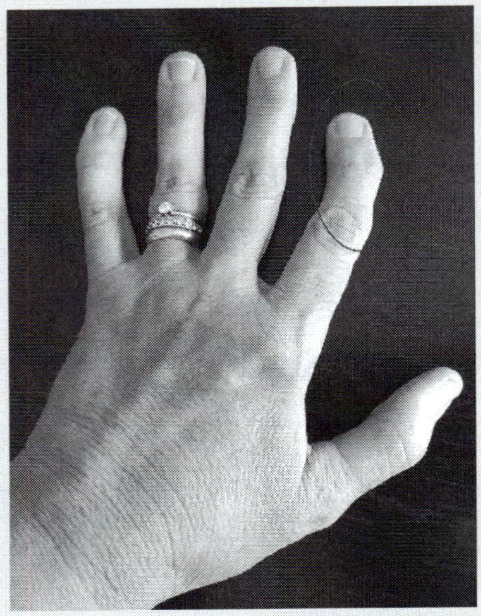

Figure 9.3. *Osteoarthritis in the left hand index finger of a 63-year-old woman.*

Source: *https://upload.wikimedia.org/wikipedia/commons/thumb/6/6e/Osteoarthritis_in_the_left_hand_index_finger.jpg/220px-Osteoarthritis_in_the_left_hand_index_finger.jpg.*

It is possible for the pain to be incapacitating, making certain activities impossible. It can be extremely painful for dogs to walk on slippery floors, climb stairs, struggle to get up after lying down, be unable to hop in and out of cars, have trouble jumping on and off furniture, and exhibit behavioral changes, among other things (e.g., hostility, trouble squatting to use the restroom). Usually, osteoarthritis affects weight-bearing joints like the hip, knee, and back. In contrast to rheumatoid arthritis, osteoarthritis primarily affects the elderly population. Growing older is the best indicator of osteoarthritis, most likely because chondrocytes are losing their capacity to preserve the structural integrity of cartilage. By the time they are 65 years old, over 30% of women have osteoarthritis to some extent. Obesity, a sedentary lifestyle, and previous joint trauma are additional risk factors for osteoarthritis.

9.2.3.2. Rheumatoid Arthritis

The condition known as rheumatoid arthritis (RA) occurs when the body's immune system begins to target bodily tissues. Numerous other body parts are also targeted by the attack in addition to the joint. The majority of damage in rheumatoid arthritis is to the cartilage and joint lining, which ultimately leads to the erosion of two opposing bones. RA is symmetrical (shows up on both sides of the body), frequently affects the fingers, wrists, knees, and elbows, and if left untreated, can cause severe deformity in a matter of years. RA primarily affects adults over the age of 20. Children with the disorder may experience skin rashes, fevers, pains, disabilities, and difficulties with day-to-day activities. Many people can have a higher quality of life with an early diagnosis and vigorous treatment than if they wait until long after RA symptoms start. The strongest risk factors for developing rheumatoid arthritis are female gender, age, obesity, prior joint damage from an injury, and tobacco smoke exposure. There is also a family history of rheumatoid arthritis (Figure 9.4).

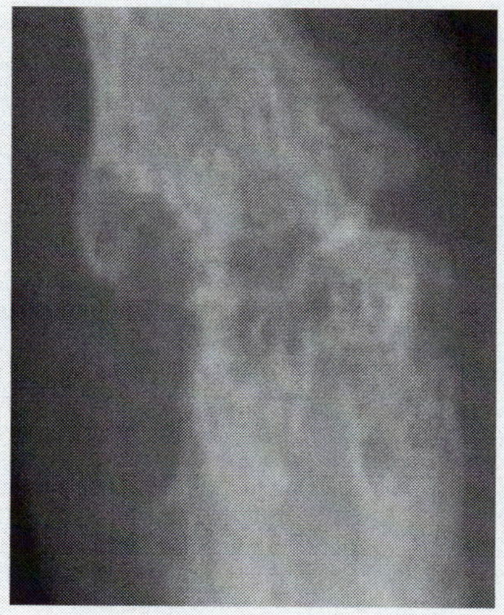

Figure 9.4. *Bone erosions by rheumatoid arthritis.*

Source: *https://upload.wikimedia.org/wikipedia/commons/6/6c/X-ray_of_right_fourth_PIP_joint_with_bone_erosions_by_rheumatoid_arthritis.jpg.*

One main characteristic of rheumatoid arthritis is bone erosion. Osteoclasts that resorb bone and osteoblasts that form new bone are constantly remodeling bone. Rheumatoid arthritis-related synovial inflammation is one of the primary causes of bone erosion in the joints. This inflammation is partly attributed to the production of pro-inflammatory cytokines and receptor activator of nuclear factor kappa B ligand (RANKL), a cell surface protein found on Th17 cells and osteoblasts. Osteoblasts can directly induce osteoclast activity via the RANK/RANKL pathway.

9.2.3.3. Systemic Lupus Erythematosus (SLE)

Lupus is a common collagen vascular disorder that can be present with severe arthritis. Other features of lupus include a skin rash, extreme photosensitivity, hair loss, kidney problems, lung fibrosis and constant joint pain.

9.2.3.4. Gout

The buildup of uric acid crystals in the joints, which results in inflammation, is the cause of gout. Pseudogout is a rare type of gouty arthritis that is brought on by the development of rhomboid calcium pyrophosphate crystals. Gouty arthritis typically affects one joint in the early stages, but over time, it can affect multiple joints and be extremely debilitating. Gout frequently causes the joints to swell and stop working. When gout is not effectively treated, gouty arthritis can become extremely painful and possibly incapacitating. When gout symptoms and uric acid levels cannot be managed with conventional gout medications that reduce uric acid production (e.g., allopurinol) or promote the kidneys' ability to remove uric acid from the body (e.g., Probenecid, for example), this condition is known as refractory chronic gout (Table 9.2).

Table 9.2. Comparison of Some Major Forms of Arthritis

	Osteoarthritis	Rheumatoid Arthritis	Gouty Arthritis
Speed of onset	Months	Weeks-months	Hours for an attack
Main Locations	Weight-bearing joints (such as knees, hips, vertebral column) and hands	Hands (proximal interphalangeal and metacarpophalangeal joint) wrists, ankles, knees and hips	Great toe, ankles, knees and elbows
Inflammation	May occur, though often mild compared to inflammation in rheumatoid arthritis	Yes	Yes
Radiologic Changes	• Narrowed joint space • Osteophytes • Local osteosclerosis • Subchondral cysts	• Narrowed joint space • Bone erosions	• "Punched out" bone erosions
Laboratory Findings	None	Anemia, elevated ESR and C-reactive protein (CRP), rheumatoid factor, anti-citrullinated protein antibody	Crystal in joints
Other Features	• No systemic signs • Bouchard's and Heberden's nodes	• Extra-articular features are common • Ulnar deviation, swan neck- and Boutonniere deformity of the hand	• Tophi • Nephrolithiasis

Source: *https://en.wikipedia.org/wiki/Arthritis.*

9.2.3.5. Other

Another severe type of arthritis is infectious arthritis. It manifests as joint pain, fever, and chills that come on suddenly. Bacteria from other parts of the body are the cause of the illness. It is imperative to diagnose and treat infectious arthritis as soon as possible to avoid irreversible joint damage. There are many different types of viruses that can cause infectious arthritis, but only about 1% of cases have this cause. The list of viruses that can cause arthritis infections now includes the SARS-CoV-2 virus, which causes COVID-19. Response to SARS-CoV-2 is reactive arthritis. Psoriatic arthritis can arise from psoriasis. Most people with psoriatic arthritis experience the skin condition first, followed by the arthritis. Constant joint pain, stiffness, and swelling are typical symptoms. While there is no known treatment for the illness, it does occasionally recur. A tiny proportion experience extremely painful and debilitating forms of arthritis that destroy the hands' tiny joints and can result in irreversible disability and hand function loss (Klippel et al., 2013; Firestein et al., 2021).

9.2.4. Treatment

Rheumatic diseases and arthritis have no known cure. Depending on the type of arthritis, there are several treatment options, such as oral and topical medications, physical therapy, diet and exercise, and orthopedic bracing. It might be necessary to have joint replacement surgery to fix damage, get function back, or get rid of pain.

9.2.4.1. Physical Therapy

Studies have generally demonstrated that engaging in physical activity for the afflicted joint can significantly enhance long-term pain relief. Additionally, it is advised to exercise the arthritic joint to preserve the health of both the individual's body as a whole and the specific joint. Physical and occupational therapy are beneficial for people with arthritis. Arthritis can cause stiff joints and restricted range of motion. It has been demonstrated that physical therapy can considerably increase function, reduce pain, and postpone the need for surgery in more advanced cases. Research has demonstrated that when treating osteoarthritis of the knee, physical therapy exercises are superior to pharmaceutical treatments. Enhancing muscular strength, endurance, and flexibility is a common goal of exercise. Exercises may occasionally be made with balance training in mind. Occupational therapy is able to help with daily tasks. With the use of assistive technology, a person's disability can be lessened and their physical limitations can be improved, usually following an amputation. Devices for assistive technology can be purchased commercially or tailored for the patient.

9.2.4.2. Medications

The treatment of arthritis involves the use of various medication types. The drugs with the fewest side effects are usually used as the first line of treatment, and if they are not sufficiently effective, other drugs may be added. The medications prescribed may vary based on the type of arthritis. For instance, acetaminophen (paracetamol) is the first-line treatment for osteoarthritis, whereas non-steroidal anti-inflammatory drugs (NSAIDs) like ibuprofen are used to treat inflammatory arthritis. NSAIDs and opioids might not be as well tolerated. On the other hand, topical NSAIDs might have safer profiles than oral NSAIDs. Injections of corticosteroids into the joint may also be an option for osteoarthritis patients with more severe symptoms. Treatment options for rheumatoid arthritis (RA) include intravenous monoclonal antibodies and corticosteroids. Owing to RA's autoimmune origin, therapies may involve anti-inflammatory and painkillers in addition to a different class of pharmaceuticals known as disease-modifying antirheumatic drugs (DMARDs). tsDMARDs, TNF biologics, and csDMARDs are particular DMARD subtypes that are advised for use in therapy. The goal of DMARD treatment is to impede the advancement of RA by inducing an adaptive immune response, which is aided by CD4+ T helper (Th) cells, particularly Th17 cells. Th17 cells produce inflammatory cytokines linked to inflammation, such as interleukin-17 (IL-17), and are more prevalent in joints where bone is being destroyed.

9.2.4.3. Surgery

A number of rheumasurgical interventions have been incorporated in the treatment of arthritis since the 1950s. Arthroscopic surgery for osteoarthritis of the knee provides no additional benefit to optimized physical and medical therapy.

9.2.4.4. Adaptive Aids

ADLs, or activities of daily living, can be difficult and painful for people with hand arthritis. Examples of these tasks include opening jars and turning a key in a lock. While assistive devices (ADs), also known as adaptive aids, are available to help with these tasks, their cost is typically higher than that of conventional products serving the same purpose. Adaptive aids, which have been made available as open-source hardware to lower patient costs, can now be 3-D printed. The great majority of people with arthritis require and make use of adaptive aids, which can greatly benefit patients with arthritis.

9.2.4.5. Alternative Medicine

The effectiveness of transcutaneous electrical nerve stimulation (TENS) for knee osteoarthritis pain management needs to be investigated further. Low-level laser therapy is a viable option for reducing arthritis-related pain and stiffness. The benefit is not conclusively shown. There is no proof that pulsed electromagnetic field therapy (PEMFT) reduces osteoarthritis pain, but there is some evidence to support improved functioning. PEMFT has not received FDA approval to treat arthritis. Health Canada has granted PEMF devices a valid license to be used in Canada for the management of arthritic pain (Klippel et al., 2013; Firestein et al., 2021).

9.3. Osteoarthritis

One form of degenerative joint disease that arises from the deterioration of joint cartilage and underlying bone is called osteoarthritis (OA). One in seven adults in the US alone are thought to be affected by it, making it the fourth most common cause of disability globally. Joint stiffness and pain are the most prevalent symptoms. Typically, the symptoms worsen gradually over many years. Additional symptoms could be decreased range of motion, swollen joints, and, in cases where the back is impacted, arm and leg weakness or numbness. The knee and hip joints, the joints in the neck and lower back, the two joints at the tips of the fingers, and the joint at the base of the thumbs are the joints that are most frequently affected. The symptoms may make it difficult to work or go about your regular activities. As opposed to some other forms of arthritis, this one affects solely the joints and not the internal organs. The causes include inherited factors, abnormal development of the joint or limb, and history of joint injury. Individuals who are overweight, have varying leg lengths, or work jobs that put a lot of strain on their joints are more at risk. Low-grade inflammatory processes and mechanical stress on the joint are thought to be the causes of osteoarthritis. It appears when the underlying bone becomes impacted by cartilage loss. Muscle loss may happen because pain may make it difficult to exercise. Medical imaging and other tests are used to confirm or rule out other issues, with signs and symptoms usually serving as the basis for the diagnosis. Unlike rheumatoid arthritis, osteoarthritis does not cause redness or heat in the joints.

Exercise, painkillers, support groups, and relieving joint stress—such as by resting or using a cane—are all part of the treatment. For those who are overweight, losing weight may be helpful. NSAIDs like ibuprofen or naproxen as well as paracetamol (acetaminophen) are examples of painkillers. Due to a lack of knowledge about the advantages of opioids as well as the risks of addiction and other side effects, long-term use is not advised. If the impairment persists after trying other therapies, joint replacement surgery might be an option. Usually, an artificial joint lasts for ten to fifteen years. The most prevalent type of arthritis, osteoarthritis, affected roughly 237 million people worldwide, or 3.3% of the total population, in 2015. As people age, it becomes more prevalent. This affects roughly 10% of men and 18% of women over the age of 60. About 2% of years that a person is disabled are due to osteoarthritis.

9.3.1. Signs and Symptoms

The primary symptom is pain, which frequently results in stiffness and loss of ability. Resting usually relieves the pain, which is usually exacerbated by prolonged activity. The stiffness usually occurs in the morning and goes away in less than 30 minutes after daily activities start, but it can come back after periods of inactivity. When a joint with osteoarthritis is moved, particularly the shoulder and knee joints, it can produce a crackling sound known as crepitus. Additionally, joint instability and locking may be complained of. Due to the pain and stiffness, these symptoms would interfere with their regular activities. Although research has produced conflicting findings, some people claim that cold temperatures, high humidity, or a drop in barometric pressure cause them to experience more pain. Though theoretically any joint in the body could be impacted, osteoarthritis typically affects the hands, feet, spine, and large weight-bearing joints like the hips and knees. Osteoarthritis usually affects movement patterns (such as gait) as it advances. The most frequent cause of a knee joint effusion is osteoarthritis (Felson & Zhang, 2018) (Figure 9.5).

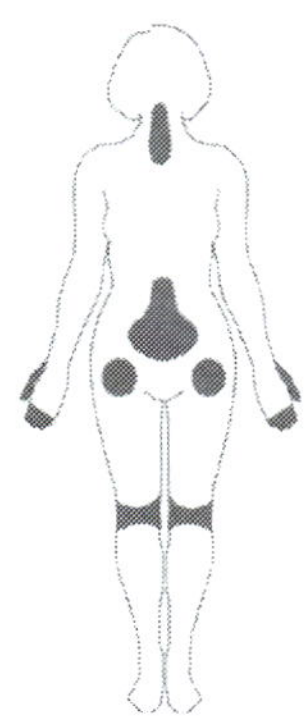

Figure 9.5. *Osteoarthritis most often occurs in the hands (at the ends of the fingers and thumbs), neck, lower back, knees, and hips.*

Source: *By US federal government – http://www.niams.nih.gov/health_info/Osteoarthritis/default.asp, Public Domain, https://commons.wikimedia.org/w/index.php?curid=40173053.*

Hard bony enlargements, known as Bouchard's nodes (on the proximal interphalangeal joints) or Heberden's nodes (on the distal interphalangeal joints), may form in smaller joints, such as the fingers. These enlargements do not always cause pain, but they do severely restrict finger movement. Bunions, which make toes red or swollen, can develop as a result of osteoarthritis.

9.3.2. Causes

The main theory for osteoarthritis is that the disease is caused by mechanical stress-related damage that the joints are unable to adequately repair. Some of the possible causes of this stress include mechanical injuries, excess body weight, loss of strength in the muscles supporting a joint, congenital or pathogenic bone misalignments, and impairment of peripheral nerves, which can result in jerky or uncoordinated movements. Exercise, including injury-free running, hasn't been linked to a higher risk of osteoarthritis in the knees, though. It hasn't been discovered that cracking one's knuckles matters either. Aging raises the risk of osteoarthritis.

9.3.2.1. Primary Osteoarthritis

Osteoarthritis is associated with obesity, particularly in relation to the knees, and a history of prior joint injuries. The higher incidence of osteoarthritis in postmenopausal women compared to men of the same age may be related to changes in sex hormone levels. There is conflicting data regarding the differences between osteoarthritis in the hips and knees between African Americans and Whites.

9.3.2.2. Occupational

Among those who work with manual handling, there is an increased risk of developing osteoarthritis in the knees and hips (e.g., lifting), engage in physically taxing work, take walks, and perform climbing tasks (e.g., climb ladders or staircases). Those who work in twisted or bent positions have a higher chance of developing osteoarthritis in general and hip osteoarthritis in particular over time. Particularly for knee osteoarthritis, people who work standing up, perform heavy lifting while maintaining a kneeling or squatting posture, and work in these positions have higher risk factors. There is no significant difference in the occupational risk of osteoarthritis between men and women.

9.3.2.3. Secondary Osteoarthritis

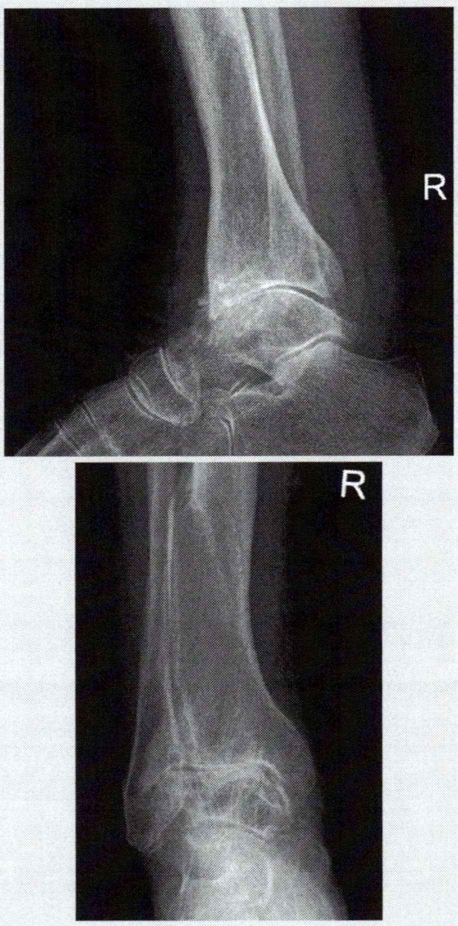

Figure 9.6. *Secondary osteoarthritis of the ankle (due to an old bone fracture) in an 82-year-old woman.*

Source: *https://en.wikipedia.org/wiki/Osteoarthritis.*

This type of osteoarthritis is caused by other factors but the resulting pathology is the same as for primary osteoarthritis (Figure 9.6):

- Alkaptonuria
- Congenital disorders of joints
- Diabetes doubles the risk of having a joint replacement due to osteoarthritis and people with diabetes have joint replacements at a younger age than those without diabetes.
- Ehlers-Danlos syndrome
- Hemochromatosis and Wilson's disease
- Inflammatory diseases (such as Perthes' disease), (Lyme disease), and all chronic forms of arthritis (e.g., costochondritis, gout, and rheumatoid arthritis). In gout, uric acid crystals cause the cartilage to degenerate at a faster pace.
- Injury to joints or ligaments (such as the ACL) as a result of an accident or orthopedic operations.
- Ligamentous deterioration or instability may be a factor.
- Marfan syndrome
- Obesity
- Joint infection (Felson & Zhang, 2018)

9.3.3. Pathophysiology

Even though osteoarthritis is a degenerative joint disease that can result in significant cartilage loss and morphological harm to other joint tissues, the disease's early stages are marked by more subtle biochemical alterations. Hydrostatic and osmotic pressures draw water in and compressive force drives it out, resulting in a delicate balance in the water content of healthy cartilage. Although cartilage proteoglycans and the Gibbs-Donnan effect produce osmotic pressure, which tends to draw water in, collagen fibers provide the compressive force (Figure 9.7).

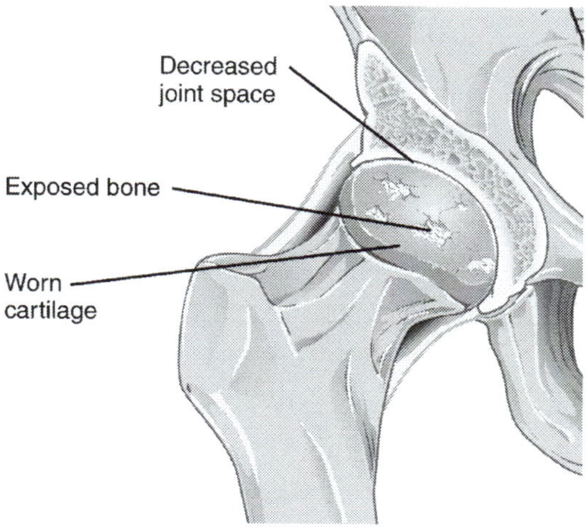

Figure 9.7. *Hip joint with osteoarthritis.*

Source: *By CFCF – Own work, CC BY-SA 4.0, https://commons.wikimedia.org/w/index.php?curid=44235706.*

On the other hand, the collagen matrix becomes more disorganized and the amount of proteoglycan in cartilage decreases when osteoarthritis starts. There is a net increase in water content as a result of the breakdown of collagen fibers. This increase happens because the overall loss of collagen outweighs the loss of proteoglycans, which lowers the osmotic pull. There may be additional joint structures that are impacted. The menisci may sustain damage and wear away, and the ligaments inside the joint may thicken and fibrose. When a person has a joint replacement, menisci may not even be present. Spurs, also known as osteophytes, are new bone outgrowths that can grow on the edge of joints. It is possible that these growths are an attempt to improve the congruence of the articular cartilage surfaces when the menisci are absent. Hypomineralization is the decrease in mineralization and increase in volume of subchondral bone. All of these modifications may result in functional issues. Lesions in the subchondral bone and thickened synovium have been linked to osteoarthritic joint pain.

9.3.4. Diagnosis

Based on the history and clinical examination, a diagnosis is made with a reasonable degree of certainty. X-rays could validate the diagnosis. Joint space narrowing, subchondral sclerosis (increased bone formation around the joint), subchondral cyst formation, and osteophytes are common X-ray abnormalities. Simple films might not be correlated with the results of a physical examination or the level of discomfort (Table 9.3).

Table 9.3. Synovial Fluid Examination

Type	WBC (per mm^3)	% Neutrophils	Viscosity	Appearance
Normal	<200	0	High	Transparent
Osteoarthritis	<5000	<25	High	Clear yellow
Trauma	<10,000	<50	Variable	Bloody
Inflammatory	2,000–50,000	50–80	Low	Cloudy yellow
Septic arthritis	>50,000	>75	Low	Cloudy yellow
Gonorrhea	~10,000	60	Low	Cloudy yellow
Tuberculosis	~20,000	70	Low	Cloudy yellow
Inflammatory: Arthritis, gout, rheumatoid arthritis, rheumatic fever				

Source: *https://en.wikipedia.org/wiki/Osteoarthritis.*

A set of criteria for the diagnosis of hand osteoarthritis based on hard tissue enlargement and swelling of specific joints was developed in 1990 by the American College of Rheumatology using data from a multi-center study. These criteria were found to be 92% sensitive and 98% specific for hand osteoarthritis in comparison to other conditions like spondyloarthropathies and rheumatoid arthritis.

- Severe osteoarthritis and osteopenia of the carpal joint and 1st carpometacarpal joint
- MRI of osteoarthritis in the knee, with characteristic narrowing of the joint space
- Primary osteoarthritis of the left knee. Note the osteophytes, narrowing of the joint space (arrow), and increased subchondral bone density (arrow).
- Damaged cartilage from sows. (a) cartilage erosion (b)cartilage ulceration (c)cartilage repair (d) osteophyte (bone spur) formation.
- Histopathology of osteoarthrosis of a knee joint in an elderly female
- In a healthy joint, the ends of bones are encased in smooth cartilage. Together, they are protected by a joint capsule lined with a synovial membrane that produces synovial fluid. The capsule and fluid protect the cartilage, muscles, and connective tissues.
- With osteoarthritis, the cartilage becomes worn away. Spurs grow out from the edge of the bone, and synovial fluid increases. Altogether, the joint feels stiff and sore.

9.3.4.1. Classification

A number of classification systems are used for gradation of osteoarthritis:

- WOMAC scale, taking into account pain, stiffness and functional limitation.
- Kellgren-Lawrence grading scale for osteoarthritis of the knee. It uses only projectional radiography features.
- Tönnis classification for osteoarthritis of the hip joint, also using only projectional radiography features.

Primary osteoarthritis comprises two subtypes: erosive osteoarthritis (EOA), also known as inflammatory osteoarthritis, and primary generalized nodal osteoarthritis. The distal interphalangeal joints of the hand are frequently affected by EOA, a much less common and more aggressive inflammatory form of osteoarthritis that is characterized by articular erosive changes on X-rays (Figure 9.8).

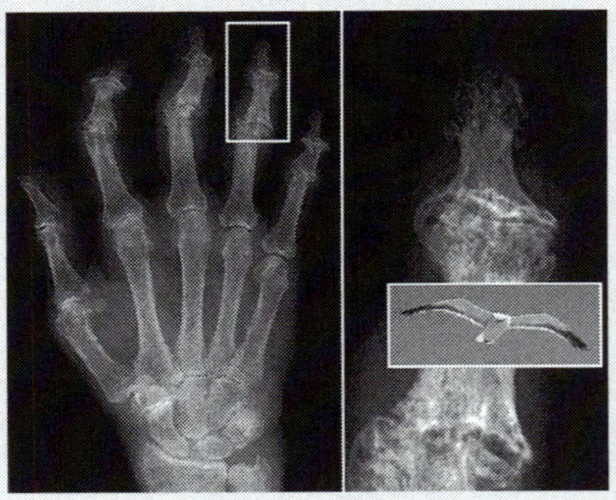

Figure 9.8. *X-ray of erosive osteoarthritis of the fingers, also zooming in on two joints with the typical "gull-wing" appearance.*

Source: *https://upload.wikimedia.org/wikipedia/commons/thumb/c/c9/Erosive_osteoarthritis_with_gull-wing_appearance%2C_with_seagull.jpg/736px-Erosive_osteoarthritis_with_gull-wing_appearance%2C_with_seagull.jpg.*

9.3.5. Management

The cornerstones of treatment include pain management drugs and lifestyle changes like exercise and weight loss. NSAIDs should only be used as supplemental therapy if acetaminophen, commonly known as paracetamol, is not enough to relieve pain. As of 2018, there are no known medications that change how the illness progresses. Losing weight can help relieve hip arthritis in those who are overweight. The following risk factors should be modified through focused interventions: 1) physical inactivity, 2) dietary exposures, 3) comorbidity, 4) obesity and overweight, 5) biomechanical factors, and 6) occupational factors. Different priorities and inadequate communication between osteoarthritis patients and clinicians frequently make successful management of the condition more difficult. By creating a common understanding of the ailment, actively listening to patient concerns, avoiding medical jargon, and customizing treatment plans to meet the patient's needs, realistic treatment goals can be accomplished (Felson & Zhang, 2018).

9.3.5.1. Exercise

For those with osteoarthritis, losing weight and exercising are recommended long-term treatments. Compared to short-term treatments, which typically carry a risk of long-term harm, weight loss and exercise are the safest and most effective long-term treatments. Low- or moderate-impact exercises, like swimming or walking, are safer for those with osteoarthritis, but high-impact exercises can raise the risk of joint injury. One study found that raising blood calcium levels had a beneficial effect on osteoarthritis. Increased calcium levels are beneficial in preventing osteoarthritis in the general population and can be achieved through regular weight-bearing exercise and an adequate dietary calcium intake. The low-density lipoprotein (LDL) cholesterol has a marginal protective effect as well. This is not advised, though, as there is a higher risk of cardiovascular comorbidities with elevated LDL levels (Figure 9.9).

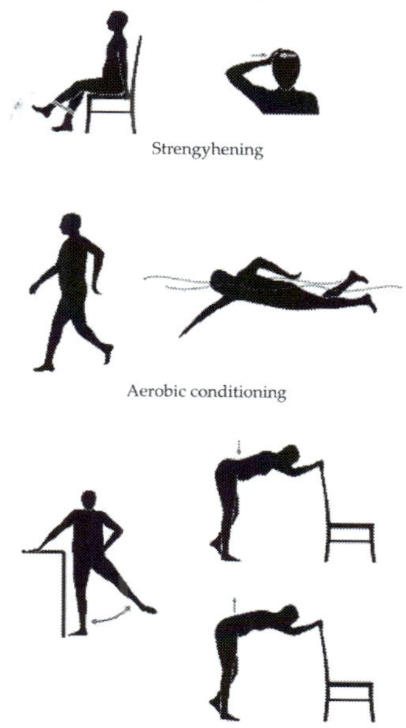

Figure 9.9. *Some kinds of exercise recommended in OA.*

Source: *https://upload.wikimedia.org/wikipedia/commons/thumb/4/43/Exercise.png/320px-Exercise.png.*

For those who have hip and knee osteoarthritis, moderate exercise may help with pain and function. These exercises, which should be performed under supervision and at least three times a week, should concentrate on particular types of exercise that have been shown to be most helpful for this type of osteoarthritis. There is little evidence in favor of a combined program, but there is some evidence in favor of some physical therapies. Greater benefit and increased participation may result from giving clear instructions, making exercise enjoyable, and reassuring people of its importance. Although supervised exercise has shown the best results for knee osteoarthritis, some evidence suggests that supervised exercise therapy may improve exercise adherence.

9.3.5.2. Physical Measures

The effectiveness of massage therapy cannot be determined due to a lack of evidence. There is conflicting evidence in support of manual therapy. According to a 2015 review, aquatic therapy can be used as an adjuvant treatment for osteoarthritis in the knee and is safe and effective. Since lower extremity arthritis can lead to impaired strength, balance, and position sense, functional, gait, and balance training has been suggested as a means of addressing these impairments, which have been linked to an increased risk of falls in the elderly population. Exercises can have a minor positive impact on hand function, pain, and stiffness in the fingers for those with hand osteoarthritis. According to a study, there is insufficient proof that having weak knee extensor muscles raises the risk of developing osteoarthritis in the knee. Osteoarthritis in the knee may be avoided by strengthening the extensor muscles in the knee.

Neutral and lateral wedge insoles don't seem to be helpful for osteoarthritis of the knee. Knee braces might be helpful, but their value has also been called into question. Heat can be applied to relieve stiffness, and cold can be applied to relieve pain and muscle spasms. Exercise in the water has been shown to temporarily improve quality of life and lessen pain and disability in those with osteoarthritis of the hips and knees. For individuals with osteoarthritis in their knees, therapeutic exercise regimens like aerobics and walking also lessen pain and enhance physical functioning for a maximum of six months following program completion. Researchers found that there was a 16% reduction in functional limitations in cases of knee osteoarthritis for every additional 1,000 steps taken daily in a 2-year study on a group of individuals. Those with osteoarthritis may find hydrotherapy beneficial for managing their pain, disability, and overall quality of life.

9.3.5.3. Thermotherapy

Ice massage was shown to significantly improve range of motion and function, but not necessarily pain relief, in a 2003 Cochrane review of 7 studies conducted between 1969 and 1999. Warm packs did not affect swelling; only cold packs could reduce it. With the potential to cause inflammation and edema, heat therapy may improve circulation and lessen pain and stiffness.

9.3.5.4. Medication

Table 9.4. Treatment Recommendations by Risk Factors

GI Risk	CVD Risk	Option
Low	Low	NSAID, or paracetamol
Moderate	Low	Paracetamol, or low dose NSAID with antacid
Low	Moderate	Paracetamol, or low dose aspirin with an antacid
Moderate	Moderate	Low dose paracetamol, aspirin, and antacid. Monitoring for abdominal pain or black stool.

Source: *https://en.wikipedia.org/wiki/Osteoarthritis.*

9.3.5.4.1. By Mouth

The first line of treatment for osteoarthritis is the painkiller paracetamol (acetaminophen). There is no difference in pain relief based on dosage. A 2015 review, however, discovered that acetaminophen had only a minor short-term benefit and raised some liver inflammation concerns in the lab. Acetaminophen and non-steroidal anti-inflammatory drugs (NSAIDs) like naproxen are equally effective for mild to moderate symptoms; however, NSAIDs may be more effective for more severe symptoms. NSAIDs are linked to more serious adverse effects, like bleeding in the stomach. In comparison to nonselective NSAIDs, COX-2 selective inhibitors, which include celecoxib, are an equally effective class of medication. They also have a lower incidence of adverse gastrointestinal side effects, but a higher incidence of cardiovascular disease, including myocardial infarction. Additionally, their cost is higher than that of generic NSAIDs. When choosing a course of treatment, patients should weigh the benefits and risks associated with each option. More objective research comparing COX-2 selective inhibitors and NSAIDS is required. For a select few, topical NSAIDS applications are successful. Since long-term use of the COX-2 selective inhibitor rofecoxib was linked to cardiovascular events, the drug was taken off the market in 2004. When it comes to managing arthritis on one's own, education can be beneficial. Coping mechanisms that involve education can reduce pain by roughly 20% more than NSAIDs alone.

In cases of osteoarthritis, if the intended level of pain relief is not obtained after two weeks, the dosage and type of painkiller should be reviewed. Oral opioids, encompassing both milder opioids like tramadol and more potent opioids, are frequently administered. The recommendation of opioids is frequently contingent upon the failure or contraindication of first-line therapies, raising questions about their appropriateness. This is because of their negligible benefit and comparatively high risk of adverse effects. Tramadol use probably has no beneficial effects on pain or physical function, and it probably increases the risk of negative side effects. When treating osteoarthritis, oral steroids are not advised. Clinical improvements in function or reduction of joint pain are not linked to the oral use of the antibiotic doxycycline in the treatment of osteoarthritis. Any possible tiny advantage of using doxycycline therapy to treat the narrowing of the joint space is unclear, and any advantages are likely to be outweighed by the negative effects that could occur. According to a 2018 meta-analysis, taking collagen supplements orally to treat osteoarthritis lessens stiffness but has no effect on pain or functional limitation.

9.3.5.4.2. Topical

Diclofenac is one of several NSAIDs that can be applied topically. According to a 2016 Cochrane review, the only application of topical diclofenac and ketoprofen for individuals with painful knee arthritis over 40 years of age is supported by reasonably reliable evidence. Osteoarthritis patients are generally not advised to use transdermal opioid painkillers. It is debatable whether topical capsaicin helps treat osteoarthritis; some reviews found it helpful, while others did not.

9.3.5.4.3. Joint Injections

In ultrasound-guided hip joint injection, the ideal needle entry point is marked with a skin indentation. For knee osteoarthritis sufferers, the use of analgesics, intra-articular cortisone injections, hyaluronic acids, and platelet-rich plasma are advised for pain management. Intra-articular injections for local drug delivery may be safer, more effective, and have higher bioavailability with less systemic exposure and fewer adverse events. The following are some of the intra-articular drugs that are marketed for the treatment of symptoms.

9.3.5.4.4. Steroids

Glucocorticoid injections into the joints, such as hydrocortisone, provide temporary pain relief that lasts a few weeks to several months. According to a 2015 Cochrane review, intra-articular corticosteroid injections of the knee did not improve quality of life or affect knee joint space; however, the quality of the studies included in the review made it difficult to determine the clinical effects one to six weeks after the injection. A 2017 trial demonstrated a decrease in cartilage thickness with intra-articular triamcinolone every 12 weeks for two years compared to placebo, and another 2015 study documented adverse effects of intra-articular corticosteroid injections at higher doses. A 2018 study discovered a correlation between intra-articular triamcinolone and elevated intraocular pressure.

9.3.5.4.5. Hyaluronic Acid

Injections of hyaluronic acid have not produced improvement compared to placebo for knee arthritis, but did increase risk of further pain. In ankle osteoarthritis, evidence is unclear.

9.3.5.4.6. Radiosynoviorthesis

Injection of beta particle-emitting radioisotopes (called *radiosynoviorthesis*) is used for the local treatment of inflammatory joint conditions.

9.3.5.4.7. Platelet-Rich Plasma

The effectiveness of injections of platelet-rich plasma (PRP) is unclear; there are suggestions that such injections improve function but not pain, and are associated with increased risk. A 2014 Cochrane review of studies involving PRP found the evidence to be insufficient.

9.3.5.5. Surgery

9.3.5.5.1. Bone Fusion

Arthrodesis (fusion) of the bones may be an option in some types of osteoarthritis. An example is ankle osteoarthritis, in which ankle fusion is considered to be the gold standard treatment in end-stage cases.

9.3.5.5.2. Joint Replacement

Joint replacement surgery or resurfacing may be advised if the symptoms of osteoarthritis significantly impair quality of life and more conservative management is not working. Joint replacement is clinically and financially beneficial, and the evidence supports this for both the knee and the hip. Individuals who underwent total knee replacement reported better feelings, higher SF-12 quality of life scores, and potential short- and long-term improvements in pain and function related to quality of life. Owing to a variety of external circumstances, comorbidities, and pain in other body parts, the advantages of these surgeries might not last for a long time. Surgical options for individuals with shoulder osteoarthritis who do not respond to medication include total shoulder arthroplasty, which replaces the entire joint, and shoulder hemiarthroplasty, which replaces a portion of the joint. Biological joint replacement is a process in which diseased tissues are replaced with healthy ones. This may come from the patient directly (autograft) or through a donor (allograft). Because the immune responses to bone and cartilage tissues are restricted, immunosuppressants are not necessary for individuals undergoing osteochondral allografts, which is a type of joint transplant. One potential procedure under investigation is the osteochondral autograft transfer system, which involves the transfer of autologous articular cartilage from a non-weight-bearing area to the damaged area.

Autologous chondrocyte implantation is an additional option if the focal defect is caused by missing cartilage.

9.3.5.5.3. Shoulder Replacement

It is occasionally recommended to have a total shoulder replacement for people with osteoarthritis in order to reduce pain and improve function. By 2030, there will be a 750% increase in demand for this treatment. Although there are various options for shoulder replacement surgeries, there is insufficient data in the form of high-quality randomized controlled trials to identify the most effective type of surgery for a given scenario, the risks associated with a given approach, or the procedure's relative effectiveness to other available treatments. Low-quality evidence suggests that there was no significant short-term clinical benefit found when comparing total shoulder arthroplasty to hemiarthroplasty. It is unclear whether a hemiarthroplasty or a total shoulder arthroplasty carries a higher risk of injury.

9.3.5.5.4. Other Surgical Options

Although osteotomy has not been thoroughly studied, it is unclear if it is more effective than other types of surgery or non-surgical treatments for individuals with knee osteoarthritis. Nevertheless, it may be helpful in these cases. In general, arthroscopic surgery is not advised because it may cause harm and has no effect on the course of osteoarthritis in the knee. It is unclear if patients with mild to moderate osteoarthritis in their knees benefit from surgery.

9.3.5.6. Unverified Treatments

9.3.5.6.1. Glucosamine and Chondroitin

There is debate regarding the efficacy of glucosamine. According to reviews, it performs about the same or marginally better than a placebo. It is possible that glucosamine hydrochloride and glucosamine sulfate are different, with the former providing benefits while the latter does not. It is not entirely clear if glucosamine sulfate slows the progression of osteoarthritis, and if it does, the evidence is probably weak. Both the National Institute for Health and Care Excellence and the Osteoarthritis Research Society International advise against using glucosamine if no benefit is seen after six months. Glucosamine is still a treatment option even though its effectiveness is difficult to determine. For knee osteoarthritis, the European Society for Clinical and Economic Aspects of Osteoporosis and Osteoarthritis (ESCEO) suggests glucosamine sulfate and chondroitin sulfate. In most cases, using it as a treatment for osteoarthritis is safe. According to a 2015 Cochrane review, the majority of chondroitin clinical trials were of poor quality, but there was some indication of a temporary reduction in pain and minimal adverse effects; the affected joints' health did not seem to be maintained or improved by the drug.

9.3.5.6.2. Supplements

Avocado-Soybean Unsaponifiables (ASU) is a dietary supplement available globally under various brand names, and in France, it is prescribed medication. It is an extract derived from avocado and soybean oils. ASU may provide some individuals with osteoarthritis with short-term pain relief, but it does not seem to preserve or improve the condition of the afflicted joints, according to a 2014 Cochrane review. According to the review, there was no difference between ASU and chondroitin, an agent with unclear efficacy in osteoarthritis, in a well-conducted two-year clinical trial. Additionally, the review concluded that there is insufficient proof of ASU safety. Boswellia serrata consistently reduces pain and improves function, according to a few excellent studies. Pain relief agents such as s-adenosyl methionine (SAMe), phytodolor, and curcumin may be useful. Since there isn't enough high-quality clinical research to support the effectiveness of SAMe, a 2009 Cochrane review advised against using it on a regular basis. The off-label use of hydroxychloroquine (HCQ) for individuals with hand or knee osteoarthritis should be discouraged, according to a 2021 review, which found that HCQ had no benefit in reducing pain and improving physical function. Colchicine has not been shown to be effective in treating arthritis pain in the hands or knees. The use of hyaluronan, methylsulfonylmethane, rose hip, capsaicin, or vitamin D is not well supported by research.

9.3.5.6.3. Acupuncture and Other Interventions

Although pain relief is improved with acupuncture, this improvement is marginal and may not be significant. Clinically meaningful benefits for peripheral joint osteoarthritis have been observed in waiting list-controlled trials; however, these may be the result of placebo effects. It doesn't appear that acupuncture has any long-term advantages. For the past 20 years, knee osteoarthritis has been treated with electrostimulation methods like TENS. But there isn't enough proof to say that it lessens discomfort or incapacity. While one Cochrane review of low-level laser therapy found no conclusive evidence of benefit, another review of the treatment found temporary relief from knee osteoarthritis. To find out if balnotherapy (mineral baths or spa treatments) for osteoarthritis enhances a person's quality of life or functional capacity, more research is required. It may be helpful to use ice packs or cold compresses, but more research is required. The use of hot packs on joints has not been shown to be beneficial. There is weak evidence to suggest that therapeutic ultrasound may be helpful for individuals with osteoarthritis of the knee; however, more investigation is required to validate and ascertain the extent and importance of this possible benefit (Scott, Wolfe, & Huizinga, 2010).

A Closer Look

Rheumatoid Arthritis: Pathogenesis and Treatment Strategies

Rheumatoid arthritis (RA) is a chronic autoimmune disorder characterized by inflammation of the synovium, the lining of the joints, leading to joint pain, swelling, stiffness, and eventually joint damage and deformity. The pathogenesis of RA involves a complex interplay of genetic, environmental, and immunological factors. Genetic predisposition plays a significant role, with certain genetic variants, particularly within the human leukocyte antigen (HLA) region, increasing susceptibility to RA. Environmental triggers such as infections, smoking, and hormonal changes may also contribute to the development of the disease in genetically predisposed individuals.

In RA, the immune system mistakenly identifies components of the synovium as foreign invaders and launches an inflammatory response, leading to the release of pro-inflammatory cytokines such as tumor necrosis factor-alpha (TNF-alpha), interleukin-1 (IL-1), and interleukin-6 (IL-6). These cytokines promote the recruitment of immune cells to the synovium, where they further perpetuate inflammation and tissue damage, resulting in the destruction of cartilage, bone erosion, and synovial proliferation known as pannus formation.

Treatment strategies for RA aim to achieve remission or low disease activity, alleviate symptoms, prevent joint damage, and improve overall quality of life. Early and aggressive intervention is key to achieving these goals. Nonsteroidal anti-inflammatory drugs (NSAIDs) and corticosteroids are commonly used to reduce pain and inflammation in the short term, but they do not alter the course of the disease or prevent joint damage.

Disease-modifying antirheumatic drugs (DMARDs) are the mainstay of treatment for RA. Traditional DMARDs such as methotrexate, sulfasalazine, and hydroxychloroquine work by suppressing the abnormal immune response and reducing inflammation. Biologic DMARDs, including TNF-alpha inhibitors (e.g., etanercept, infliximab, adalimumab), interleukin-6 (IL-6) inhibitors (e.g., tocilizumab), and other targeted therapies (e.g., rituximab, abatacept), specifically target key molecules involved in the inflammatory cascade, offering more effective disease control and slowing joint damage progression.

In recent years, Janus kinase (JAK) inhibitors have emerged as another class of targeted therapy for RA. These oral medications inhibit the Janus kinase enzymes involved in cytokine signaling pathways, thereby reducing inflammation and joint damage. Tofacitinib and baricitinib are examples of JAK inhibitors approved for the treatment of RA.

In addition to pharmacological interventions, lifestyle modifications such as regular exercise, physical therapy, and joint protection techniques can help improve joint function and reduce pain in RA patients. Patient education and psychological support are also important components of comprehensive RA management, empowering patients to actively participate in their treatment and cope with the challenges of living with a chronic autoimmune disease (Scott, Wolfe, & Huizinga, 2010)

Summary

- Osteoarthritis, the most prevalent form of joint disease, typically occurs with aging or as a result of joint injury or overuse. It involves the gradual breakdown of cartilage, the tissue that cushions the ends of bones within the joint, leading to pain, stiffness, and reduced range of motion.
- Joint disease is any of the diseases or injuries that affect human joints. Arthritis is no doubt the best-known joint disease, but there are also many others.
- Arthritis is a generic term for inflammatory joint disease. Regardless of the cause, inflammation of the joints may cause pain, stiffness, swelling, and some redness of the skin about the joint.
- Inflammation of a synovial bursa, the lubricating sac located over a joint or between tendons and muscles or bones, is called bursitis (or bursal synovitis). Bursas sometimes are affected along with the joints and tendon sheaths in rheumatoid arthritis and gout.
- Joint cartilage may be damaged rapidly by the formation of pus in infections by such bacteria as staphylococci, hemolytic streptococci, and pneumococci. Tuberculosis of the joint can result in extensive destruction of the adjacent bone and open pathways to the skin.
- The collagen diseases are so called because in all of them, abnormalities develop in the collagen-containing connective tissue. These diseases are primarily systemic and are frequently accompanied by joint problems.
- Blunt injuries to joints vary in severity from mild sprains to overt fractures and dislocations. A sprain is ligament, tendon, or muscle damage that follows a sudden wrench and momentary incomplete dislocation (subluxation) of a joint.
- Osteoarthritis is a ubiquitous disorder affecting all adults to a greater or lesser degree by the time they have reached middle age. The name osteoarthritis is a misnomer insofar as its suffix implies that the condition has an inherently inflammatory nature.

References

1. Felson, D. T., & Zhang, Y. (2018). An update on the epidemiology of knee and hip osteoarthritis with a view to prevention. *Arthritis & Rheumatology, 41*(8), 1343–1355. https://doi.org/10.1002/art.40831.
2. Firestein, G. S., Budd, R. C., Gabriel, S. E., McInnes, I. B., & O'Dell, J. R. (2021). *Kelley and Firestein's Textbook of Rheumatology*. Philadelphia, PA: Elsevier.
3. Hochberg, M. C., Silman, A. J., Smolen, J. S., Weinblatt, M. E., & Weisman, M. H. (2014). *Rheumatology*. Philadelphia, PA: Mosby.
4. Klippel, J. H., Stone, J. H., Crofford, L. J., & White, P. H. (2013). *Primer on the Rheumatic Diseases*. New York, NY: Springer.
5. Schumacher Jr., H. R. (2010). *Primer on the Metabolic Bone Diseases and Disorders of Mineral Metabolism*. Hoboken, NJ: Wiley-Blackwell.

6. Scott, D. L., Wolfe, F., & Huizinga, T. W. J. (2010). *Rheumatoid Arthritis*. New York, NY: Oxford University Press.

7. Singh, J. A., & Cleveland, J. D. (2020). *Gout & Other Crystal Arthropathies*. New York, NY: Springer.

8. Smith, H. S. (2017). *Current Therapy in Pain*. Philadelphia, PA: Elsevier.

Chapter

10

SYMPTOMS OF EATING DISORDERS AND WEIGHT PROBLEMS

Contents

Introduction

Weight issues and eating disorders are complicated conditions that can have a major negative impact on a person's physical and mental health. Early intervention and successful treatment for these disorders depend on the ability to recognize their symptoms. Anorexia nervosa, which is typified by a warped body image and an acute fear of gaining weight, is one of the most well-known eating disorders. Anorexics frequently severely restrict their food intake, which causes severe weight loss and malnourishment. To manage their weight, they might also overdo it on their workouts. Its physical manifestations include extreme thinness, exhaustion, lightheadedness, and hair loss. An obsession with food, an obsession with body weight, and social disengagement are examples of psychological symptoms. Bulimia nervosa is another prevalent eating disorder characterized by episodes of binge eating that are followed by purging behaviors like overindulging in exercise, throwing up, or abusing laxatives. Bulimia is more difficult to identify than anorexia because its sufferers may maintain a relatively normal weight. Bulimia can manifest physically as gastrointestinal disorders, dental issues, and swollen glands. Individuals who suffer from bulimia may feel low self-esteem, guilt, and shame psychologically.

The hallmark of binge eating disorder is frequent episodes of heavy food consumption without purging. During these episodes, people with this disorder frequently feel out of control and may eat quickly until they are uncomfortable full. Obesity and conditions like diabetes, heart disease, and elevated blood pressure are linked to binge eating disorder. Emotions of distress regarding eating habits, anxiety, and depression are examples of psychological symptoms.

Weight problems include a broad range of problems relating to body weight and shape, aside from clinical eating disorders. Being obese is defined as having too much body fat, and it is a major global health concern. It raises the risk of a number of illnesses, such as heart disease, type 2 diabetes, and some cancers. A poor diet and sedentary lifestyle are two examples of behavioral, environmental, and genetic factors that can contribute to obesity. Conversely, underweight people may also be at risk for health issues. In particular in children and adolescents, chronic undernourishment can result in nutrient deficiencies, weakened immune systems, and impaired growth and development. Inadequate calorie intake, illnesses, or eating disorders like anorexia nervosa can all lead to underweight.

There are many ways that eating disorders and weight issues present themselves, and they can have a serious negative impact on both mental and physical health. Treating these problems and averting long-term consequences require early identification and action. In order to support healing and recovery, treatment frequently takes a multidisciplinary approach and includes medical, nutritional, and psychological support.

Orientation and Directional Terms

Term	Definition	Illustration
Binge eating disorder	Binge eating disorder is a mental illness that manifests as a behavioral disorder. It causes chronic, compulsive overeating.	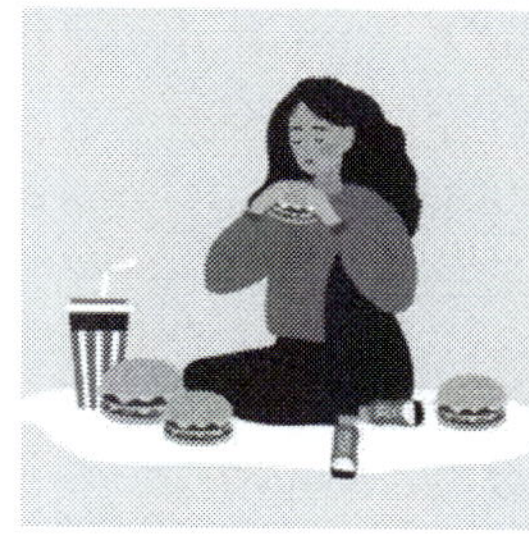
Stereotypes	A stereotype is a generalized belief about a particular category of people. It is an expectation that people might have about every person in a particular group.	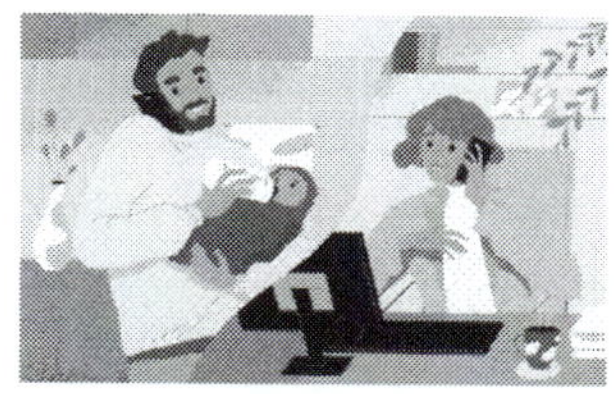
Anorexia nervosa	Anorexia nervosa is also called anorexia. It is a serious medical illness It is not a lifestyle choice. This eating disorder makes you obsess about your weight and food.	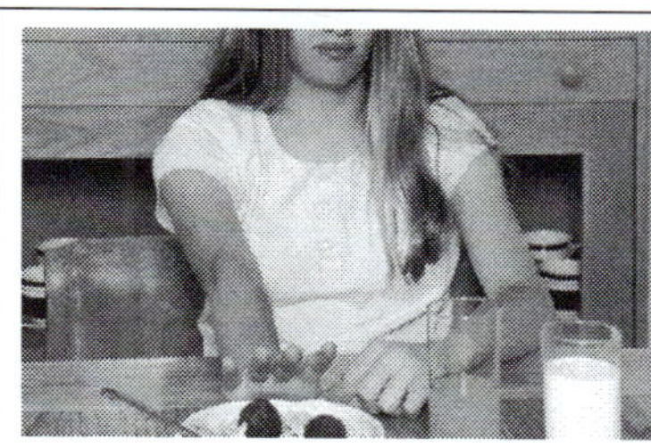
Bulimia	Bulimia is a serious illness that causes severe problems with a person's eating behaviors.	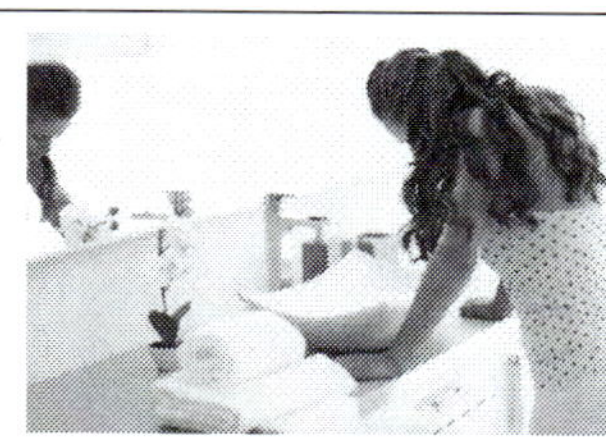
Eating disorders	An eating disorder is a mental disorder defined by abnormal eating behaviors that adversely affect a person's physical or mental health.	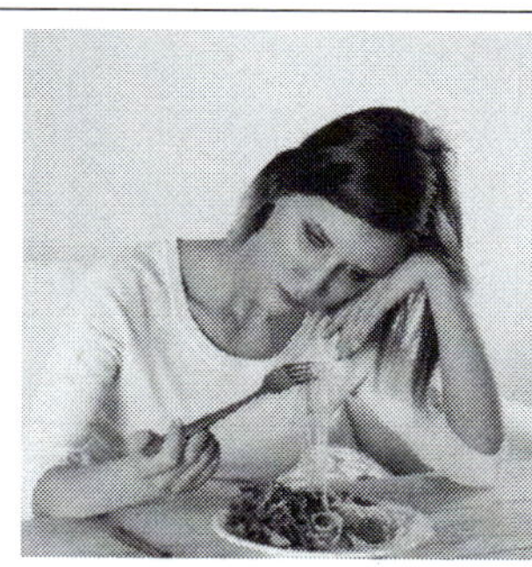

10.1. Overview of Symptoms of Eating Disorders

Complex mental health conditions known as eating disorders are typified by abnormal eating habits that have a detrimental effect on a person's emotional and physical health. These conditions are frequently accompanied by unhealthy eating and food-related behaviors, a skewed perception of one's own body, and intense concern over one's weight and form. Comprehending the indications of eating disorders is essential for prompt intervention and efficacious therapy. One of the most well-known eating disorders is anorexia nervosa. Even though they are severely underweight, anorexics usually have a severe fear of gaining weight or getting fat. To control their weight, they might follow strict eating regimens, drastically reduce their caloric intake, or exercise excessively. Severe weight loss, emaciation, exhaustion, weakness, and amenorrhea (female menstruation absence) are among the physical signs of anorexia. Additionally, they might display behavioral indicators like eating in private, developing eating rituals, and avoiding social settings where food is involved.

Bulimia nervosa is defined by repeated instances of overeating, followed by actions taken to prevent weight gain. Overeating involves consuming a large amount of food in a short period, often feeling like losing control. People with bulimia may resort to purging methods like self-induced vomiting, misusing laxatives or diuretics, fasting, or excessive exercising. Physical signs of bulimia can include swollen glands, teeth enamel erosion, digestive issues, and imbalances in electrolytes. Mentally, those with bulimia might feel ashamed, guilty, and have low self-esteem due to their eating habits.

While bulimia nervosa and binge eating disorder (BED) are similar, BED does not involve the compensatory purging behaviors. BED sufferers usually eat a lot of food quickly, usually in reaction to emotional distress or as a coping mechanism for unpleasant emotions. Anxiety, shame, and guilt are frequently experienced during binge eating episodes. BED sufferers do not frequently engage in inappropriate compensatory behaviors, which can result in substantial weight gain and health issues related to obesity, unlike bulimia sufferers.

Previously known as eating disorder not otherwise specified (EDNOS), other specified feeding or eating disorders (OSFED) cover a spectrum of eating behaviors that do not fit the diagnostic criteria for anorexia, bulimia, or binge eating disorder but nevertheless have a substantial negative impact on an individual's life. Atypical anorexia nervosa, in which patients display anorexic symptoms but do not fit the low weight criteria, purging disorder, in which patients engage in purging behaviors without binge eating, and night eating syndrome, in which patients consume a large portion of their daily food intake at night, are all included in this category.

A relatively recent term, orthorexia nervosa, refers to an obsessive fixation on eating pure or healthful foods to the detriment of one's physical and mental well-being. People who suffer from orthorexia may avoid social situations where food is involved, limit their diet to only foods they believe to be healthy, and feel guilty or anxious when they stray from their eating regimen. Though orthorexia is not officially classified as a separate eating disorder in diagnostic manuals such as the DSM-5, it is similar to other eating disorders in that it is characterized by compulsive food-related thoughts and behaviors. A range of conditions are included in the category of eating disorders, and they are distinguished by disordered eating patterns, skewed body image, and psychological distress. Early intervention and the right kind of treatment depend on the ability to identify the symptoms of these disorders. Given the complexity of eating disorders, a multidisciplinary approach involving medical, nutritional, and psychological support is frequently required to address the condition and aid in healing (Yager et al., 2005; Herpertz-Dahlmann, 2008).

10.1.1. Importance of Eating Disorders

Eating disorders are severe mental illnesses characterized by abnormal eating patterns. This could entail cutting back on food intake, consuming enormous amounts of food at once, or eliminating food that was consumed in an unhealthy way (e.g., purging, abusing laxatives, fasting, or engaging in excessive physical activity), or a mix of these. It is critical to keep in mind that emotions, not just food, play a role in eating disorders. The way a person engages with food may increase their sense of control or ability to cope.

Eating disorders include:

- anorexia
- bulimia
- binge eating disorder

Additionally, "other specified feeding or eating disorder" (OSFED) diagnoses are frequently given to patients. This is simply a case of an eating disorder that does not precisely match the list of symptoms that a specialist will look for in order to diagnose someone with anorexia, bulimia, or binge eating disorder. It is not a less serious form of eating disorder. Since there is frequently significant overlap between various eating disorders, it is also possible for someone to switch between diagnoses if their symptoms change. Making sure the patient is receiving the best care possible for their condition is the goal of diagnosis.

Among all mental illnesses, anorexia has the highest mortality rate. Eating disorders can be extremely harmful and even deadly. However, eating disorders are treatable conditions despite being serious medical conditions. From our daily interactions with those impacted, we at Beat are aware that a full recovery is highly achievable. Recovery from an eating disorder is more likely the earlier it is treated, just like with any other illness. The most crucial thing is to get evaluated and into treatment as soon as possible for yourself or the person you're supporting.

- **Who Gets Eating Disorders?:** Many misconceptions exist regarding the people who can suffer from eating disorders. These can be extremely damaging! It is crucial to keep in mind that there's always a chance that someone may acquire an eating disorder. Anybody, regardless of age, gender, or ethnic or cultural background, can develop an eating disorder, although young women are more likely to do so, especially those between the ages of 12 and 20. It is estimated that approximately 25% of those affected are men. In actuality, the number of victims may be higher than we currently believe among men and boys, the elderly, and members of racial or cultural minorities. This is due to the possibility that these individuals will be less likely to seek assistance for a condition that is already very taboo to discuss.

10.1.2. Types of Eating Disorders

Eating disorders are a group of conditions marked by an unhealthy relationship with food. The main types of eating disorders are:

1. *Anorexia Nervosa:* This is typified by weight loss that is frequently brought on by overindulgent

exercise and dieting, sometimes to the point of starvation. Even after drastically cutting their weight, anorexics believe they will never be thin enough and still consider themselves to be "fat."

2. *Bulimia Nervosa:* A severe, potentially fatal eating disorder marked by a pattern of binge eating followed by self-induced vomiting or other compensatory behaviors meant to counteract the effects of the binge eating. Bulimia nervosa patients experience episodes of binge eating, which is followed by purging (vomiting or taking laxatives), fasting, or excessive exercise to make up for the overindulgence. In contrast to anorexia, bulimia patients frequently maintain a normal weight. However, their distorted body image and severe fear of gaining weight are the same. They fervently want to reduce weight because they perceive themselves as "fat." People who suffer from bulimia often develop an intense ability to conceal their bulimic behaviors because they feel ashamed and disgusted with themselves.

3. *Binge Eating Disorder (BED):* A severe eating disorder marked by frequent episodes of binge eating without the employment of healthy coping mechanisms to regulate weight. Those who suffer from binge eating disorder experience frequent episodes of eating excessive amounts of food, as opposed to simply being overeaters all the time. Similar to bulimics, they frequently experience these episodes feeling out of control, which leads to feelings of guilt and shame afterwards. The more upset they are about bingeing, the more likely they appear to do it, which turns the behavior into a vicious cycle. People who suffer from binge eating disorder are typically overweight or obese because they do not fast, purge, or exercise after their binges. In contrast to other eating disorders, binge eating disorder affects men almost as frequently as it does women. The National Institute of Mental Health reports that binge eating disorder typically manifests at age 25, with a higher incidence in individuals under 60.

4. *Avoidant/Restrictive Food Intake Disorder (ARFID):* A serious eating disorder characterized by eating and feeding disturbances resulting in significant weight loss and other medical complications.

5. *Other Specified Feeding or Eating Disorder (OSFED):* Most people with eating disorders are categorized as OSFED because they do not meet the criteria for anorexia, bulimia, or binge eating disorder. A person must exhibit feeding or eating behaviors that impair functioning in certain areas and cause clinically significant distress in order to be diagnosed with OSFED, even if they do not fully meet the criteria for any other feeding or eating disorder. Then, a diagnosis that identifies a particular explanation for why the presentation does not match the features of another disorder (e.g., bulimia nerveosa: rare cases).

The following are further examples for OSFED:

- **Atypical Anorexia Nervosa:** All criteria are met, except despite significant weight loss, the individual's weight is within or above the normal range.
- **Binge Eating Disorder (of Low Frequency and/or Limited Duration):** All of the criteria for BED are met, except at a lower frequency and/or for less than three months.
- **Bulimia Nervosa (of Low Frequency and/or Limited Duration):** All of the criteria for Bulimia Nervosa are met, except that the binge eating and inappropriate compensatory behavior occurs at a lower frequency and/or for less than three months.
- **Purging Disorder:** Recurrent purging behavior to influence weight or shape in the absence of binge eating
- **Night Eating Syndrome:** Recurrent episodes of night eating. Eating after awakening from sleep, or by excessive food consumption after the evening meal. There is an awareness and recall of the eating. The behavior is not better explained by environmental influences or social norms. The behavior causes significant distress/impairment, and is not better explained by another mental health disorder (e.g., BED).

6. *Rumination Disorder:* After eating, rumination disorder is characterized by frequent regurgitation of food. People who have this illness regurgitate food they have already swallowed into their mouths without showing any symptoms of nausea, vomiting fits, or disgust. After that, the food is usually chewed again, spit out, or swallowed. It is possible to characterize the regurgitating behavior as automatic or uncontrollable. The characteristics of rumination disorder include:

- Repeated regurgitation of food over a period of at least one month
- The repeated regurgitation is not a result of an associated gastrointestinal or other medical condition
- Weight loss and failure to make expected weight gains in children
- Malnutrition
- Attempts to hide the regurgitation behavior by placing a hand over the mouth or coughing
- Avoidance of eating before social situations, such as work or school

It is possible for ruminating disorder to start in early life, childhood, adolescence, or adulthood. Babies that suffer from this condition often strain, arch their back, hold their heads back, and make tongue-sucking motions. Even if a lot of food is consumed, malnutrition can still happen, especially if food is regurgitated and spat out. Like other repetitive motor behaviors (i.e., rumination and regurgitation), it appears that these behaviors serve a self-stimulating or self-soothing purpose in both infants and older individuals with intellectual disabilities. e. head banging and rocking).

7. *Pica:* Eating one or more nonfood, nonnutritive substances on a regular basis is what defines pica. People

who have pica frequently eat things like paper, soap, hair, gum, ice, paint, pebbles, soil, and chalk. Generally speaking, those who have pica do not have a food aversion. The eating of nonfood, nonnutritive substances must occur for at least one month in order to diagnose Pica. PICA is usually not diagnosed in children under two years old in order to rule out the developmentally normal mouthing of objects by babies that could lead to ingestion. Medical issues like intestinal blockage and bowel issues can arise as a result of pica. Infections can also occur if someone eats dirt or excrement. Although the exact prevalence of pica is unknown, individuals with intellectual disabilities are more likely to experience it. Some pregnant women experience pica in response to cravings for particular foods, like ice or chalk (Yager et al., 2005; Herpertz-Dahlmann, 2008).

10.1.3. Causes of Eating Disorders

The development of an eating disorder is a complex process that cannot be explained by a single factor. Numerous variables come together, encompassing genetic, psychological, environmental, social, and biological effects. For the chance of any one person developing the condition to increase, a number of risk factors must come together. Although we are still unsure of the exact causes of eating disorders and which treatments are best for each individual, we do know that there are effective treatments out there. World-class research is being conducted, with a large portion of it taking place in the UK and involving collaboration with global centers of excellence. Because eating disorders are complicated, different people will have different symptoms. Individuals can vary in how they react to treatment and how long it takes them to recover. Some people may experience symptoms from multiple eating disorders, or as they recover, they may experience different types of symptoms. In addition to their eating disorder, people with eating disorders may also struggle with other mental or physical health conditions. These may occasionally develop concurrently with the eating disorder or as a result of it, or they may contribute to its development. In addition to treating eating disorders, medical professionals should consider the patient's overall health.

10.1.3.1. Genetics

Several research indicate that eating disorders may be inherited due to Mendelian inheritance. When examining the various criteria of both bulimia nervosa and anorexia nervosa as endophenotypes contributing to the disorders overall, twin studies have discovered a small amount of genetic variance. A genetic connection has been discovered on a chromosome in several relatives of an anorexic. A person's likelihood of developing an eating disorder is seven to twelve times higher if they are a first-degree relative of someone who has had or is currently suffering from an eating disorder. Additionally, twin studies demonstrate that a hereditary component may contribute to the development of eating disorders, and evidence points to a genetic locus associated with anorexia nervosa susceptibility. Biological and genetic factors account for about 60% of cases of eating disorders. Other cases are brought on by outside factors or issues with development. Binge and purging behaviors may also be caused by other neurobiological variables related to emotional reactivity and impulsivity.

- **Epigenetics:** Through processes like DNA methylation, environmental factors can modify gene expression through epigenetic mechanisms, which are separate from and unaffected by underlying DNA sequence changes. They may happen at any point in a person's life and have the potential to be reversible. They are also inherited. Ethnic mechanisms causing dysregulation of dopaminergic neurotransmission have been linked to a number of eating disorders. According to one study, women with eating disorders have known changes in ANP homeostasis, which may be attributed to epigenetic mechanisms. Additional genes under investigation for epigenetic research on eating disorders are brain-derived neurotrophic factor (BDNF), pro-opiomelanocortin (POMC), and leptin.

10.1.3.2. Psychological

The Diagnostic and Statistical Manual of Mental Health Disorders (DSM-IV), published by the American Psychiatric Association, lists eating disorders as Axis I disorders. Other psychological problems can also contribute to eating disorders; some of these meet the criteria for a diagnosis of their own under Axis I, while others fall under Axis II and are therefore classified as comorbid conditions with eating disorders. Three subtypes of Axis II disorders are distinguished: A, B, and C. It is still unclear if eating disorders and personality disorders are causally related. A prior eating disorder may make some people more susceptible to developing an eating disorder in the future. Some people develop them later. It has been demonstrated that comorbidity is influenced by the type and severity of eating disorder symptoms. Even when used by professionals, there has been significant debate over the diagnostic criteria for a number of diagnoses, including eating disorders, so the DSM-IV should not be used by laypeople to self-diagnose.

10.1.3.3. Personality Traits

The emergence of eating disorders is linked to a number of childhood personality traits. These characteristics may intensify during adolescence as a result of a range of physiological and cultural factors, including the hormonal changes brought on by puberty, the stress of approaching adult demands, and sociocultural factors and perceived expectations, particularly in relation to body image. Mentalization disorders and a brittle sense of self have been linked to eating disorders. Numerous personality traits are highly heritable and have a genetic component. Anoxic or traumatic brain injury, neurodegenerative illnesses like Parkinson's disease, neurotoxicity from lead exposure, bacterial or parasitic infections like Lyme disease or Toxoplasma gondii, and hormonal fluctuations can all result in the acquisition of maladaptive levels of specific traits. These features have been linked to the amygdala and the prefrontal cortex, among other brain regions; research using different imaging modalities, including fMRI, is still ongoing. It has been demonstrated that abnormalities in the prefrontal cortex and executive functioning system influence eating behavior.

10.1.3.4. Celiac Disease

Compared to the general population, people with gastrointestinal disorders may be more susceptible to developing disordered eating behaviors, particularly restrictive eating disturbances. There is evidence linking celiac disease and anorexia nervosa. It appears that gastrointestinal symptoms have a complicated role in the emergence of eating disorders. According to some writers, individuals with unresolved symptoms before being diagnosed with gastrointestinal disease may develop a food aversion and change their eating habits. According to other writers, increased symptoms during the course of their diagnosis increased risk. It has been shown that some sufferers of inflammatory bowel disease, celiac disease, or irritable bowel syndrome decide to eat their trigger foods in order to aid in weight loss because they are unaware of how important it is to adhere to their diet. Conversely, people who maintain a healthy diet may experience anxiety, aversion to certain foods, and eating disorders due to worries about cross-contamination of their food. According to some authors, medical professionals should assess whether any patient with an eating disorder has an undiagnosed case of celiac disease, particularly if they exhibit any gastrointestinal symptoms (e.g., decreased appetite, bloating, distension, vomiting, diarrhea, or constipation), weight loss, or growth failure. They should also routinely inquire about dieting, vomiting for weight control, or concerns about weight or body shape in order to assess the possibility of eating disorders, particularly in women.

10.1.3.5. Environmental Influences

10.1.3.5.1. Child Maltreatment

It has been demonstrated that child abuse, which includes neglect and physical, psychological, and sexual abuse, roughly triples the risk of eating disorders. The risk of bulimia appears to be roughly doubled by sexual abuse; the correlation with anorexia is less clear.

10.1.3.5.2. Social Isolation

It has been demonstrated that social isolation negatively impacts a person's mental and physical health. Individuals with established social relationships tend to have a lower mortality rate than those who are socially isolated. Individuals with pre-existing medical or mental health conditions have a significantly higher mortality rate; this effect has been observed more in cases of coronary heart disease.

The level of risk linked to social isolation is on par with the risk associated with smoking cigarettes and other significant biomedical and psychosocial risk factors. Being alone can naturally cause stress, depression, and anxiety. An individual may engage in emotional eating, wherein food is used as a comfort, in an effort to lessen these upsetting feelings. Binge eating has also been linked to the loneliness of social isolation and the stressors that come with it as triggers.

10.1.3.5.3. Parental Influence

It has been demonstrated that parental influence plays a fundamental role in how children develop their eating behaviors. Numerous diverse factors, including familial genetic predisposition, dietary choices influenced by cultural or ethnic preferences, the parents' own body type and eating habits, their level of involvement and expectations regarding their children's eating behavior, and the interpersonal relationship between parent and child, all manifest and shape this influence. This is in addition to the overall psychosocial atmosphere of the house and whether a stable, nurturing environment exists or not. Research has demonstrated the significant contribution of maladaptive parental behavior to the emergence of eating disorders. Regarding the more nuanced facets of parental influence, research indicates that eating habits are formed in early life and that, as early as age two, children should be given the freedom to determine when they are full. Research has demonstrated a clear connection between parental pressure to eat more and obesity.

Dietary coercion has not been shown to be an effective means of regulating a child's eating habits. Studies have demonstrated that a child's level of pickiness and their willingness to try a more diverse diet are influenced by affection and attention.

Research has indicated that parents' perceptions of their child's body are shaped by stereotypes. The way these unfavorable stereotypes are presented has an impact on the child's satisfaction with and body image. An expert in the field of eating disorder research claims that girls who are high achievers, obedient, and constantly trying to please their parents are at risk of developing anorexia nervosa. Daughters are unable to accept their own feelings and desires because their parents tend to be overly controlling and do not support emotional expression. Adolescent girls in these controlling households are unable to be independent from them even though they know they should, which frequently leads to rebellion. They may feel more in control of their eating because it gives them a sense of control.

10.1.3.5.4. Cultural Pressure

Particularly in western society, there is a cultural emphasis on thinness. A child's perception of outside pressure to attain the ideal body that the media portrays is a predictor of eating disorders, body dysmorphic disorder, and unsatisfactory body image. One significant risk factor for eating disorders is the cultural pressure placed on both men and women to be "perfect." Furthermore, eating disorders become more common when women of all races base their self-evaluation on the culturally idealized body. Non-Western nations where thinness is not viewed as the ideal are seeing an increase in eating disorders, indicating that social and cultural pressures are not the only factors contributing to eating disorders. Anorexia, for instance, has been observed in every non-Western region of the world, indicating that the disorder is not as culturally restricted as previously believed. Studies on bullemia rates, however, indicate that the condition may be culturally specific. Although bulimia is less common than anorexia in non-Western nations, it can be assumed that these nations have undoubtedly been exposed to or impacted by Western ideology and culture.

Socioeconomic status (SES) has been considered a risk factor for eating disorders because it is assumed that having more resources enables one to consciously decide to diet and lose weight. Additionally, some research has linked rising SES to rising levels of body dissatisfaction. But after achieving a high socioeconomic status, this relationship becomes weaker and sometimes even disappears.

Apart from socioeconomic status, the realm of sports is also regarded as a cultural risk factor. Eating disorders and athletes often coexist, particularly in sports where weight is a competitive factor. This category includes weight-dependent sports like body building, dancing, horseback riding, gymnastics, and wrestling. Competitive athletes, particularly women, are more likely to suffer from eating disorders, which can cause biological and physical changes related to weight that are similar to prepubescent phases. Women frequently lose their competitive edge as their bodies change, which pushes them to take drastic measures to keep their younger body shape. In an attempt to gain muscle rather than lose fat, men frequently struggle with binge eating followed by excessive exercise; however, the desire to gain muscle is just as much an eating disorder as the obsession with thinness.

The estimated percentage of athletes that struggle with eating disorders based on the category of sport.

- Aesthetic sports (dance, figure skating, gymnastics) – 35%
- Weight dependent sports (judo, wrestling) – 29%
- Endurance sports (cycling, swimming, running) – 20%
- Technical sports (golf, high jumping) – 14%

- Ball game sports (volleyball, soccer) - 12%

Some of these athletes use exercise to maintain their weight and figure, but the majority turn to eating disorders in an attempt to maintain their competitive edge. This is equally as serious as controlling nutrition in order to compete. Despite conflicting data regarding the threshold for eating disorder diagnosis in athletes, research indicates that all athletes, regardless of level of competition, are more likely than non-athletes to suffer from eating disorders, particularly those who play sports where being thin is a factor.

Societal pressures within the homosexual community contribute to a higher risk of eating disorder symptoms in homosexual men compared to heterosexual men. In the gay culture, muscularity is associated with social and sexual desirability as well as power. This pressure to have a thin or muscular body to attract potential partners can lead to the development of eating disorders. Individuals with higher eating disorder symptom scores are more concerned about how others perceive them and engage in more frequent and excessive exercise. Body dissatisfaction is also linked to external motivation for working out and is more prevalent among younger homosexual males striving for a thin and muscular physique.

Understanding some of the restrictions and difficulties associated with numerous research attempts to investigate the functions of culture, ethnicity, and SES is crucial. First off, it should be noted that the majority of cross-cultural research employ DSM-IV-TR definitions, which have come under fire for being perceived as having a Western cultural bias. As a result, certain cultural variations linked to various disorders may not be picked up by tests and questionnaires. Furthermore, not many studies have tried to quantify the extent to which people living in areas potentially impacted by Western culture have assimilated into mainstream society or maintained the traditional cultural values of their community (Yager et al., 2005; Herpertz-Dahlmann, 2008).

10.1.4. Diagnosis of an Eating Disorder

A variety of experts, including doctors and mental health specialists like social workers, psychologists, and psychiatrists, can diagnose eating disorders. A pediatrician or family practice physician may make an eating disorder diagnosis based on symptoms observed during routine examinations or inquiries from the patient or parent. Sometimes a patient or family member will schedule an assessment with a mental health professional because they are concerned. Eating disorders can cause a person to overeat or undereat. They might also be obsessed with their weight or form.

There are four main types of eating disorders:

i. **Anorexia Nervosa:** People with this condition don't eat enough. And they may have an extremely thin appearance.

ii. **Bulimia Nervosa:** People with this condition overeat and then purge to avoid gaining weight. They may also abuse laxatives and diet pills.

iii. **Binge Eating:** People with this condition eat uncontrollably and don't purge.

iv. **Other Specified Feeding or Eating Disorder (OSFED):** This condition was originally called "eating disorders not otherwise specified" (EDNOS).

It is unclear what specifically causes eating disorders. However, the illness can be caused by a number of factors. Teenage and early adulthood can be the onset years for eating disorders. These days, a lot of people are preoccupied with how they see themselves. Additionally, the illness may run in families. An eating disorder is more likely in people with certain emotional disorders, such as depression and obsessive-compulsive disorder. Substance abuse disorders can lead to severe and potentially fatal consequences.

Therefore, it is critical to seek treatment for these conditions. However, a physician must first diagnose an eating disorder in order to begin treatment.

Certain people might contest an issue. However, some signs may indicate that a person has a food problem. Physicians diagnose eating disorders based on psychological and physical examinations. Additionally, they will confirm that you fit the diagnostic requirements for an eating disorder.

10.1.4.1. Physical Evaluations

10.1.4.1.1. Physical Exam

During a physical exam, your doctor will check your height, weight, and vital signs. Your doctor will also listen to your lungs and heart since eating disorders can cause:

- high or low blood pressure
- slow breathing
- slow pulse rates

Your doctor may examine your abdomen. They may also check your skin and hair for dryness, or look for brittle nails. And they may ask about any other possible problems, like a sore throat or intestinal issues. These can be complications of bulimia.

10.1.4.1.2. Laboratory Tests

Eating disorders can damage the body and cause problems with vital organs. So, doctors may run lab tests, including:

- a complete blood count
- liver, kidney, and thyroid function tests
- urinalysis

Your doctor may also order an X-ray to look for broken bones, which can be a sign of bone loss from anorexia or bulimia. And an electrocardiogram can check your heart irregularities. Your doctor may also examine your teeth for signs of decay. This is another symptom of an eating disorder.

10.1.4.2. Psychological Evaluations

Doctors don't diagnose eating disorders based on a physical exam. A psychological evaluation by a mental health doctor is also required.

- Your mental health doctor will ask you questions about your eating habits. The goal is to understand your attitude toward food and eating. The doctor also needs to get an idea of how you perceive your body.
- The questions can be personal, especially when talking about dieting, binging, purging, or extreme exercise habits. It is important to answer honestly so your doctor can make an accurate diagnosis and recommend a treatment plan.

10.1.4.3. Reviewing Diagnostic Criteria for Eating Disorders

To be diagnosed with an eating disorder, you must meet the criteria for a specific type of disorder. Symptoms of eating disorders vary depending on the type of eating disorder. They may include:

1. Anorexia Nervosa
    - thin appearance

- insomnia
- extreme tiredness
- dizziness or fainting spells
- bluish nails
- brittle hair and nails
- constipation
- dry skin
- irregular heart rhythm

2. Bulimia Nervosa
    - fear of gaining weight
    - extreme use of weight loss supplements
    - forced vomiting
    - extreme exercising
    - regularly using laxatives, diuretics, or enemas
3. Binge Eating
    - eating unusually large portions of food
    - eating until uncomfortably full
    - insistence on eating alone
    - constantly dieting but not losing weight
    - depression and anxiety

10.1.5. Warning Signs of an Eating Disorder

There are many different ways that anorexia nervosa, bulimia, and overeating disorders can present with signs, symptoms, and causes. Anorexia and bulimia are also closely linked to a number of other eating and body image disorders, such as orthorexia, body dysmorphic disorder, and exercise addiction. Many eating disorder sufferers have overwhelming internal feelings that drive them to rely on symptoms to manage severe pain, anxiety, or other troubling emotions, even though they do not exhibit any outward symptoms. Eating disorders are neither a sign of vanity nor a stage of adolescence. At the first indication of symptoms, it is imperative that an eating disorder sufferer seek medical attention. Based on research, the best clinical outcomes are achieved with early and sufficient intervention.

An individual with disordered eating behaviors is unable to lead a complete life and obstructs their ability to experience healthy emotional, social, and spiritual development. These efforts to "eat healthy" are not "normal," and professional treatment for eating disorders is necessary.

Behaviors associated with eating disorders may include:

- Constant adherence to increasingly strict diets, regardless of weight
- Habitual trips to the bathroom immediately after eating
- Secretly bingeing on large amounts of food
- Hoarding large amounts of food
- Increase in consumption of laxatives, diuretics or diet pills
- Exercising compulsively, often several hours per day
- Using prescription stimulant medications (like Adderall) and/or illicit stimulant drugs (like cocaine) to suppress appetite

Despite different symptoms, eating disorders share common roots that depend on genetics, environmental factors, medical history, life experiences, and the presence of co-occurring psychiatric and addictive disorders. Common signs of the emotional changes associated with having an eating disorder are:

- Withdrawal from friends and family, particularly following questions about her disease or visible physical/medical side effects

- Avoidance of meals or situations where food may be present
- Preoccupation with weight, body size and shape, or specific aspects of one's appearance
- Obsessing over calorie intake and calories burned via exercise, even as one may be losing significant amounts of weight

10.1.5.1. Self-Injury / Self-Harm

The intentional, direct injury of bodily tissue, usually without suicidal intent, is referred to as self-injurious behavior. In the ED, self-harm that is not fatal is common—roughly 25% of cases. Self-harm typically first manifests between the ages of 12 and 24 and is most prevalent in adolescence and early adulthood. Roughly 25% of eating disorder sufferers who also self-harm also fit the profile for borderline personality disorder.

To effectively treat co-occurring disorders, management and prevention of eating disorder behaviors are typically required. It is ineffective to pursue treatment for anxiety or depression on its own while abusing one's eating disorder. Additionally, balanced eating and a sufficient nutritional intake may occasionally be very helpful in reducing the symptoms of other behavioral disorders like depression (Yager et al., 2005; Herpertz-Dahlmann, 2008).

10.1.6. Eating Disorders and Common Co-Occurring Disorders

When an individual is impacted by two or more psychiatric disorders simultaneously, this is known as co-occurring disorders or dual diagnoses. If an eating disorder occurs alongside another diagnosis and is not recognized or treated, it can hinder the recovery process and lead to relapses. Proper evaluation and evidence-based treatment that is personalized to the individual's specific needs is essential for managing co-occurring disorders. This can be especially challenging when eating disorders are involved, as malnourishment and low body weight can exacerbate psychiatric symptoms that may resemble anxiety and depression.

We offer comprehensive evaluations at the Center for Eating Disorders, including formal psychological testing when required, in order to accurately identify and rule out co-occurring disorders. Ensuring that a person's treatment plan can effectively address any intersection of co-occurring disorders and promote holistic healing requires taking this necessary step.

Some of the most common co-occurring disorders in individuals with eating disorders include:

- **Depression:** The majority of studies suggest that between 50 and 75% of individuals with eating disorders will go through a major depressive episode at some point in their lives. Nonetheless, it is still unknown what percentage of major depressive disorder diagnoses can be attributed to starvation rather than an independent disorder because malnourishment can exacerbate depressive symptoms. It is crucial to remember that people who have eating disorders and a history of depression may also be more vulnerable to suicide.
- **Anxiety Disorders:** Approximately two-thirds of individuals with eating disorders will experience one or more anxiety disorders in their lifetime. Common anxiety disorders that co-occur with eating disorders include Obsessive Compulsive Disorder (OCD) and Social Phobia. Other anxiety disorders that may

co-occur are Generalized Anxiety Disorder, specific phobias, and PTSD. Research indicates that early-onset anxiety disorders could be a potential risk factor for the development of anorexia nervosa and bulimia nervosa in the future.

- **Post-Traumatic Stress Disorder (PTSD):** The prevalence of eating disorders and trauma together is high. Anxiety disorders such as post-traumatic stress disorder (PTSD) can arise after being exposed to a traumatic event that puts your safety in jeopardy or leaves you feeling powerless. Natural disasters, military conflict, and sexual or physical abuse are examples of such occurrences. For additional information on trauma symptoms and our specialized treatment plan for patients with co-occurring eating disorders and trauma disorders, click this link.
- **Alcoholism / Substance Abuse**

  The Center for Eating Disorders offers a specialty treatment track for individuals with both substance use disorders and eating disorders, as it is vital to address both issues together. Approximately half of those with eating disorders also experience substance abuse disorders.
- **Borderline Personality Disorder (BPD):** One of the many personality disorders that can affect and interfere with a person's day-to-day activities is borderline personality disorder (BPD). It is linked to issues with self-image, emotion regulation, impulsive behavior, interpersonal relationship issues, and thought changes brought on by stress. Approximately 6–11% of individuals with eating disorders also have BPD, which is a slightly higher rate than the 2-4% of the general population. On the other hand, eating disorders are more common in those with BPD; according to one study, 53.8% of patients with BPD also satisfied the criteria for an eating disorder.

10.1.7. Specialized Treatment Tracks: The Right Therapy for Each Patient

Providing targeted, efficient therapy that is appropriate for each patient is the aim of treatment at The Center for Eating Disorders. This entails depending on solid research and therapies that are supported by evidence and linked to long-term, successful recovery outcomes. It also entails making use of those therapies and putting them to specific uses based on the goals and strengths that are particular to each person.

10.1.7.1. Individual Therapy Tracks

All patients in higher levels of care are guided along one of five targeted therapy paths or a combination of them, that best supports their unique treatment goals after a thorough intake evaluation, feedback from the treatment team, and input from the individual and family. Throughout the hospital stay, individual therapy sessions are guided by the path that has been identified.

The five tracks include:

i. Symptom Management

ii. Body image and self-esteem

iii. Motivation for change

iv. Interpersonal difficulties

v. Emotion regulation

It is the goal for every patient to cultivate an undestanding of the development, maintenance and purpose of their eating disorder regardless of the identified therapeutic track.

10.1.7.2. Dual Diagnosis: Specialty Treatment Tracks

It is not uncommon for people who suffer from eating disorders to also experience co-occurring disorders like mood and personality disorders, anxiety and depression, or both. At The Center for Eating Disorders, co-occurring disorders, also known as "dual diagnoses," are directly addressed at every stage of treatment because they frequently impact the thoughts and symptoms of eating disorders. Furthermore, we provide two specialized treatment tracks in the inpatient and partial hospital programs to assist people who have an eating disorder in addition to trauma and/or substance abuse disorders.

10.1.7.2.1. Substance Abuse Disorders

Substance abuse disorders involve maladaptive patterns of substance use that lead to significant impairment or distress in one or more of the following ways:

- A failure or inability to fulfill major role obligations at work, school or home
- Recurrent use of a substance in situations that would be hazardous such as while driving, supervising small children, or operating machinery
- Recurrent substance-related legal problems
- Continuing to use a substance despite persistent interpersonal or social problems that result from using the substance

Substance abuse and eating disorders are similar in that people frequently struggle mightily to abstain from the substance or behavior, even when doing so has detrimental social, physical, and psychological effects. Illegal substances and the misuse or abuse of over-the-counter and prescription medication are two factors that can contribute to substance abuse disorders.

These are just some of the common drugs of abuse:

- Alcohol
- Nicotine
- Inhalants
- Marijuana
- Club drugs (i.e., Ecstasy, LSD, PCP)
- Heroin
- Cocaine
- Depressants
- Anabolic Steroids
- Caffeine
- Diet Pills
- Diuretics
- Laxatives
- Prescription Medications
- Over-the-counter medications

Laxative and diuretic abuse is a fairly common occurrence in people with eating disorders. Misguided beliefs that these substances will aid in weight loss are frequently the starting point for their use. These drugs not only don't work to help people lose weight, but abusing them can lead to some extremely serious health issues, including increased bloating, weight gain, and chronic abdominal pain. Abuse of these substances frequently results in physical dependency, as is the case with many of the substances mentioned above. The cycle of addiction and abuse intensifies as the body grows tolerant to the substance and a greater quantity is needed to produce the same effects.

10.1.7.2.2. Dual Diagnosis: Eating Disorders and Substance Abuse

Roughly 50% of people who suffer from eating disorders also have a substance use disorder. Although bulimia nervosa sufferers and those who engage in binge/purge behaviors are most at risk for substance use disorders, substance abuse can coexist with any kind of eating disorder. Diverse viewpoints exist regarding the similarities and causes of these two disorders co-occurring so frequently. Both substance abuse and eating disorders are typically regarded as bio psychosocial illnesses, which means that a variety of factors, such as biology, personality traits, social experiences, family history, and culture, may contribute to their development. Examining the unique and personal elements that may be causing the person's illnesses may be a step in the recovery process for both disorders.

It is crucial to comprehend how the two disorders interact throughout this healing process. For instance, substance abuse frequently exacerbates innate personality traits like impulsivity and mood instability, which can exacerbate the difficulties associated with eating disorder recovery. In patients with eating disorders, substance abuse exacerbates the neurological, gastrointestinal, hepatic, and cardiovascular effects of malnutrition. Additionally, there is a significant risk of symptom substitution for people who receive treatment for eating disorders without also receiving treatment for substance abuse, or vice versa. When a person is able to avoid acting on eating disorder symptoms but increases substance use as a coping mechanism for feelings or situations that used to trigger eating disorder behaviors, it can lead to symptom substitution, or moving from one problematic behavior to another. This can happen during the recovery process. The substitution of symptoms can pose substantial obstacles to the healing process. At The Center for Eating Disorders, we support the growth of constructive coping mechanisms and resources so that people can treat their eating disorders and substance abuse at the same time.

10.1.7.2.3. PTSD and Trauma Symptoms

Any traumatic event that puts your safety in jeopardy or leaves you feeling helpless can lead to the development of post-traumatic stress disorder, or PTSD. It is common for someone to experience fear, sadness, anxiety, or even numbness following a traumatic event. With time, these emotions usually pass and one can resume their regular activities. But occasionally, trauma can be so severe that the distressing emotions persist and worsen to the point where they seriously disrupt daily life and keep the victim mired in the traumatic event. Risky eating disorder behaviors are frequently adopted by people with PTSD as a coping mechanism for these upsetting memories.

Some of the signs and symptoms of PTSD are:

- Intrusive, upsetting memories of the event
- Flashbacks and/or Nightmares
- Feelings of intense distress when reminded of the trauma
- Intense physical reactions to reminders of the event (e.g., pounding heart, rapid breathing, nausea, muscle tension, sweating)
- Avoiding activities, places, thoughts, or feelings that remind you of the trauma

- Inability to remember important aspects of the trauma
- Loss of interest in activities or life in general
- Feeling detached from others and emotionally numb
- Sense of a limited future
- Difficulty falling or staying asleep
- Irritability or outbursts of anger
- Difficulty concentrating
- Hypervigilance (on constant "red alert")
- Feeling jumpy and easily startled
- Anger and irritability
- Guilt, shame, or self-blame
- Substance abuse
- Feelings of mistrust and betrayal
- Depression and hopelessness
- Suicidal thoughts and feelings
- Feeling alienated and alone
- Physical aches and pains

10.1.7.2.4. Eating Disorder and Effects of Trauma

The foundation of trauma treatment is empirically supported techniques that adhere to consensus recommendations from experts. That is to say, trauma treatment is predicated on an approach that emphasizes the significance of biological, psychological, and social factors, just like the treatment of eating disorders in general.

In addition to receiving individualized eating disorder interventions, The Center's trauma specialty track offers the following therapeutic components:

- Specific CBT-based trauma work during individual psychotherapy
- Weekly participation in trauma group therapies including psychoeducation, skills training and art therapy.
- Individualized nutritional counseling around trauma-related fear of foods
- Daily psychiatric assessment and treatment of trauma symptomatology.
- Individualized trauma work during art therapy and other expressive therapies
- All individual and group trauma work is specially tailored to address the individual's age and developmental needs.

Like all patients in the program, the therapy focus will be decided upon with consideration for each patient's unique needs while keeping the trauma in perspective. Furthermore, it should be mentioned that the aim of individual therapy for all patients, irrespective of their course of treatment, is to reduce and eradicate eating disordered behaviors while fostering an understanding of the genesis, maintenance, and purpose of their eating disorder. Understanding the significance of the trauma on a personal level must therefore be a part of the unique conceptualization of the eating disorder. Additionally, managing the symptoms of an eating disorder and trauma happens simultaneously.

Overall, the therapy will allow for an understanding of the links in meaning between the trauma and the eating disorder while developing and practicing adaptive coping skills. At the Center for Eating Disorders, trauma therapy is CBT-based and includes the following 5 stages:

- **Stage 1:** Education about trauma symptoms and reactions

- **Stage 2:** Learning about and practicing behavioral coping skills such as grounding, containment, stimulus control, distraction and stress management
- **Stage 3:** Identification and modification of thoughts related to the trauma that are perpetuating symptoms
- **Stage 4:** Identification of core assumptions and beliefs related to the trauma
- **Stage 5:** Restoration of functional beliefs and adaptive coping patterns.

10.1.8. Connection Between Eating Disorders and Infertility

10.1.8.1. The Power of Nourishment

It is common knowledge that a person's ability to conceive is greatly influenced by their diet—that is, what they eat—and nutrition—what they get from eating. One of the most effective lifestyle adjustments a man or woman can make to increase fertility, reduce the risk of miscarriage, and have a healthy pregnancy is to feed the body properly. Consuming a "fertility diet" before becoming pregnant is not unusual, and many medical professionals advise it as a way to assist the body's reproductive processes.

Infertility affects about 1 million married women in the United States between the ages of 15 and 44, according to the Centers for Disease Control and Prevention (CDC), despite the growing awareness of fertility treatments and prenatal care. The inability to become pregnant after a year of trying to conceive is referred to as infertility. It is perhaps not surprising that there is a connection between eating disorders and infertility given the relationship between dietary intake and fertility.

Devastating mental illnesses known as eating disorders are characterized by significant disruptions in eating patterns and/or weight control. In addition to the many psychological, physical, and emotional repercussions these disorders are linked to, one important health effect is reproductive system damage.

Regardless of the type of eating disorder, it is not uncommon for individuals who struggle with an eating disorder or disordered eating tendencies to experience the following complications with reproductive health:

- Amenorrhea, or an abnormal absence of menstruation
- Oligomenorrhea, or infrequent menstrual periods
- Failure to ovulate
- Low egg or sperm production
- Reduced sex drive
- Higher risk of developing Polycystic Ovarian Syndrome (PCOS)

The reproductive system is clearly weakened in these circumstances, which could raise the risk of infertility. Not only can eating disorders have detrimental physical effects, but their correlates, such as stress, anxiety, and depression, can also be harmful to fertility. Sadly, some people who battle eating disorders are unaware of these repercussions until they encounter difficulties attempting to conceive.

It is important to remember that people who are battling eating disorders can still become pregnant, even though it might be more difficult in the situations listed above. Research indicates that eating disordered women are among the most likely to become pregnant unintentionally, possibly as a result of the myth that ovulation cannot occur without menstruation. To minimize complications for both the mother and the fetus, those who do become pregnant while their eating disorder is still active should seek out additional support from medical professionals right away.

10.1.8.2. The Power of Healing

Up to 80% of women who recover from eating disorders are able to conceive, despite the concerning risks to reproductive health that may arise from being in the grip of an eating disorder. Periods can return to normal after recovery, and fertility issues may persist, illustrating the body's amazing resiliency.

Pregnancy has far better odds when there is a healthy relationship with food, the soul, and oneself. Infertility and eating disorders are associated with a great deal of social stigma and shame, which may prevent people from seeking treatment. When thinking about becoming a parent, it is important to be open and honest with your medical professionals about your healing process so that you can get the right care before, during, and after pregnancy. Certain eating disorder-related problems, like body dissatisfaction or fear of gaining weight, frequently resurface. However, pregnancy can also improve a person's attitude and sense of appreciation for their body and self for some eating disorder survivors (Yager et al., 2005; Herpertz-Dahlmann, 2008).

10.1.9. Postpartum Depression Can Increase the Risk of an Eating Disorder

Postpartum depression (PPD) raises awareness of a distressing illness that many new mothers frequently experience in private. After giving birth to her daughter, a 31-year-old mother is just one of many women who will struggle with postpartum depression. One in seven mothers will receive a diagnosis of PPD, a serious mental health illness that can cause severe symptoms of anxiety and depression, according to Postpartum Support International.

10.1.9.1. Understanding Postpartum Depression

Some of the symptoms related to PPD and anxiety include but are not limited to:

- Feeling irritable or angry with those around you
- Having difficulty bonding with your baby
- Experiencing feelings of anxiousness or panic
- Feeling depressed and sad
- Having difficulty eating and/or sleeping
- Ideations or intentions of hurting yourself or your baby

Unfortunately, a lot of recently arrived mothers may mistake these indications or symptoms for a lack of maternal competence; however, PPD is a legitimate mental health condition for which there are useful and successful treatments. The experience of PPD can act as a stressor for newlyweds who have previously battled eating disorders or have a history of disordered eating, potentially leading to the recurrence of an eating disorder. PPD can increase a woman's risk of resuming abnormal and compensatory behaviors with food and body, even after years of remission from eating disorders.

10.1.9.2. Connection between Postpartum Depression and Eating Disorders

The Eating Disorder Program discovered that roughly 35% of women who received treatment for anxiety in different studies had previously struggled with an eating disorder. Eating disorders are thought to be a risk factor during pregnancy, and the postpartum and pregnancy years can be extremely vulnerable for women, particularly those who have a history of mental health problems. Mothers are dealing with biological, emotional, and environmental changes, all of which have the potential to set off triggers for a mother who is predisposed to mental illness.

10.1.9.3. Effective Treatment and Intervention

Undiagnosed and untreated PPD can have serious repercussions for the mother and her family as a whole. Establishing proper treatment for moms with mental health issues is a crucial first step in creating effective interventions, as children of mothers with active eating disorders may be more likely to experience eating disorders themselves. Regular prenatal and postpartum screenings can give doctors and midwives a valuable window of time to look for a history of mental illness. When an eating disorder is detected in a pregnant woman, medical professionals can support early treatment approaches that could break a recurrent cycle.

Because women are typically motivated to make the necessary changes that will support healthy outcomes for their babies, pregnancy is often an ideal time to intervene with treatment that will help improve the prognosis for both the mother and the baby. Including mental health services in routine prenatal health screenings can also assist medical professionals in determining the likelihood of PPD and/or pregnancy-related depression. Pregnant women with a history of eating disorders who are aware of their increased risk of developing postpartum depression (PPD) can set up prenatal protocols, such as working with a support group or consulting a therapist, to better support them after giving birth.

Speak with your doctor and/or treatment team about proactive measures you can take to make sure you and your child receive support during the postpartum phase of your motherhood journey if you are a woman with a history of eating disorders and are currently pregnant (Yager et al., 2005; Herpertz-Dahlmann, 2008).

10.2. Weight Problems of Eating Disorders

Eating disorders such as anorexia nervosa, bulimia nervosa, and binge eating disorder all involve unhealthy relationships with food, which can lead to serious weight problems. Anorexia often involves restricting food intake to dangerous levels, resulting in severe underweight and malnutrition. Bulimia consists of cycles of binge eating followed by purging behaviors, which can cause weight fluctuations and potential harm to organs. Binge eating disorder is characterized by consuming large amounts of food in short periods, often leading to obesity and health issues. These disorders not only impact physical health but also mental and emotional well-being, requiring comprehensive treatment that addresses both the body and mind.

It is common for the majority of us to occasionally gain or lose weight. Some individuals with eating disorders, like bulimia or anorexia nervosa, develop a major medical problem related to their obsession with weight.

Signs and symptoms of eating or weight problems include:

1. Extreme thirst, dehydration, or hunger
2. Losing weight without trying or abnormal weight loss
3. Desire to binge on food excessively
4. Desire to vomit on purpose
5. Desire to starve (not eat at all)
6. A preoccupation with food and weight

7. Distorted body image
8. Excessive fear of gaining weight
9. Refusing to eat or eating tiny portions or eating alone
10. Compulsive exercise
11. Sensitivity to cold
12. Menstruation ceases
13. Abuse of laxatives, diuretics, or diet pills
14. Depression

Eating disorders are extremely dangerous and can cause fatalities as well as serious medical complications. Speak with a medical professional about your problems with food and weight, or seek assistance if a loved one has these problems. You might also need to see a dietitian, a psychiatrist, and an eating disorder therapist in addition to a physician who specializes in treating eating disorders.

10.2.1. Extreme Thirst, Dehydration, or Hunger

Severe thirst, dehydration, or hunger may indicate a variety of medical issues, ranging from mild to severe. These symptoms can point to problems with fluid balance, blood sugar levels, or underlying health conditions. Extreme thirst, dehydration, and hunger are often connected, as they can stem from imbalances in the body's regulatory systems. Polydipsia, or extreme thirst, is a feeling of needing more fluids than usual and can be a sign of conditions like diabetes mellitus or diabetes insipidus. In diabetes mellitus, high blood sugar levels can lead to increased thirst as the body attempts to dilute excess glucose by pulling water from tissues. Conversely, diabetes insipidus is characterized by the kidneys' inability to retain water, resulting in excessive urination and subsequent thirst.

When the body loses more fluids than it takes in, it becomes dehydrated, which can have dangerous effects on electrolyte balance and overall health. Dehydration can cause extreme thirst, dry mouth, dark urine, exhaustion, lightheadedness, and disorientation. Dehydration can be caused by not drinking enough water, perspiring too much (e.g., as a result of strenuous exercise or warm weather), nausea, diarrhea, or specific illnesses like kidney disease. Polyphagia, also known as extreme hunger, is a strong feeling of hunger that can cause overindulgence in food. It may indicate a number of diseases, such as hyperthyroidism, diabetes mellitus, or psychological issues like depression or anxiety. Despite eating enough food, people with diabetes mellitus may experience increased hunger because of their body's incapacity to properly utilize glucose. An overactive thyroid gland is a defining feature of hyperthyroidism, which can also result in weight loss and increased appetite.

In certain instances, intense feelings of thirst, dehydration, and hunger could be attributed to lifestyle choices like over-exercising, unhealthy eating habits, or the side effects of certain medications. Nonetheless, if these symptoms persist or become severe, it is important to seek medical attention from a healthcare provider to rule out any potential underlying health issues and prevent any complications. Treatment for extreme thirst, dehydration, or hunger may involve addressing the root cause, such as managing blood sugar levels for individuals with diabetes, replenishing fluids and electrolytes using oral rehydration solutions or intravenous fluids, and making necessary adjustments to one's diet and lifestyle in order to promote overall health and wellbeing.

10.2.2. Losing Weight Without Trying or Abnormal Weight Loss

Unintentional weight loss or abnormal weight loss can be a cause for concern as it could indicate underlying health issues, including eating disorders. Factors like increased physical activity, changes in diet, or stress can occasionally lead to unintentional weight loss. However, it is important to be able to distinguish between normal weight fluctuations and those that are associated with eating disorders.

Eating disorders, such as anorexia nervosa and bulimia nervosa, involve deliberate attempts to control food intake and body weight, resulting in significant and sustained weight loss. Individuals with anorexia nervosa often have a fear of gaining weight despite being underweight, and may severely restrict their food intake, engage in excessive exercise, or misuse laxatives or diuretics to achieve weight loss. This can lead to rapid and substantial weight loss, along with physical and psychological symptoms like fatigue, weakness, dizziness, thinning hair, and mood disturbances.

Individuals with bulimia nervosa may engage in binge eating followed by behaviors like self-induced vomiting, fasting, or excessive exercise to avoid gaining weight. While some may maintain a steady weight or have fluctuations within a healthy range, others may experience gradual weight loss due to their bingeing and purging habits. Other eating disorders like binge eating disorder (BED) or other specified feeding or eating disorders (OSFED) may involve overeating or loss of control around food, leading to weight gain or weight fluctuations. However, individuals with BED or OSFED may also adopt restrictive eating patterns or compensatory behaviors, which can result in weight loss or challenges in maintaining a stable weight over time.

It is crucial to remember that not all weight loss is a sign of an eating disorder. Unintentional weight loss can have a variety of causes, including gastrointestinal problems, cancer, thyroid disorders, and mental health conditions like anxiety or depression. However, it is critical to seek assessment and assistance from a healthcare provider if an individual is exhibiting noticeably and inexplicably decreased body weight in addition to symptoms suggestive of disordered eating or concerns about their body image. In order to address eating disorders and support recovery, early intervention and appropriate treatment are essential because, if left untreated, these conditions can have serious physical and psychological repercussions.

10.2.3. Desire to Binge on Food Excessively

One of the main signs of binge eating disorder (BED), which is included under the category of eating disorders in psychiatric diagnostic manuals like the DSM-5, is the urge to overindulge in food. BED sufferers frequently go through episodes of binge eating, in which they feel out of control and eat a lot of food in a short amount of time. Guilt, humiliation, or distress are frequently felt in conjunction with this behavior.

Some common features of the desire to binge excessively in BED include:

1. **Loss of Control:** During binge eating episodes, individuals often feel unable to stop eating or control their intake, even when they are uncomfortably full.
2. **Rapid Consumption:** Binge eating episodes typically involve consuming food rapidly, without regard for hunger or fullness cues.
3. **Eating in Secret:** Many individuals with BED feel embarrassed or ashamed of their binge eating behaviors and may eat in secret to hide their consumption from others.
4. **Preoccupation with Food:** Between

episodes of binge eating, individuals with BED may experience persistent thoughts about food, eating, or body weight.

5. **Emotional Triggers:** Binge eating episodes in BED are often triggered by negative emotions such as stress, anxiety, depression, or boredom. Food becomes a coping mechanism for dealing with uncomfortable feelings.
6. **Use of Food as Comfort:** Some individuals with BED use food as a source of comfort or emotional support, turning to binge eating to cope with difficult situations or emotions.
7. **Lack of Purging Behaviors:** Unlike bulimia nervosa, individuals with BED do not engage in compensatory behaviors such as vomiting, fasting, or excessive exercise following binge eating episodes.

Although binge eating is a major aspect of borderline eating disorder (BED), not everyone who indulges in occasional overindulgence or overeating fits the criteria for this disorder. BED is diagnosed based on a pattern of binge eating that has been present for three months or more, at least once a week, and is accompanied by distress or impairment from the behavior.

Obesity, diabetes, heart disease, depression, and other serious physical and psychological effects can result from binge eating disorder. Therapy for borderline eating disorder (BED) typically combines nutritional counseling with psychotherapy, such as cognitive-behavioral therapy (CBT) or interpersonal therapy, to address disordered eating patterns, enhance body image, and create healthier coping mechanisms for handling emotions. In some situations, a prescription for medication may also be given to address underlying anxiety or mood disorders (Yager et al., 2005; Herpertz-Dahlmann, 2008)

10.2.4. Desire to Vomit on Purpose

Self-induced vomiting, or the desire to intentionally throw up, is a defining symptom of bulimia nervosa, an eating disorder marked by frequent episodes of binge eating followed by compensatory behaviors to avoid gaining weight. It is crucial to remember, though, that people who suffer from other eating disorders, like anorexia nervosa or other specified feeding and eating disorders (OSFED), may also experience self-induced vomiting. This is especially true for those who follow restrictive eating habits interspersed with periods of overeating.

Some key features of the desire to vomit on purpose as a symptom of eating disorders include:

1. **Compensatory Behavior:** Individuals who engage in self-induced vomiting typically do so as a way to compensate for the perceived or actual consumption of a large amount of food during binge eating episodes. Vomiting is used as a means to rid the body of food and calories consumed during these episodes, with the goal of avoiding weight gain or alleviating feelings of guilt or shame associated with overeating.
2. **Secretive Behavior:** Many individuals who engage in self-induced vomiting may do so in secret, hiding their behavior from others due to feelings of embarrassment, shame, or fear of judgment. This secretive behavior can contribute to feelings of isolation and further perpetuate the

cycle of the eating disorder.

3. **Frequency:** In bulimia nervosa, self-induced vomiting typically occurs following episodes of binge eating, which may happen several times a week or even daily. The frequency of vomiting can vary depending on individual factors, such as severity of the disorder and level of distress experienced.
4. **Physical Consequences:** Self-induced vomiting can have serious physical consequences, including electrolyte imbalances, dehydration, erosion of tooth enamel (dental erosion), inflammation or rupture of the esophagus, and disruption of gastrointestinal function. Over time, repeated vomiting can lead to long-term health complications and medical emergencies.
5. **Psychological Impact:** The desire to vomit on purpose is often driven by underlying psychological factors, such as body image dissatisfaction, low self-esteem, perfectionism, or difficulties in coping with stress or negative emotions. Individuals may use vomiting as a maladaptive coping mechanism to regulate emotions or exert control over their body and weight.

It is crucial to understand that self-induced vomiting can signify severe distress and functional impairment and is a serious symptom of eating disorders. Addressing the underlying problems causing this behavior and fostering recovery require early intervention and appropriate treatment. Bulimia nervosa and other eating disorders are commonly treated with a mix of medical supervision, nutritional counseling, psychotherapy, and, in certain situations, medication to treat co-occurring mental health issues.

10.2.5. Desire to Starve (Not Eat at All)

One of the main symptoms of anorexia nervosa, an eating disorder marked by severe dietary restriction and a crippling fear of gaining weight or getting fat, is the desire to starve or abstain from eating completely. Even though they are significantly underweight, people with anorexia may have a skewed perception of their bodies and believe they are overweight. A number of psychological issues, such as an obsession with one's weight and body shape, low self-esteem, perfectionism, and a need for control, can lead to the desire to starve oneself.

Restricting their food intake helps anorexics feel more in control of their bodies and lives and helps them deal with underlying emotional distress or feelings of inadequacy. They might associate thinness with success or worthiness and see starvation as a kind of self-control. The promotion of thinness as a sign of beauty and desirability by cultural norms and societal pressures may also contribute to the desire to starve.

People with anorexia may continue their restrictive eating habits despite the serious psychological and physical effects of starvation, frequently downplaying or denying the severity of their illness. Prolonged starvation can cause a number of health problems in the long run, such as electrolyte imbalances, cardiovascular disease, gastrointestinal disorders, malnutrition, and cognitive decline. Anorexia nervosa can have potentially fatal effects if left untreated.

An all-encompassing treatment strategy that takes into account the disorder's psychological and physical components is necessary to address the urge to starve and encourage anorexia nervosa recovery. In order to manage co-occurring psychiatric symptoms, this may involve medication, nutritional rehabilitation, psychotherapy (such as cognitive-behavioral therapy or family-based therapy), and medical monitoring. Improving outcomes and assisting those suffering from anorexia in regaining a healthy relationship with food and their bodies depend heavily on early intervention and continued support (Yager et al., 2005; Herpertz-Dahlmann, 2008).

10.2.6. A Preoccupation With Food and Weight

Anorexia nervosa, bulimia nervosa, binge eating disorder, and other specified feeding and eating disorders (OSFED) are among the eating disorders characterized by an obsession with food and weight. Obsessive behaviors and thoughts about food, eating, and body image are common in people with these conditions, and they can have a serious negative influence on their everyday lives and general wellbeing. The obsession with food and weight in anorexics is marked by a relentless pursuit of thinness and a skewed perception of body size and shape. They may plan their meals carefully, count calories carefully, or completely avoid certain foods, which frequently leads to severe dietary restriction and noticeable weight loss. When someone suffers from anorexia, they associate being thin with acceptance and self-worth, so eating becomes a source of fear and anxiety for them.

Differently, those who suffer from bulimia nervosa also have an obsession with food and weight. Strong cravings or emotional distress are common causes of binge eating episodes, which result in an inability to control eating behavior. Motivated by guilt and a desire to repair the perceived harm caused by overindulging, people may participate in compensatory behaviors like self-induced vomiting, excessive exercise, or fasting after a binge. The obsession with food that characterizes binge eating disorder (BED) is typified by recurrent episodes of compulsive overeating, usually in reaction to stressful situations or unpleasant emotions. Food turns into a coping method for handling uncomfortable emotions, but binge eating's associated guilt and shame only serve to feed the cycle of overeating.

A major obsession with food and weight can occur in even those with OSFED, which is a broad category of eating disorder symptoms that do not neatly fit into any one diagnostic category. This obsession can show up as binge eating episodes, restrictive eating patterns, or other eating disorders that affect regular eating and wellbeing. All things considered, the obsession with food and weight in eating disorders is a result of a complicated interaction between biological, psychological, and social factors.

Treatment strategies for these conditions frequently combine medical supervision, nutritional counseling, psychotherapy, and support from a multidisciplinary treatment team to target these underlying causes. Encouraging people to have a better relationship with food and their bodies is crucial to fostering long-term healing and overall wellbeing.

10.2.7. Distorted Body Image

Many eating disorders, such as anorexia nervosa, bulimia nervosa, and binge eating disorder, often involve a distorted perception of body image. This means individuals may see themselves as either overweight when they are actually underweight, or too thin when they are at a healthy weight or overweight. Various factors, like societal pressures to be thin and media's portrayal of ideal body types, can influence individuals to internalize unrealistic beauty standards and lead to dissatisfaction with their own bodies.

Distorted body image is also significantly influenced by psychological factors. Negative body image perceptions are often linked to low self-esteem, perfectionism, anxiety, and depression. Experiences that are traumatic, like being teased or bullied about one's appearance, can make one feel even more unhappy and self-conscious.

A skewed perception of one's body frequently motivates eating disorders in people. For instance, the false notion that one is overweight drives severe dietary restriction and weight loss initiatives in anorexia nervosa. The belief that one is overweight can cause binge eating episodes in bulimia nervosa, which are then followed by compensatory purging behaviors to avoid gaining weight. A distorted body image can fuel feelings of shame and self-loathing, which in turn feeds the cycle of binge eating, even in cases of binge eating disorder in people who may be overweight or obese.

Managing distorted body image is a key aspect of treating eating disorders. Psychotherapy, specifically cognitive-behavioral therapy (CBT) and interventions focused on body image, can assist individuals in confronting negative thoughts about their bodies and cultivating a healthier and more positive self-perception. Furthermore, educating individuals on media literacy and the diversity of body types can aid in identifying and resisting unrealistic beauty standards imposed by society. Ultimately, encouraging body acceptance and self-kindness are vital for achieving sustained recovery from eating disorders and enhancing overall quality of life (Yager et al., 2005; Herpertz-Dahlmann, 2008).

10.2.8. Excessive Fear of Gaining Weight

An intense fear of gaining weight is a key feature of many eating disorders, especially anorexia nervosa. Those affected by this fear often experience significant anxiety and distress when faced with the idea of putting on even a small amount of weight, even if they are already underweight or at a healthy weight. This fear can completely consume their thoughts and behaviors regarding food, eating, and body image. In the case of anorexia nervosa, the fear of gaining weight drives individuals to adopt restrictive eating habits and extreme measures to manage their food consumption. This can include meticulously tracking calorie intake, avoiding foods perceived as fattening, or engaging in excessive exercise to burn off any calories consumed. Additionally, individuals may develop specific rituals around food, such as cutting their meals into small pieces or arranging them in certain ways, to exert control over their eating habits.

Anorexia nervosa often involves a fear of gaining weight based on a distorted perception of body size and shape. Despite being underweight, individuals with this disorder may see themselves as overweight or fat, which reinforces their fear of weight gain and leads to disordered eating behaviors. This fear of gaining weight can also be present in other eating disorders like bulimia nervosa and binge eating disorder. Those with bulimia nervosa may fear weight gain after binge eating episodes and may resort to self-induced vomiting or excessive exercise to prevent it. Likewise, individuals with binge eating disorder may fear gaining weight from recurrent episodes of overeating and may feel distressed or guilty as a result.

In eating disorders, the fear of gaining weight is frequently accompanied by severe psychological distress, such as depression, anxiety, and low self-esteem. Serious health effects may also result from it, such as electrolyte imbalances, malnutrition, and organ damage. Treatment for eating disorders must address the excessive fear of gaining weight. Individuals can develop healthier attitudes toward food, eating, and body image and challenge illogical beliefs about weight gain with the aid of psychotherapy, especially cognitive-behavioral therapy (CBT) and exposure therapy. Restoring physical health and treating nutritional deficiencies also require medical supervision and nutritional counseling. In the end, helping those with eating disorders recover and enhance their general well-being requires them to get over their fear of gaining weight (Yager et al., 2005; Herpertz-Dahlmann, 2008).

10.2.9. Refusing to Eat or Eating Tiny Portions or Eating Alone

Common behaviors seen in people with eating disorders, especially anorexia nervosa and avoidant/restrictive food intake disorder (ARFID), include refusing to eat, eating small portions, or eating by themselves. These behaviors can have detrimental effects on one's physical and mental well-being and are frequently motivated by a complex interaction of psychological, social, and biological factors. One of the main characteristics of anorexia nervosa is eating infrequently or not at all. Even if they are severely underweight, people with anorexia usually have a strong fear of gaining weight or getting fat. They frequently severely restrict their food intake as a result of this fear, almost to the point of starvation. To exercise control over their eating, they could keep a close eye on their calorie intake, abstain from foods they believe to be unhealthy or high in calories, or follow special mealtime rituals. Anorexics frequently eat by themselves because it conceals their disordered eating patterns and keeps others from seeing them.

Similar to this, people with ARFID may show extreme selectivity or pickiness when it comes to food, which causes them to eat in tiny amounts or not at all. In contrast to anorexia, sensory sensitivity, fear of unpleasant outcomes (like choking or vomiting), or lack of interest in food are the main causes of avoidance in ARFID. For ARFID, eating by yourself may be preferred over social pressure or uncomfortable situations involving food.

Refusing to eat or eating tiny portions can have major physical effects in both anorexia nervosa and ARFID, especially in children and adolescents. These effects include malnutrition, nutrient deficiencies, dehydration, weakened immune systems, and impaired growth and development. In addition, these actions may result in strained relationships, social isolation, and decreased functioning in a variety of spheres of life.

Refusing to eat, eating small portions, or eating by yourself necessitates a thorough approach to treatment that takes care of the underlying causes of these behaviors. Psychotherapy, in particular exposure therapy and cognitive-behavioral therapy (CBT), can assist people in improving their relationship with food, challenging illogical beliefs about eating and food, and developing healthier coping mechanisms. Restoring physical health and encouraging regular eating patterns also require nutritional counseling and meal assistance. Family involvement may be very important, particularly when it comes to young adults or adolescents. In the end, treating these behaviors and encouraging recovery in people with eating disorders require early intervention and continued support.

10.2.10. Compulsive Exercise

Exercise addiction or exercise dependence, other names for compulsive exercise, is a pattern of behavior defined by an overwhelming need to exercise, usually at the expense of one's physical and mental well-being. Though it can happen on its own, this behavior is frequently linked to eating disorders, especially bulimia nervosa and anorexia nervosa. People who suffer from compulsive exercise may feel driven to work out more than is necessary for their health or fitness and may become upset or anxious if they are unable to exercise. They might put exercise above all other commitments and activities, putting in a lot of time and effort into their workouts, and finding it difficult to take days off or rest periods. Exercise may also be used by compulsive exercisers as a way to cut calories, make up for lost food, or get to a target weight or body type.

Exercise addiction can have detrimental effects on one's body and mind. Physically, overtraining and excessive exercise can result in weariness, exhaustion, aches and pains in the muscles, injuries, and weakened immunity. In females, it can also upset the balance of hormones and menstrual cycles, resulting in amenorrhea, or the absence of menstruation. Psychological factors such as control issues, low self-esteem, perfectionism, and body image concerns frequently motivate compulsive exercise. It can exacerbate relationship problems and social isolation, as well as feelings of guilt, shame, anxiety, and depression.

Promoting recovery and general well-being requires recognizing and treating compulsive exercise. A multidisciplinary approach is usually used in treatment, involving medical monitoring, nutritional counseling, and psychotherapy. Acceptance and commitment therapy (ACT) and cognitive-behavioral therapy (CBT) are frequently used to assist people in overcoming erroneous beliefs regarding exercise, creating more balanced relationships with physical activity, and developing healthier coping mechanisms. Involving the family may also be advantageous, particularly when dealing with teenagers or young adults.

It is critical to understand that, when done sensibly and in moderation, exercise can be a constructive and joyful activity. Exercise does, however, require professional assistance and intervention when it becomes obsessive and harmful to one's health and ability to function. People who suffer from compulsive exercise can develop healthier habits and attitudes toward physical activity with the right support and treatment, which will ultimately improve their general health and quality of life.

10.2.11. Sensitivity to Cold

One common physical symptom of many eating disorders, especially anorexia nervosa, is sensitivity to cold. Those who suffer from anorexia frequently have trouble controlling their body temperature because of their abnormally low body weight and decreased body fat percentage. Even in relatively mild conditions, this can result in increased sensitivity to cold temperatures.

Several factors contribute to sensitivity to cold in individuals with anorexia nervosa:

1. **Low Body Weight:** Anorexia nervosa is characterized by severe weight loss and malnutrition, which can lead to a decrease in body fat and muscle mass. Body fat serves as insulation and helps retain heat, so individuals with low body weight have less insulation against cold temperatures.
2. **Reduced Metabolic Rate:** Severe calorie restriction and malnutrition in anorexia can lead to a decreased metabolic rate, which affects the body's ability to generate heat. As a result, individuals with anorexia may have difficulty maintaining a normal body temperature, especially in cold environments.
3. **Impaired Circulation:** Malnutrition and dehydration can impair

circulation and blood flow to the extremities, making hands and feet particularly prone to feeling cold. This reduced blood flow can contribute to sensations of coldness and discomfort, even when ambient temperatures are not exceptionally low.

4. **Hormonal Imbalances:** Anorexia nervosa can disrupt hormonal balance, including alterations in thyroid function and reproductive hormones, which play roles in regulating metabolism and body temperature. Dysregulation of these hormones can contribute to sensitivity to cold.

For people suffering from anorexia nervosa, being sensitive to cold can have serious repercussions on their quality of life, comfort, and ability to go about their everyday lives. Additionally, it can intensify already present psychological and physical symptoms of the illness, like depression, weakness, and exhaustion.

In order to address cold sensitivity in anorexics, comprehensive treatment plans that improve metabolic function, restore weight and nutritional balance, and address underlying psychological issues that contribute to disordered eating behaviors must be implemented. Treatment must include psychotherapy, medical supervision, nutritional rehabilitation, and assistance from a multidisciplinary team. Over time, improving thermoregulation and lowering cold sensitivity can be achieved by gaining weight and returning the body to its normal state.

10.2.12. Menstruation Ceases

Amenorrhea, or the cessation of menstruation, is a serious health issue that is frequently linked to eating disorders, especially anorexia nervosa. Severe calorie restriction, quick weight loss, and low body fat cause hormonal imbalances in anorexics, particularly affecting the hypothalamic-pituitary-ovarian axis. Because the body perceives starvation, it prioritizes survival over reproductive function, resulting in irregular or absent menstrual cycles.

Menstruation cessation indicates the severity of the eating disorder in addition to being a physical sign of the body's malnourishment and hormonal imbalance. Long-term effects of amenorrhea on reproductive health may include infertility, osteoporosis (low bone density), fractures, and other problems relating to the bones. Furthermore, in addition to causing psychological distress, amenorrhea can also make a person feel inadequate, ashamed, and less feminine.

When treating amenorrhea in patients with eating disorders, a comprehensive treatment strategy is needed to address the disorder's psychological and physical components. The promotion of menstrual recovery and the restoration of hormonal balance depend on nutritional rehabilitation, weight restoration, and medical supervision. Psychotherapy, in particular family-based therapy and cognitive-behavioral therapy (CBT), can assist people in addressing underlying psychological factors that contribute to disordered eating behaviors, developing healthier coping mechanisms, and challenging distorted beliefs about food, weight, and body image. Promoting menstrual recovery and general well-being in people with eating disorders requires early intervention and extensive support (Yager et al., 2005; Herpertz-Dahlmann, 2008).

10.2.13. Abuse of Laxatives, Diuretics, or Diet Pills

Abuse of diet pills, laxatives, or diuretics is a

ha4rmful behavior that is frequently linked to eating disorders, specifically bulimia nervosa and some anorexia nervosa subtypes. These drugs are used as purging techniques to reduce feelings of guilt or anxiety related to food consumption, regulate weight, or flush calories from the body after eating. However, abusing them can have detrimental effects on one's physical and mental health.

Laxatives are drugs that cause bowel movements, and people with bulimia nervosa frequently abuse them to purge after binge eating episodes. Overuse of laxatives can cause long-term harm to the colon and digestive system, electrolyte imbalances, dehydration, and gastrointestinal problems (such as persistent constipation or diarrhea).

Diuretics are drugs or chemicals that cause the production of more urine; they are frequently used to treat edema and hypertension. Diuretics may be misused in the context of eating disorders in order to get rid of water weight and momentarily lessen bloating or swelling. On the other hand, overuse of diuretics can cause kidney damage, cardiovascular issues, electrolyte imbalances (especially potassium and sodium), and dehydration. People with eating disorders frequently abuse diet pills, including over-the-counter and prescription supplements, to suppress appetite, speed up metabolism, or aid in weight loss. On the other hand, a lot of diet pills include stimulants, appetite suppressants, or other potentially dangerous substances that can negatively impact the nervous system, the cardiovascular system, and general health. When diet pills are misused, they can cause major side effects such as agitation, high blood pressure, insomnia, increased heart rate, and even potentially fatal events like strokes or heart attacks. They can also cause addiction, tolerance, and dependence. Abuse of laxatives, diuretics, or diet pills is frequently caused by psychological issues that are beneath the surface, such as issues with body image, low self-esteem, perfectionism, and a need for control. People who engage in these behaviors often experience feelings of shame, guilt, and secrecy because they may try to conceal their purging habits from others.

When it comes to treating laxative, diuretic, or diet pill abuse in people with eating disorders, a thorough treatment strategy that takes into account the disorder's psychological and physical components is necessary. Psychotherapy, in particular, dialectical behavior therapy (DBT) and cognitive-behavioral therapy (CBT), can assist people in learning new techniques to manage stress and emotions, developing healthier coping mechanisms, and challenging false beliefs about food, weight, and body image. In addition, medical supervision and dietary guidance are necessary to address the physical effects of purging behaviors and to support general health and wellbeing. In the end, breaking the cycle of purging behaviors and fostering recovery in people with eating disorders require early intervention and continued support (Yager et al., 2005; Herpertz-Dahlmann, 2008).

10.2.14. Depression

Eating disorders and depression frequently co-occur, and depression can make eating disorders worse and make them more chronic. Depression symptoms, such as protracted melancholy, hopelessness, low self-esteem, and a loss of interest in or enjoyment from once-enjoyed activities, are frequently experienced by people with eating disorders. Eating disorders and depression have a complicated, reciprocal relationship in which one illness influences and feeds the other in a vicious cycle. An eating disorder may develop before depression does, acting as a risk factor that encourages the emergence of disordered eating habits. In certain cases, depressive symptoms like low self-esteem and trouble managing stress or emotions can lead to the adoption of unhealthy coping strategies like purging, binge eating, or restrictive eating as a means of numbing painful emotions or coping with upsetting feelings.

On the other hand, starvation, health issues, and social isolation linked to eating disorders can worsen depressive symptoms and prolong the cycle of both illnesses. Malnutrition brought on by fasting or purging can mess with the brain's neurotransmitter system and hormonal balance, which can lead to mood swings and depressive symptoms. Furthermore, the shame, guilt, and social disengagement that people with eating disorders frequently go through can make them feel even more alone and worsen depressing and hopeless emotions.

When treating eating disorders and depression together, a comprehensive treatment strategy is needed to address both issues at the same time. Psychotherapy, in particular, dialectical behavior therapy (DBT) and cognitive-behavioral therapy (CBT), can assist people in recognizing and challenging harmful thought patterns, creating more effective coping mechanisms, and enhancing their self-worth and ability to regulate their emotions. In certain situations, a doctor may prescribe medication to treat depression and stabilize mood, such as antidepressants or mood stabilizers.

In addition to being crucial elements of treatment for eating disorders, nutritional rehabilitation and medical monitoring can also help restore physical health and address underlying biological factors that contribute to depression. A multidisciplinary treatment team's support and family involvement is essential for delivering comprehensive care and encouraging long-term recovery from eating disorders and depression. To end the cycle of co-occurring eating disorders and depression and to enhance general wellbeing and quality of life, early intervention and continued support are essential.

A Closer Look

Challenges of Weight Maintenance

How many times have you seen yourself gaining weight the instant you attempt to resume your previous routine after experiencing rapid and successful weight loss? This phenomenon, known as the "Yo-Yo effect," occurs when an individual experiences rapid weight loss or gain as a result of crash diets and intense exercise, followed by a period of inactivity and an attempt to resume their previous routine.

Let us find out the reasons why it is difficult to maintain weight

- **Crash Diet**

Most people who follow a crash diet do so to lose weight quickly. Crash diets come in many forms, such as following a one-food diet plan for every meal (such as the soup, salad, juice, egg, chicken, or cabbage diets). These diets cause a sharp decrease in calories, which leads to weight loss in four to six weeks. These diets are hard to stick to for very long, and they usually cause you to crave sweets and fried foods a lot, which makes you go back to your old habits and gain weight again.

- **Extreme Exercise with No Dietary Modification**

Exercising for at least 150 minutes per week can assist in reaching weight loss goals. Research indicates that individuals who engage in physical activity for over 60 minutes daily while burning 700 calories can potentially lose over 7kg in just 3 months. However, maintaining weight loss becomes challenging without changes to diet, as even a small decrease in physical activity can hinder progress.

- **Increase in Calorie Intake**

According to studies, the amount of calories burned each day decreases by 20–30 KCal for every kilogram of weight loss. Losing weight also causes an increase in appetite. This could cause an unconscious bias toward portion sizes and a gradual daily increase of 20–30% in energy intake. This will make it even harder to maintain one's weight.

- **Behavioral Changes**

Achieving quick weight loss can boost your confidence and prevent you from gaining weight. People usually return to their usual habits of consuming high-calorie foods and engaging in little physical activity. They eventually return to the same weight, of course. Stress levels rise when one regains the weight they have lost, along with feelings of guilt and low self-worth. As a result, making long-term lifestyle changes that combine exercise and dietary changes becomes crucial.

- **Lack of Sleep**

The length and quality of sleep are crucial factors in maintaining a healthy weight. Research presented at the European Congress on Obesity found that longer sleep duration, particularly with adequate deep sleep, can contribute to weight maintenance. The study revealed that individuals who sleep for less than six hours have a higher BMI, with an increase of 1.3 compared to those who sleep for more than six hours. Inadequate sleep quality also raises the risk of high blood pressure, high cholesterol, and the accumulation of fatty deposits in the arteries.

Furthermore, there are certain hormonal and genetic variables that make it difficult to maintain weight. It is possible to maintain weight with lifestyle modifications, even though it is a challenging task. All you need to do is maintain your diet, exercise routine, and behavioral adjustments over the long term (Yager et al., 2005; Herpertz-Dahlmann, 2008).

Summary

- Eating disorders and weight problems are complex conditions that can have serious physical and psychological effects on individuals. Recognizing the symptoms of these disorders is crucial for early intervention and effective treatment.
- Eating disorders are complex there is no one single reason why someone develops an eating disorder. A whole range of different factors combine, including genetic, psychological, environmental, social and biological influences.
- Anorexia nervosa, bulimia, and overeating disorders can have numerous combinations of signs, symptoms and causes. Additionally, several other eating and body image disorders are closely related to anorexia and bulimia, including orthorexia, body dysmorphic disorder, and exercise addiction.
- Extreme thirst, dehydration, or hunger can be symptoms of various medical conditions, ranging from mild to severe. These symptoms can indicate issues with fluid balance, blood sugar levels, or underlying health conditions.
- Losing weight unintentionally or experiencing abnormal weight loss can be concerning and may indicate underlying health issues, including eating disorders.
- The desire to starve, or avoid eating altogether, is a significant symptom often associated with anorexia nervosa, an eating disorder characterized by extreme restriction of food intake and an intense fear of gaining weight or becoming fat
- A preoccupation with food and weight is a hallmark feature of various eating disorders, including anorexia nervosa, bulimia nervosa, binge eating disorder, and other specified feeding and eating disorders (OSFED).

References

1. Austin, S. B., Ziyadeh, N. J., Forman, S., Prokop, L. A., Keliher, A., & Jacobs, D. (2008). Screening high school students for eating disorders: Results of a national initiative. *Preventing Chronic Disease, 5*(4), A114. https://doi.org/10.5888/pcd5.080063.
2. Briere, J., & Scott, C. (2007). Assessment of trauma symptoms in eating disordered populations. *Eating Disorders: The Journal of Treatment and Prevention, 15*(4), 347–358.
3. Bulik, C. M., & Mazzeo, S. E. (2009). Child and adolescent psychiatric clinics of North America. *Child and Adolescent Psychiatric Clinics of North America, 18*(1).
4. Franko, D. L., Keshaviah, A., Eddy, K. T., et al. (2013). A longitudinal investigation of mortality in anorexia nervosa and bulimia nervosa. *American Journal of Psychiatry, 170*(8), 917–925. https://doi.org/10.1176/appi.ajp.2013.12101259.
5. Herpertz-Dahlmann, B. (2009). Adolescent eating disorders: Definitions, symptomatology, epidemiology and comorbidity. *Child and Adolescent Psychiatric Clinics of North America, 18*(1), 31–47. https://doi.org/10.1016/j.chc.2008.07.003.
6. Pinhas, L., McVey, G., Walker, K. S., Norris, M., Katzman, D., & Collier, S. (2013). Trading health for a healthy weight: The uncharted side of healthy weights initiatives. *Eating Disorders, 21*(2), 109–116. https://doi.org/10.1080/10640266.2013.769616.

7. Pinhas, L., Morris, A., Crosby, R. D., & Katzman, D. K. (2011). Incidence and age-specific presentation of restrictive eating disorders in children: A Canadian Pediatric Surveillance Program study. *Archives of Pediatrics & Adolescent Medicine, 165*(10), 895–899. https://doi.org/10.1001/archpediatrics.2011.147.

8. Rosen, D. S. (2003). Eating disorders in children and young adolescents: Etiology, classification, clinical features, and treatment. *Adolescent Medicine: State of the Art Reviews, 14*(1), 49–59.

9. Weaver, L., & Liebman, R. (2011). Assessment of anorexia nervosa in children and adolescents. *Current Psychiatry Reports, 13*(2), 93–98. https://doi.org/10.1007/s11920-010-0177-7.

10. Yager, J., Devlin, M. J., Helmi, K. A., Herzog, D. B., Mitchell, J. E., Powers, P. S., & Zerbe, K. J. (2005). Eating disorders. *Focus, 3*.

INDEX

C

D

E

F

G

H

I

FSC
www.fsc.org
MIX
Papier | Fördert gute Waldnutzung
FSC® C083411

Kolibri 360 GmbH
Ferdinand-Jühlke-Straße 7
99095 Erfurt, Deutschland
produktsicherheit@kolibri360.de